INJECTABLE DRUG DEVELOPMENT

TECHNIQUES TO REDUCE PAIN AND IRRITATION

Edited by

Pramod K. Gupta

and

Gayle A. Brazeau

informa

healthcare

New York   London

First published in 1996 by Interpharm Press.

Simultaneously published in the USA by Informa Healthcare, 52 Vanderbilt Avenue, 7th Floor, New York, NY 10017, USA.

Informa Healthcare is a trading division of Informa UK Ltd. Registered Office: 37–41 Mortimer Street, London W1T 3JH, UK. Registered in England and Wales number 1072954.

A CIP record for this book is available from the British Library.

Library of Congress Cataloging-in-Publication Data available on application

ISBN-13: 9781574910957

Orders may be sent to: Informa Healthcare, Sheepen Place, Colchester, Essex CO3 3LP, UK
Telephone: +44 (0)20 7017 5540
Email: CSDhealthcarebooks@informa.com
Website: http://informahealthcarebooks.com/

For corporate sales please contact: CorporateBooksIHC@informa.com
For foreign rights please contact: RightsIHC@informa.com
For reprint permissions please contact: PermissionsIHC@informa.com

Contents

B: METHODS TO ASSESS PAIN, IRRITATION, AND MUSCLE DAMAGE FOLLOWING INJECTIONS

8. A Primer on In Vitro and In Vivo Cytosolic Enzyme Release Methods   155

Gayle A. Brazeau

9. Histological and Morphological Methods   177

Bruce M. Carlson and Robert Palmer

Preface

Parenteral formulations administered via intravenous, subcutaneous, and intramuscular injections are critical routes of administration when the oral ingestion of drugs is contraindicated. The increasing importance of biotechnology and the development of increasing numbers of therapeutic peptides and/or gene products during the next century will necessitate a better understanding of the interactions between parenteral formulations and the site of injection. A common limitation with the injection of numerous parenteral formulations is the occurrence of pain and/or tissue damage that may result from the active drug, the formulation components, or the total formulation. While there is information discussing the mechanisms of pain or tissue damage and methods to evaluate the extent of tissue irritation associated with parenteral administration scattered throughout the medical literature, we felt that a compilation of this material would be beneficial for pharmaceutical formulators as well as regulatory personnel involved with the development and approval of parenteral products.

Consequently, the focus of this book is on providing parenteral formulation scientists with the requisite scientific background and techniques to evaluate parenteral formulations with respect to their potential to cause pain, irritation, and muscle damage. More important, this reference will provide the formulator with various strategies that can be used in the pharmaceutical industry to minimize these adverse effects. It is important for the parenteral formulator to understand and characterize the magnitude and mechanisms by which key components can contribute to the irritation, pain, and damage. If severe, these issues could limit the clinical acceptance of a formulation, particularly for those formulations requiring multiple or repeated injections over a long period of time. Finally, it will be important for the formulator to be knowledgeable in various strategies by which parenteral products could be developed with reduced tissue toxicity, either pain on injection or tissue damage. This text is designed to provide an overview of the basics related to irritation or tissue damage, methods to evaluate pain or tissue damage, and strategies to reduce or negate pain or tissue damage associated with parenteral administration.

An understanding of this complex area necessitates an interdisciplinary approach. To achieve this goal, we have solicited chapters from an interdisciplinary team of experts in the United States and Europe in the areas of pharmaceutics, physiology, anatomy, toxicology, and product formulation. We believe this book will be useful for graduate students, parenteral formulation scientists, pharmacists, medical practitioners, and individuals involved with clinical and regulatory approval of parenteral products.

ACKNOWLEDGMENTS

We would like to thank the numerous individuals without whose support and assistance this book would not have been possible. We also would like to thank our families for their patience and support during the long hours in the editing and writing of this book. We sincerely acknowledge our dissertation advisors for their scientific and professional guidance throughout the years. Equally important, we appreciate the support of our professional colleagues at TAP, Abbott Laboratories, and the University of Florida College of Pharmacy.

A contributed book of this nature would not have been possible without concerted efforts of the individual authors and our publishers. They have assisted us and contributed more than they will ever know, and for that we are most grateful.

Pramod Gupta
Gayle Brazeau
May 1999

Editors and Contributors

Pramod K. Gupta, Editor

Pramod K. Gupta is Manager of Pharmaceutical Development at TAP Holdings Inc. (a joint venture between Abbott Laboratories and Takeda Chemical Industries of Japan) based in Deerfield, Illinois. His current responsibilities include preformulation and formulation development, analytical methods, scale-up and manufacturing, stability, and interaction with the FDA. Previously, he held Project Leader and Senior Scientist positions at Abbott Laboratories in North Chicago, Illinois.

Dr. Gupta earned his BS in pharmaceutical sciences from the University of Saugar, India, and his PhD in pharmaceutics from the University of Otago, New Zealand. He has published more than 50 papers and book chapters in the area of formulation development, holds 5 patents, and is a recipient of numerous awards for his efforts in this area of research. He is coeditor of *Inhalation Delivery of Therapeutic Peptides and Proteins*. Dr. Gupta is a member of the American Association of Pharmaceutical Sciences, the Controlled Release Society, and the Australasian Society of Clinical and Experimental Pharmacologists.

Gayle A. Brazeau, Editor

Gayle A. Brazeau, PhD, is Associate Professor/Assistant Dean for Curricular Affairs and Accreditation at the University of Florida College of Pharmacy. She graduated from the University of Toledo with a BS in pharmacy and an MS in pharmaceutical sciences. She received her PhD from SUNY Buffalo in pharmaceutics. Dr. Brazeau has been active in professional organizations, including AACP and AAPS, and in 1992 she received an AFPE Gustavus A. Pfeiffer Faculty Development Research Fellowship. She has been a member of the FDA Advisory Committee for Pharmaceutical Sciences.

Dr. Brazeau's research interests focus on understanding the biochemical and toxicological interactions of compounds with skeletal muscle. In this work, she has investigated the myotoxicity of various compounds and formulation excipients and strategies to reduce tissue damage and pain associated with the injection of parenteral formulations. She has received research funding from the PDA, pharmaceutical companies, and the NIDA.

Michael J. Akers

Michael J. Akers received a BA in biology from Wabash College (Crawfordsville, Ind.) and a PhD in pharmaceutics from the University of Iowa College of Pharmacy. He was a Senior Scientist at Searle Laboratories (Skokie, Ill.) and Alcon Laboratories (Fort Worth, Tex.) and Associate Professor at the University of Tennessee College of Pharmacy (Memphis, Tenn.). In late 1981 he joined Eli Lilly and Company as a Research Scientist in the Parenteral Products Development Department. Currently, he is a Senior Research Scientist in the Biopharmaceutical Products Development Department, focusing on the commercial development of new parenteral dosage forms. He has significantly contributed to the development of 11 marketed pharmaceutical products.

Dr. Akers is author or coauthor of 58 publications, 3 U.S. patents, and 16 book chapters, primarily in the field of parenteral science and technology. He is also Director of a short course on parenteral products technology at the Center for Professional Advancement. He is on the editorial advisory board of the *PDA Journal of Pharmaceutical Science and Technology* and a founder of the newest AAPS journal, *Pharmaceutical Development and Technology*. He is active in the AAPS, the PDA, and the USP.

Robert M. Beihn

Robert M. Beihn, PhD, is vice president of Scintiprox, Inc., of Indianapolis, Ind. He spent 20 years in the department of nuclear medicine at the University of Kentucky and VA Medical Centers and 10 years at Oak Ridge Associated Universities in Oak Ridge, Tenn. His primary research interests involve the scintigraphic evaluation of pharmaceutical dosage forms and the subsequent interpretation of the resulting scintigraphic images.

Marcus E. Brewster

Marcus E. Brewster received his BS degree (1978) from Mercer University and his PhD from the University of Florida (1982) in the area of pharmaceutical sciences (medicinal chemistry). After a postdoctoral fellowship at the University of Florida, he joined Pharmatec, Inc., in 1983, where he served as a Senior Scientist, Group Leader, Associate Director of Research, Director of Research, and, finally, Senior Director of Research and Discovery. In 1997, he joined Janssen Pharmaceutica, a Johnson and Johnson company, as Director of Drug Delivery Research. Dr. Brewster's research interests are in drug targeting; the development of pharmaceutical excipients, including cyclodextrins; and semi-empirical molecular orbital models to address problems of biological, chemical, and pharmaceutical importance.

John B. Cannon

John B. Cannon received a BS in chemistry in 1970 from Duke University and a PhD in chemistry from Princeton University. He is currently Associate Research Fellow in the Pharmaceutical Products Division of Abbott Laboratories (North Chicago, Ill.). Previously he was a postdoctoral research fellow at the University of California at San Diego, an instructor at Northern Illinois University (Dekalb, Ill.), Assistant Professor of Chemistry at Cleveland State University (Cleveland, Ohio), and a research chemist in veterinary formulations development at American Cyanamid Company (Princeton, N.J.) His fields of specialization include pharmaceutical formulation, drug delivery, preformulation, topical and transdermal delivery, liposomes, emulsions, and heme and porphyrin chemistry and formulation.

Bruce M. Carlson

Bruce M. Carlson received his MD and PhD degrees from the University of Minnesota in 1965 and has been at the University of Michigan since 1966. He is presently Professor and Chairman of the Department of Anatomy and Cell Biology and a Research Scientist in the Institute of Gerontology. He is completing a term as president of the American Association of Anatomists.

Daan J. A. Crommelin

Daan J. A. Crommelin is a professor in the Department of Pharmaceutics at Utrecht University. He is also Scientific Director of the Utrecht Institute for Pharmaceutical Sciences (UIPS), Adjunct Professor in the Department of Pharmaceutics and Pharmaceutical Chemistry at the University of Utah, and Scientific Director of OctoPlus B.V., a company specializing in drug formulation. His research is focused on advanced drug delivery and drug targeting strategies. He has published over 200 articles in peer-reviewed journals.

Elias Fattal

Elias Fattal received his pharmacy degree in 1983 and a PhD in 1990 from the University of Paris-XI (Châtenay-Malabry, France). From 1990 to 1991, he had a postdoctoral fellowship in the Department of Pharmaceutical Chemistry at the University of California, San Francisco. Since 1992, he has been Associate Professor of Pharmaceutical Technology at the University of Paris-XI. His research activity deals with the design of polymeric nano- and microparticles and liposomes for the delivery of peptides/proteins and nucleic acids. Fattal has published over 70 scientific papers in these areas.

Agatha Feltus

Agatha Feltus is a graduate student in pharmaceutical sciences at the University of Kentucky. She has a BS degree in chemistry from the University of Kentucky and currently holds a fellowship from the National Science Foundation.

Carol A. Brister Gatlin

Carol A. Brister Gatlin received a BS in pharmacy from Oregon State University. She has experience as a retail and hospital pharmacist and as a medical information specialist. She has worked as a Medical Information Consultant and a Medical Writer for the National Institutes of Health Clinical Center, the University of Kentucky Medical Center, Duke University, Ask the Pharmacist (ATP), and Genzyme. She has contributed to several publications and coauthored a physicochemical review of sweetening agents.

Larry A. Gatlin

Larry A. Gatlin received a BS in pharmacy from Oregon State University and a PhD in pharmaceutical science from the University of Kentucky. He was an officer in the Public Health Service at the National Institutes of Health Clinical Center in Bethesda, Md., and has worked at the Upjohn Company, Genentech, Glaxo Wellcome, and Biogen. Dr. Gatlin has published and lectured in the areas of filtration, preformulation, parenteral product development, macromolecules formulation, and lyophilization.

Malcolm J. Jackson

Malcom J. Jackson was trained in biochemistry at the University of Surrey and University College, London. He currently is Professor and Head of the

Department of Medicine at the University of Liverpool. He has published over 100 scientific papers and 60 review articles, mainly relating to the role of oxidative stress in tissue damage and its prevention by antioxidants. Dr. Jackson currently holds research grants from several major UK and international agencies.

Michael Jay

Michael Jay, PhD, is Director of the Center for Pharmaceutical Science and Technology and Professor of Pharmaceutical Sciences at the University of Kentucky College of Pharmacy. Previously he served on the faculty in the department of nuclear medicine at the University of Connecticut. He has authored over 80 peer-reviewed publications, primarily in the area of radiopharmaceutics.

Farida Kadir

Farida Kadir studied pharmacy at Utrecht University and received her pharmacy degree in 1988. She then worked as a part-time pharmacist in a community pharmacy. After obtaining her PhD at Utrecht University in 1992, she was a Clinical Research Scientist until 1996. Dr. Kadir is now director of POA, an institute specializing in organizing postacademic courses and congresses. Her main interest is in the field of drug delivery systems in pharmaceutical practice.

Wolfgang Klement

Wolfgang Klement studied medicine and earned his PhD in 1985 from the University Erlangen-Nuernberg, Germany. From 1985 to 1992, he trained as an anesthesiology physician at the Institute for Clinical Anesthesiology and Intensive Care at the University of Duesseldorf, Germany. He also received scientific training in the Department of Experimental Anesthesiology, with an emphasis on the function of the nociceptive system of subcutaneous veins in humans. After receiving postdoctoral qualification in 1992, he supervised anesthetists in various operative departments at the Institute of Clinical Anesthesiology and Intensive Care. Dr. Klement is now Head of the Department of Anesthesiology and Intensive Care of the Ev. Jung-Stilling-Hospital in Siegen, Germany.

Joseph F. Krzyzaniak

Joseph F. Krzyzaniak received his BS in chemistry (1992) from Missouri Western State College and his PhD in pharmaceutical sciences (1997) from the University of Arizona. In 1997, he accepted a position in the

Pharmaceutics group at G. D. Searle & Company, where he is involved in physical/chemical characterization and formulation development of new chemical entities. Dr. Krzyzaniak is a member of the American Association of Pharmaceutical Scientists and has presented/published research involving the prediction of physical properties of organic molecules, the development of hemolytically safe parenteral formulations, and the physical/chemical characterization of pharmaceutical solids.

Thorsteinn Loftsson

Thorsteinn Loftsson received his MSPharm degree in 1975 from the Royal Danish School of Pharmacy in Copenhagen and his MS (1978) and PhD (1979) degrees from the Department of Pharmaceutical Chemistry at the University of Kansas in Lawrence. At the University of Iceland in Reykjavik, Iceland, he was appointed Assistant Professor (1979), Associate Professor (1983), and, most recently, Professor of Physical Pharmacy (1986). His main research interests have been the pharmaceutical application of cyclodextrins, but other research interests include drug stability, prodrugs, soft drugs, and drug delivery through biological membranes. He has authored or coauthored over 110 papers in peer-reviewed journals, 10 book chapters, 14 patents and patent applications, and over 100 abstracts.

John M. Marcek

John M. Marcek received his BS in animal science from the University of New Hampshire in 1980 and his MS in animal science from Oregon State University in 1983. He was employed at the University of Minnesota in the Department of Animal Science, supervising an endocrinology laboratory, from 1983 to 1987. He was then employed as Research Associate in toxicology at Pharmacia & Upjohn from 1987 to 1998. Currently, he is in Worldwide Regulatory Toxicology at Pharmacia & Upjohn, writing and compiling regulatory submissions.

Anne McArdle

Anne McArdle, PhD, is a biochemistry graduate from the University of Liverpool. She is a lecturer in the Department of Medicine at the University of Liverpool and currently holds a Queen Elizabeth and Queen Mother Fellowship funded by the UK charity *Research into Ageing*. She is using molecular biological approaches to study the mechanisms by which muscles of the aged are more susceptible to damage and are less able to recover successfully.

Christien Oussoren

Christien Oussoren studied pharmacy at Utrecht University and received her pharmacy degree in 1990. From October 1990 to September 1991, she worked as a pharmacist in a hospital and a community pharmacy. Dr. Oussoren received her PhD from Utrecht University in 1996. In January 1997, she was appointed a faculty member at the University of Utrecht. Her main research interests are in the field of biodistribution and in vivo application of colloidal drug carrier systems.

Robert Palmer

Robert Palmer, presently a medical student at the Medical College of Ohio, worked in Dr. Bruce Carlson's laboratory after his graduation from college.

Katalin Prokai-Tatrai

Katalin Prokai-Tatrai received a BS (1979) and an MS (1981) in chemical engineering and a PhD in organic chemistry (1986) from the University of Veszprem, Hungary. She held a faculty position and did research in organometallic chemistry and organic synthesis in the Department of Organic Chemistry at the University of Veszprem before emigrating to the United States in 1987. She worked as a Research Scientist and later as Senior Research Scientist at Pharmatech, Inc. (Alacuha, Fla.), before transferring to the Department of Pharmacology and Therapeutics in the College of Medicine at the University of Florida in 1989 to develop potential drugs against Alzheimer's disease. In 1993, Dr. Prokai-Tatrai joined the Center for Drug Discovery, where she became Associate Scientist. Her primary research is in the design and development of brain-targeted delivery of neuropeptides. She is the coauthor of over 30 publications, including a patent.

Laszlo Prokai

Laszlo Prokai received his BS (1978) and MS (1980) degrees in chemical engineering and a PhD (1983) in radiochemistry from the University of Veszprem, Hungary. He worked for the Hungarian Oil and Gas Research Institute in Veszprem and was an Adjunct Lecturer in the Department of Organic Chemistry at the University of Veszprem until 1986. Then he joined the Center for Drug Design and Delivery in the Department of Medicinal Chemistry at the College of Pharmacy at the University of Florida (Gainesville) to pursue postdoctoral research. He became Assistant Research Scientist in 1989 in the Department of Medicinal Chemistry. In 1991, he was appointed Assistant Professor in the Center for Drug Discovery and the Department of Pharmaceutics at the College of Pharmacy at the University of Florida (Gainesville), with a promotion to Associate Professor in 1996.

Dr. Prokai's research interests include metabolism-based drug design and discovery, peptide drug delivery into the central nervous system, biochemistry, and the pharmacology of neuropeptides. He is also an expert in analytical mass spectrometry. Dr. Prokai has authored a book, coauthored 5 book chapters, and written over 60 scientific articles. He is a member of the American Chemical Society, the Hungarian Chemical Society, and the American Society for Mass Spectrometry.

Fabiana Quaglia

Fabiana Quaglia is a postdoctoral fellow in the Department of Pharmaceutical and Toxicological Chemistry at the University of Naples, Italy. She received her degree in pharmacy in 1992 and a PhD in pharmaceutical sciences in 1997 from the University of Naples. In 1997, she had a postdoctoral fellowship at the University of Paris-Sud-France. Her research interests include the investigation of in vitro models that mimic interactions between drugs/biological structures and carriers for the controlled release of drugs and biomacromolecules.

Steven C. Sutton

Steven C. Sutton served as a summer intern at Ayerst Labs (Rouses Point, N.Y.), which led to a BS in pharmacy from the Massachusetts College of Pharmacy and a retail pharmacy position. He then received a PhD in pharmaceutical sciences from the State University of New York at Buffalo and was a researcher in oral drug delivery at CIBA-Geigy (Ardsley, N.Y.) and oral permeation enhancers and in vitro–in vivo correlations (IVIVC) at INTERx Research Labs (Lawrence, Kan.).

Dr. Sutton is Principal Research Investigator in the Pharmaceutical R&D Dept. at Pfizer Central Research (Groton, Conn.), where he is pursuing the solubility and permeability limitations of drug candidates, computer modeling of complex gastrointestinal and pharmacokinetic problems, and IVIVC of extended-release formulations. Dr. Sutton was a founder of the AAPS Hudson Valley and Kansas City Pharmaceutics Discussion Groups and the Oral Absorption Focus Group. He has chaired the AAPS Midwest Regional Meeting and was the AAPS representative on the Biopharmaceutics Classification System Expert Panel. Dr. Sutton has written over 70 articles, abstracts of work in progress, and presentations.

Susan L. Way

Susan L. Way received her BS in chemistry and biology from Georgetown College, Kentucky, in 1983 and her PhD in pharmaceutical sciences from the University of Kentucky in 1992. She has been working in the pharmaceutical industry since 1992 and is experienced in both solid and nonsolid dosage form development. She is currently employed at Boehringer Ingelheim Pharmaceuticals, Inc. (Ridgefield, Conn.), where her responsibilities include preclinical and clinical formulation development and preformulation activities.

Samuel H. Yalkowsky

Samuel H. Yalkowsky received his BS in pharmacy from Columbia University in 1965 and his PhD in pharmaceutical chemistry from the University of Michigan in 1969. He was associated with the Upjohn Company from 1969 until 1982, when he joined the faculty at the University of Arizona.

Dr. Yalkowsky is currently involved in basic research on the relationships between chemical structure and physical phenomena. He has developed a state-of-the-art algorithm for estimating the aqueous solubility of organic compounds. He has also made great progress in developing an algorithm for estimating the melting points of organic compounds. In addition, Dr. Yalkowsky is studying the alteration of solubility by physical means, including the development of formulations for insoluble drugs and the improved dissolution of environmentally important solutes from soil. This formulation work has been extended to include the development of novel dosage forms and the pharmaceutical evaluation of parenteral formulations. His work has led to over 100 scientific publications and patents and 3 books.

Section A

Background of Pain, Irritation, and/or Muscle Damage with Injectables

1

Challenges in the Development of Injectable Products

Michael J. Akers

Biopharmaceutical Products Development
Lilly Research Laboratories
Indianapolis, Indiana

The injection of drugs is necessary either because a need exists for a very rapid therapeutic effect, or the drug compound is not systemically available by non-injectable routes of administration. Early use of injections led to many adverse reactions because the needs for sterility and freedom from pyrogenic contamination were poorly understood (Avis 1992). Although Pasteur and Lister recognized the need for sterilization to eliminate pathogenic microorganisms during the 1860s, sterilization technologies did not advance until much later. For example, the autoclave was discovered in 1884, membrane filtration in 1918, ethylene oxide in 1944, high efficiency particulate air (HEPA) filters in 1952, and laminar airflow in 1961. Increases in body temperature and chills in patients receiving injections were observed in 1911, which were found in 1923 to be due to bacteria-produced pyrogens. The science and technology of manufacturing and using injectable products have both come a long way since their inception in the mid-1850s. However, the assurance of sterility, particularly with injectable products manufactured by aseptic manufacturing processes, continues to be tremendously challenging to the parenteral drug industry.

Injectable products have some very special characteristics unlike any other pharmaceutical dosage form (Table 1.1). Each of these characteristics offers unique challenges in the development, manufacture, testing, and use of these products. These will be discussed more specifically in later sections of this chapter.

Table 1.1. Special Characteristics of and Requirements for Injectable Dosage Forms

---

- Toxicologically safe—many potential formulation additives are not sufficiently safe for injectable drug administration

- Sterile

- Free from pyrogenic (including endotoxin) contamination

- Free from foreign particulate matter

- Stable—not only physically and chemically but also microbiologically

- Compatible with intravenous admixtures if indicated

- Isotonic

GENERAL CHALLENGES

From a formulation development standpoint, the injectable product formulation must be as simple as possible. As long as there are no major stability, compatibility, solubility, or delivery problems with the active ingredient, injectable product formulation is relatively easy to accomplish. Ideally, the formulation will contain the active ingredient and water in a vehicle (e.g., sodium chloride or dextrose) that is isotonic with bodily fluid. Unfortunately, most active ingredients to be injected do not possess these ideal properties. Many drugs are only slightly soluble or are insoluble in aqueous media. Many drugs are unstable for extended periods of time in solution and even in the solid state. Some drugs are very interactive with surfaces such as the container/closure surface, surfaces of other formulation additives, or surfaces of administration devices.

There are three interesting phenomena that make injectable drug formulation, processing and delivery so complicated compared to other pharmaceutical dosage forms:

1. There are relatively few safe and acceptable formulation additives that can be used. If the drug has significant stability, solubility, processing, contamination, and/or delivery problems, the formulation scientist does not have a plethora of formulation materials that can be used to solve these problems.

2. In non-parenteral processing, because of the frequent potential for powder toxicology concerns, the process is set up to protect personnel from the product. In injectable product processing, the opposite exists—the process is set up to protect the product from personnel because the major sources of contamination are people.

3.   When a manufacturer releases a non-injectable dosage form to the marketplace, the ultimate consumer takes that dosage form from its package and consumes it. Because there is little manipulation of the non-injectable dosage form, potential problems created by the consumer of these products are infrequent. However, most injectable dosage forms experience one or several extra manipulations before administration to the patient. Injectable drug products are withdrawn from vials or ampoules, placed in administration devices, and/or combined with other solutions, and they are sometimes combined with other drugs. The point here is that something is usually done to the injectable product that can potentially affect its stability or solubility, or another performance factor; such manipulations are done beyond the control of the manufacturer. Yet when problems occur, e.g., stability or solubility issues, the manufacturer is responsible for solving them even though the manufacturer did not cause them.

SAFETY CONCERNS

Drug products administered by injection must be safe from two standpoints: (1) the nature of the formulation components of the product and (2) the anatomical/physiological effects of the drug product during and after injection.

Compared to other pharmaceutical dosage forms, there are relatively few formulation additives a formulation scientist can choose from to solve solubility and/or stability problems, maintain sterility, achieve and maintain isotonicity, extend or control the release of drugs from depot injections, or accomplish some other need from a formulation standpoint (e.g., bulking agent, viscosity agent, suspending/emulsifying agent). Because of the irreversibility of the injectable route of administration and the immediate effect and contact of the drug product with the bloodstream and systemic circulation, any substance that has potential toxic properties, either related to the type of substance or its dose, will either be unsuitable for parenteral administration or will have restrictions for the maximum amount to be in the formulation. For example, the choices of antimicrobial preservative agents for parenteral administration are very limited, and even those agents that are acceptable have limits on how much of the agent can be contained in a marketed dosage form. Similar restrictions exist for antioxidant agents, surface active agents, solubilizers, cosolvents, and other stabilizers (e.g., disodium ethylenediaminetetraacetic acid [EDTA]).

There are many potential clinical hazards that may result from the administration of drugs by injection (Duma et al. 1992) (Table 1.2). Several of these hazards (e.g., hypersensitivity reactions, particulate matter, phlebitis)

Table 1.2. Clinical Hazards of Parenteral Administration

Air emboli

- Limited to IV or IA (intra-arterial) usage

Bleeding

- Usually related to patient's condition

Fever and Toxicity

- Local or systemic
- Secondary to allergic or toxic reaction

Hypersensitivity

- Immediate and delayed

Incompatibilities

- Can be most threatening if occurring in the vascular compartment

Infiltration and extravasation

- Limited to IV or IA usage

Overdosage

- Drugs or fluids

Particulate matter

- Most serious in IV or IA administration
- Can cause foreign body reaction

Phlebitis

- Usually with IV administration

Sepsis

- May be localized, systemic, or metastatic

Thrombosis

- Limited to IV or IA administration

---

can be directly related to formulation and/or packaging components. For example, some well-known hypersensitivity reactions exist with the use of bisulfites, phenol, thimerosal, parabens, and latex rubber.

MICROBIOLOGICAL AND OTHER CONTAMINATION CHALLENGES

There are three primary potential contamination issues to deal with. The first is to achieve and maintain *sterility*. Sterility, obviously, is the uniquely premier attribute of a sterile product. The concept of sterility is intriguing because it is an absolute attribute, i.e., the product is either sterile or not sterile. The achievement, maintenance, and testing of sterility involve challenges that occupy the time, energy, and money of thousands of people and numerous resources. Sterility, by definition, is simple—the absence of microbial life. However, how does one prove sterility? Compendial sterility tests use a very small sample from a much larger product population. How confident can one be of the sterility of each and every unit of product based on the test results of a very small sample size? Sterility essentially cannot be proved; it can only be assured. This is a huge challenge to the parenteral drug and device industry.

Sterility can be achieved by a variety of methods, including saturated steam under pressure (the autoclave), dry heat, gases such as ethylene oxide and vapor phase hydrogen peroxide, radiation such as cobalt 60 gamma radiation, and aseptic filtration through at least 0.2 μm filters. Different types of materials and products are sterilized by different methods. For example, glass containers are usually sterilized by dry heat; rubber closures and filter assemblies by saturated steam under pressure; plastic and other heat labile materials by gaseous or radiation methods; and final product solutions either by saturated steam under pressure (if the product can withstand high temperatures), or, more commonly, by aseptic filtration. Each of these sterilization procedures must undergo significant study (process validation) in order to ensure that the method is dependable to a high degree of assurance to sterilize the material/product in question under normal production conditions. Great challenges exist in performing sterilization process validation and monitoring. There are also continuous efforts to find newer or better sterilization methods to increase the convenience and assurance of sterility (Akers et al. 1997).

Injectable products must be *free from pyrogenic contamination*. Pyrogens are metabolic by-products of microbial growth and death. Pyrogenic contamination must be prevented since the most common sterilization methods (e.g., steam sterilization, aseptic filtration) cannot destroy or remove pyrogens. Prevention can occur using solutes prepared under pyrogenic conditions, pyrogen-free water produced by distillation or reverse osmosis, pyrogen-free packaging materials where glass containers have been depyrogenated by validated dry heat sterilization methods, and rubber closures and plastic materials that have been sufficiently rinsed with pyrogen-free water. The reason for Good Manufacturing Practice (GMP) requirements for time limitations during parenteral product processing is to eliminate the potential for pyrogenic contamination, since subsequent sterilization of the product will remove microbial contamination but not necessarily pyrogens.

In sufficient injected amounts, pyrogens can be very harmful to humans. Pyrogens are composed of lipopolysaccharides that will react with the hypothalamus of mammals, producing an elevation in body temperature (hence its Greek roots [*pyro* means fire and *gen* means beginning]).

Depending on the amount of pyrogen injected, other physiological problems can occur, including death. Compendial tests, both in vivo (rabbit model) and in vitro (Limulus amebocyte lysate), are established to ensure that products used in humans are tested and do not contain levels of pyrogens that will do any harm.

Injectable products, if injected or infused as solutions, must be *free from particulate matter contamination*. Particulate matter in injectables connotates at least three important perceptions:

1.   The degree of product quality and the subsequent reflection of the quality of the product manufacturer.

2.   The degree of product quality in the "customer's" view (patient, medical professional, regulatory agency).

3.   The clinical implications of the potential hazards of particulate matter.

The first two perceptions—related to the manufacturer and to the user or customer—are relatively well-defined and understood in that evidence of particulate matter will trigger a series of reactions, ranging from product complaints to product recalls and other regulatory actions. However, the third perception, that particulate matter is clinically hazardous, begs more questions and discussion. There is substantial evidence of the adverse physiological effects of injected particulate matter, but still much conjecture regarding the relationship between the clinical hazard and the type, size, and number of particulates (Groves 1993).

STABILITY CHALLENGES

Injectable drugs are administered either as solutions or as dispersed systems (suspensions, emulsions, liposomes, other microparticulate systems). The majority of injectable drugs have some kind of instability problem. Many drugs that are sufficiently stable in ready-to-use solutions have some stability restrictions such as storage in light-protected packaging systems or storage at refrigerated conditions, or there may be formulation ingredients that stabilize the drug but can themselves undergo degradation.

The *chemical stability* of injectable products generally involves two primary routes of degradation—hydrolytic and oxidative. Other, less predominant, chemical degradation mechanisms of injectable drugs involve racemization, photolysis, and some special types of chemical reactions occuring with large molecules. A majority of injectable drug products are too unstable in solution to be marketed as ready-to-use solutions. Instead, they are available as sterile solids produced by lyophilization (freeze-drying) or sterile crystallization/powder filling technologies. Drugs that can be marketed as ready-to-use solutions or suspensions still offer the challenge of needing suitable buffer systems or antioxidant formulations for long-term storage stability. Freeze-dried products can undergo degradation during the freezing and/or freeze-drying process and, therefore, require formulation additives to minimize degradation or other physical-chemical instability problems. Drugs sensitive to oxidation require not only suitable antioxidants and chelating agents in the formulation, but they also require special precautions during manufacturing (e.g., oxygen-free conditions), and special packaging and storage conditions to protect the solution from light, high temperature, and any ingress of oxygen. Stabilization of injectable drugs against chemical degradation offers a huge challenge to formulation scientists.

Physical stability problems are well-known for protein injectable dosage forms as proteins tend to self-aggregate and eventually precipitate. Many injectable drugs are poorly soluble and require cosolvents or solid additives to enhance and maintain drug solubility. However, improper storage conditions, temperature cycling, or interactions with other components of the product/package system can all contribute to incompatibilities resulting, usually, in the drug falling out of solution (manifested as haze, crystals, or precipitate). Again, the formulation scientist is challenged with finding solutions to physical instability problems. Such solutions can be found with either creative formulation techniques or special handling and storage requirements.

Microbiological issues arise with storage stability related to the container-closure system being capable of maintaining sterility of the product; the antimicrobial preservative system, if present, still meeting compendial microbial challenge tests; and the potential for inadvertent contamination of non-terminally sterilized products and the degree of assurance that such products will not become contaminated. The concern for microbiological purity as a function of product stability has caused the Food and Drug Administration (FDA) and other worldwide regulatory bodies to require manufacturers of injectable products to perform sterility tests at the end of the product shelflife or to have sufficient container-closure integrity data to ensure product sterility over the shelf life of the product.

The *compatibility* of injectable drugs when combined with one another and/or combined with intravenous fluid diluents can create significant issues for formulation scientists. Unlike solid and semisolid dosage forms, which are used as they were released from the manufacturer, injectable dosage forms are usually manipulated by people (pharmacist, nurse, physician) other than the ultimate consumer (patient) and are combined with other drug products and/or diluents before injection or infusion. These manipulations and combinations are beyond the control of the manufacturer and can potentially lead to an assortment of problems. For example, faulty aseptic techniques during manipulation (e.g., reconstitution, transfer, admixture) can lead to inadvertent contamination of the final product. In addition, drug combinations and additions to certain intravenous diluents can lead to physical and chemical incompatibilities. It is a great challenge to the injectable product formulator and Quality Control (QC) management to anticipate these potential problems and do whatever can be done to avoid or eliminate them.

SOLUBILITY CHALLENGES

Many drugs intended for injectable administration are not readily soluble in water. Classic examples include steroids, phenytoin, diazepam, amphotericin B, and digoxin. While most insolubility problems can be solved, they usually require a great amount of effort from the formulation development scientist. If a more soluble salt form of the insoluble drug is not available (e.g., poor stability, difficulty in manufacture, cost, etc.), then two basic formulation approaches can be attempted. One involves using formulation additives such as water miscible cosolvents, complexating agents (such as cyclodextrin derivatives), and surface active agents. If none of these additives work, then the other approach involves the formulation of a more complex dosage form such as an emulsion or liposome. Table 1.3 lists the most common approaches for solving solubility problems with injectable drugs.

Table 1.3. Approaches for Increasing Solubility

Salt formation (~1000× increase)

pH adjustment

Use of cosolvents (~1000× increase)

Use of surface-active agents (~100× increase): e.g., polyoxyethylene sorbitan monooleate (0.1 to 0.5%) and polyoxyethylene-polyoxypropylene ethers (0.05 to 0.25%)

Use of complexing agents (~500× increase): e.g., β-cyclodextrins and polyvinyl pyrrolidone (PVP)

Microemulsion formulation

Liposome formulation

Mixed micelle formulation (bile salt + phospholipid)

"Heroic" measures: e.g., for cancer clinical trial formulations, use dimethylsulfoxide (DMSO), high concentrations of surfactants, polyols, alcohols, fatty acids, etc.

PACKAGING CHALLENGES

A formulator can create an excellent injectable formulation that is very stable, easily manufacturable, and elegant. Yet the formulation must be compatible with a packaging system. Currently, the most common injectable packaging systems are glass vials with rubber closures and plastic vials and bottles with rubber closures. Glass-sealed ampoules are not as popular as in the past because of concerns with glass breakage and particulates. Other packaging systems include glass and plastic syringes, glass bottles, glass cartridges, and plastic bags.

The formulation scientist must recognize that rubber closures are formulations in themselves and, thus, contain several components that can either leach out of the rubber material or be responsible for adsorbing drug molecules or other components like antimicrobial preservatives from the product solution. A great amount of effort must take place to ensure that the rubber closure is compatible with the drug formulation. Studies that must be conducted include long-term stability tests, where the container is inverted so that the product experiences maximum contact with the rubber closure.

Packaging materials are known to be primary sources of particulate matter contamination due to either inadequate cleaning of the packaging material or substances leaching from the material. Examples include glass particles, polymeric particles, and rubber leachates such as zinc, aluminum, and other rubber component materials.

MANUFACTURING CHALLENGES

The greatest manufacturing challenge, assuming the drug product cannot withstand terminal sterilization, is the achievement, maintenance, and assurance of sterility. Examination of a typical process flowchart in Figure 1.1 reveals many potential opportunities for contamination if the manufacturing process is not well controlled.

Table 1.4 lists all of the factors that must be in control for sterility assurance in manufacturing drug products by aseptic processing. Each of these factors requires significant resources to do the job correctly. Because of the great concerns for potential contamination of products produced by aseptic processing and the fact that the primary source of such contamination originates from people working in the aseptic environment, new technologies such as barrier isolator technology and blow-fill-seal filling systems are being developed. These technologies allow products to be manufactured aseptically in sterile environments without the need for direct contact of product and people.

Figure 1.1. Typical process flowchart.

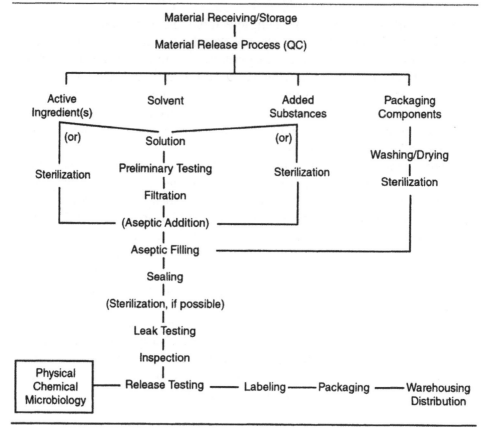

Table 1.4. Factors Involved in Sterility Assurance

Environmental monitoring	Sanitization
Operator involvement	Media fills
Facilities	Sterile filtration validation
HVAC (heating, ventilation, and air-conditioning) system monitoring and maintenance	Bioburden and microbial limits testing
Validation of sterilization cycles	Container-closure integrity
Contingency plans for unusual events during manufacturing	Adherence to and enforcement of established programs
Compendial sterility testing	Compendial preservative efficacy testing

Besides sterility assurance, other manufacturing challenges include

1. Minimizing formation of particulate matter during processing

2. Maintaining product stability, particularly of protein products, during processing

3. Special processing requirements for processing sterile powders, dispersed systems (e.g., suspensions and emulsions), and advanced formulations such as microspheres, liposomes, and devices.

4. Development, control, and validation of freeze-drying cycles

5. Sorting and labeling operations to ensure that no lot reaches the market that has significant quality defects, and that all product labels are accurate.

6. Proper handling of the finished product before release to and distribution throughout the world.

DELIVERY/ADMINISTRATION CHALLENGES

There are many potential hazards in the administration of drugs by the injectable route. These are presented in Table 1.2. Pain and tissue irritation are caused by a variety of factors covered throughout this volume. The formulation scientist must ensure that the formulation ingredients and packaging materials are non-toxic qualitatively and quantitatively, and that the final formulation is isotonic or as close to being isotonic as possible. The challenge lies in formulating a final injectable drug product that is soluble, stable, and compatible while using a minimal number of well-known formulation additives and known packaging materials (glass, rubber, plastic). This is a challenge far easier said than done because of the severe limitations in the type and quantity of formulation additives acceptable for use in injectable products. There are, however, a number of resources available to the scientist responsible for sterile drug dosage form development that provide guidance and examples of acceptable formulation additives to solve problems with solubility, stability, maintenance of sterility, and minimization of pain and tissue irritation (Boylan et al. 1995; Akers 1995; Ahern and Manning 1992; Pearlman and Wang 1996).

REFERENCES

Ahern, T. J., and M. C. Manning, eds. 1992. *Stability of protein pharmaceuticals, Part A and Part B*. New York: Plenum Press

Akers, M. J. 1995. Parenterals: Small volume. In *Encyclopedia of pharmaceutical technology*, edited by J. Swarbrick. and J. C. Boylan. New York: Marcel Dekker.

Akers, M. J., S. L. Nail, and M. J. Groves. 1997. Top 10 current technical issue in parenteral science revisited. *Pharm. Tech.* 21:126–135.

Avis, K. E. 1992 The parenteral dosage form and its historical development. In *Pharmaceutical Dosage Forms: Parenteral Medications*, vol. 1, 2nd ed., edited by K. E. Avis, H. A. Lieberman, and L. Lachman. New York: Marcel Dekker, pp. 1–15.

Boylan, J. C., A. L. Fites, and S. L. Nail. 1995. Parenteral products. In *Modern pharmaceutics*, edited by G. S. Banker and C. T. Rhodes. New York: Marcel Dekker.

Duma, R. J., M. J. Akers, and S. J. Turco. 1992. Parenteral drug administration: Routes, precautions, problems, complications, and drug delivery systems. In *Pharmaceutical dosage forms: Parenteral medications*, vol. 1, 2nd ed., edited by K. E. Avis, H. A. Lieberman, and L. Lachman. New York: Marcel Dekker, pp. 17–58.

Groves, M. J. 1993. Particulate matter: Sources and resources for healthcare manufacturers. Buffalo Grove, Ill., USA: Interpharm Press, Inc.

Pearlman, R., and Y. J. Wang. 1996. *Formulation, characterization, and stability of protein pharmaceuticals*. New York: Plenum Press.

2

Pain, Irritation, and Tissue Damage with Injections

Wolfgang Klement

Department of Anesthesiology and Intensive Care
Ev. Jung-Stilling-Hospital
Siegen, Federal Republic of Germany

MUST INJECTIONS HURT?

Parenteral administration of drugs is common in medical practice, especially for drugs with little or no bioavailability following gastrointestinal absorption, with more rapid onset times than possible with oral administration, or with desired local effects. Since needles are used to penetrate the skin, some amount of pain is tolerated by the physician (who does not feel it) and by the patient (who preferably wants to get help). Pain, however, is an essential sensation warning the organism against possible tissue damage. Scrutiny of knowledge about the possibility of irritation and damage with certain drugs and their formulations reveals that the physician's knowledge of irritation and damage is often small compared to the increasing numbers of injections and infusions he or she applies.

This chapter's point of view derives from the author's experiences with years of intravenous (IV) administration of infusions and anesthetic drugs with relatively high incidences of pain, itching, edema, and thrombotic complications; often, there is little knowledge about the underlying mechanisms and tolerance of the "usual" problems. Anesthesiologists, in particular, are confronted with problems associated with injections, especially with IV routes, for the following reasons:

- Anesthesia, regional or general, is usually performed through an IV line.

- By means of their daily training, anesthesiologists are considered "IV specialists" and are often called in case of problems with IV lines and administration.

- Most of the anesthetic drug formulations, minimally, have the potency to evoke pain.

Thus, most of the studies dealing with pain and discomfort on injection are related to data from anesthesia-related drugs.

Systematic studies in humans about serious sequelae of injections are lacking. This may be due to ethical reasons or to the scarcity of such complications, since new drug formulations have been tested extensively in animals before administration in humans is allowed. Nevertheless, there are numerous case reports dealing with thrombotic complications, tissue damage, and necrosis after drug injections. This helps us keep in mind that pain, irritation, and damage are still problems with injectable products and that we must not diminish our efforts to design safer drug formulations.

MECHANISMS OF PAIN AND DAMAGE

From a theoretical point of view, there are a number of factors that can lead to pain and damage.

Pain is mediated by the stimulation of nociceptors, which are spread throughout the whole organism in different densities. Nociceptors can be stimulated by strong mechanical pressure, low or high temperatures, and/or chemical irritants. The possible chemical agents are numerous and may be released from noxious cellular damage (e.g., potassium and hydrogen ions, adenosine triphosphate [ATP]) or they may be a chain link in the inflammation cascade that takes place after a noxious stimulus (e.g., kinines, histamine, serotonin, etc.; see Figure 2.1).

Thus, injections may cause pain mechanically by forcing a nonfitting volume of injection into tissue or a small vessel, by low (< 20°C) or high (> 40°C) temperature of the injected solution, or by chemical activation (directly or by causing cellular damage). Remember that pain not only warns of possible tissue damage, but that serious and noxious stimuli also cause the nociceptors to release mediators for starting the inflammatory cascade (e.g., substance P, calcitonin gene-related peptide, etc.), which in turn causes weal, flare reaction, and edema. In sum, chemical irritants may cause not only pain but also morphological changes like inflammation via excessive stimulation of nociceptors.

Cellular and tissue damage can be caused by cellular or tissue specific toxicity or by aggressive physicochemical properties (e.g., acidity, basicity, high or low osmolality) leading to cellular membrane destabilization. In both cases, the extent of possible damage depends on the local peak concentration of the irritant, as well as on the time course of local

Figure 2.1. Interactions of nociceptor, tissue, and vessels during inflamation following trauma.

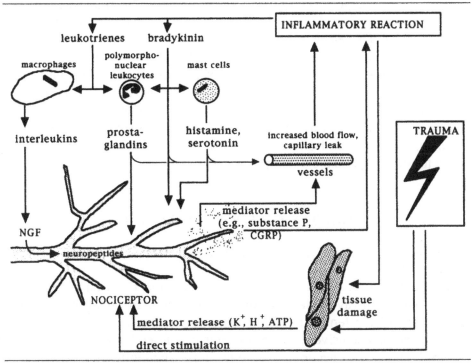

Trauma causes cellular damage and thus direct and indirect noxious stimulation of the nociceptor. The mediators released by the activated nociceptor start the inflammation cascade, leading to an increase in nociceptor activation, mediator release, and vascular and tissue reactions.

concentration. The peak concentration in the tissue or blood is determined by the concentration and volume of the injection and the speed of injection. Immediate processes like dilution in blood, local binding (e.g., proteins, fat), enzymatic degradation, and chemical reactions all contribute to the effective peak concentration during injections.

The time course of local concentration depends on the distribution (diffusion) of the substance in the tissue and the velocity of chemical reactions with the surrounding tissue. This, in turn, depends on the supply of reacting substances and thus is often determined by local blood flow. Thus, the possibility for serious sequelae is highest with injections of noxious formulations designed for specific areas into the wrong area (e.g., solutions for artery embolization of arteriovenous malformations into the wrong vessel or paravascularly; paravascular administration of chemotherapy; injection of a solution for an intramuscular [IM] route into subcutaneous fat).

Various kinds of *allergic reactions* can also cause complications, both at the site of injection as well as systemically. The reason for damage is based on the molecular structure of all substances. Aspects of a drug formulation other than the actual drug (vehicles, diluents, stabilizers) are also able to cause allergic reactions. This mixture should be tailored to the patient's disposition and allergies. In most cases, local reactions are moderate and transient. Therefore, allergic reactions will only be discussed when their likelihood is high or there is a possibility for severe damage.

This chapter presents an overview of the problems and sequelae that can occur using different routes of injection, primarily IV. Certain drugs and formulations will serve as examples (where possible sequelae with injections were observed and studied). If known, reasons and mechanisms for pain, irritation, and damage are described, and suggestions are provided to prevent possible damage.

ROUTES OF DRUG INJECTION

Cutaneous/Subcutaneous Injections

Subcutaneous and, in particular, paravascular injections have been performed where intravascular injections were intended. Since it is unclear whether or not inattentive paravascular injections will occur with incorrect needle position exclusively, this problem is discussed later.

Subcutaneous injections are done more frequently into tissues with relatively low blood flow like fat and connective tissue. On the one hand, this would hopefully produce the desired effect of slow absorption and longer duration of action. Irritant drug formulations, on the other hand, also form long acting subcutaneous deposits and stay in contact with the tissue, vessels, and nerve fibers, slowly decreasing in concentration. Therefore, the theoretical possibility of causing damage is high, and this is the reason that some drug formulations designed for injection into the muscles with a good blood supply may cause severe damage when injected into subcutaneous fat.

A review of possible cutaneous reactions to injectables was published recently (Morgan 1995a; Morgan 1995b). It included special aspects of skin pathology and histopathology. In most of the cutaneous and subcutaneous injections three groups of drugs were administered: insulins, heparins, and local anesthetics. Therefore, these drugs will serve as examples for sequelae of cutaneous injections for the following discussion.

In the case of *insulin,* local reactions to injection are frequently immunologic problems. In early formulations, pain, itching, flare, edema, and indurations occurred in more than 50 percent of the patients during therapy. These preparations were impure and acidic (pH 3.5), which may explain the high incidence of allergic reactions and pain on injection. The incidence of allergic reactions decreased with highly purified insulins and is minimal with human insulin produced using recombinant DNA (deoxyribonucleic acid) technology (Goldfine and Kahn 1994). Since the incidence of latex allergies seems to be increasing, care should be taken that the sealing compounds of vials and syringes used in insulin therapy do not contain rubber. This may exert an allergic reaction that does not depend on insulin allergy (Towse et al. 1995). A special case of damage to the cutis and subcutis is caused by insulin-induced lipatrophy, which occurs with repeated injections at the same injection site. The incidence is said to be up to 3 percent in adults and even higher in children. The underlying mechanism is thought to be immunologic (Reeves et al. 1980). The addition of corticosteroids (Kumar et al. 1977), use of highly purified insulins, regular change of injection site, and intramuscular administration should prevent its development.

With subcutaneous *heparin* injection, a heparin-induced skin necrosis may occur days after the drug administration (starting with edema, flare, and pain at the injection site) and lead to necrotic lesions of the cutis and subcutis. An impressive image of such a reaction was recently published (Christiaens and Nieuwenhuis 1996). This complication is rare and its causes are unknown, but the delay between first injections and necrosis does not indicate a direct chemical reaction to the drug formulation. Since heparin-induced skin necrosis is often accompanied by thrombocytopenia, it may represent a localized form of the heparin-induced thrombocytopenia syndrome (Mar et al. 1995) and cause local thrombotic lesions of small vessels followed by tissue necrosis.

Local anesthetics, usually administered intra- or subcutaneously for minor surgical procedures, were known to cause pain on injection, especially in the case of lidocaine. That pain on injection occurs with the application of local anesthetics, which the patient is told will minimize his or her pain during surgery, does not help improve the patient's confidence in modern medicine. Numerous studies have been performed, examining how to avoid pain on injection (see Table 2.1).

Since the pH of various formulations of lidocaine varies between 4 and 5 (author's unpublished data; Lugo-Janer et al. 1993), the acidity was believed to cause pain, thus, the solutions were buffered, usually with small amounts of 8.4 percent sodium bicarbonate. With the use of buffered versus plain lidocaine, the intensity of pain on intra- and subcutaneous injection decreased by 40 to 80 percent (Brogan et al. 1995; Matsumoto et al. 1994; Christoph et al. 1988). Similar results were obtained with buffered lidocaine in digital nerve blocks (Bartfield et al. 1993), buffered prilocaine in IV regional anesthesia (Armstrong et al. 1990), and intracutaneously injected buffered mepivacaine (Christoph et al. 1988).

Some authors tried to use warmed plain lidocaine (37 to 40°C) to minimize pain on injection. While pain intensity sometimes decreased by 40 to 70 percent (Brogan et al. 1995; Davidson and Boom 1992), others failed to evoke beneficial effects with warming (Mader et al. 1994; Dalton et al. 1989). Buffered lidocaine provoked the same low pain intensity with 37°C

Table 2.1. Studies Reflecting Efforts to Minimize Pain on Injection with Local Anesthetics

Reference	Local Anesthetic	Block	Method and Success in Reducing Pain			
			Warm	Buffered	Warm and Buffered	Diluted
Martin et al. (1996)	Lidocaine (buffered)	s.c.	Ø			
Waldbillig (1995)	Lidocaine	digital nerve	→			
Brogan et al. (1995)	Lidocaine	s.c.	↓↓	↓↓		
Farley et al. (1994)	Lidocaine, mepivacaine	i.c.		↓↓		→
Matsumoto et al.(1994)	Lidocaine	i.c.		↓↓		Ø
Mader et al. (1994)	Lidocaine	s.c.	Ø	Ø	↓↑	
Lugo-Janer et al (1993)	Lidocaine, epinephrine	i.c.		↓↓		
Bartfield et al. (1993)	Lidocaine	digital nerve				→
Davidson and Boom (1992)	Lidocaine	s.c.	↓↓	↓↓		
Armstong et al. (1990)	Prilocaine	Bier's block	↓↓	↓↓		
Christoph et al. (1988)	Lidocaine, mepivacaine	i.c.		↓↓		

Ophthalmologic and urologic blocks were omitted. Methods for reduction of pain were warming to 37°C, buffering with sodium bicarbonate, both, and dilution in salt solutions. Results are encrypted as Ø = no effect, ↓ = reduced pain, and ↓↓ = markedly reduced pain. Due to acid pH, buffering of local anesthetics is the most promising method for alleviation of pain on injection.

s.c. = subcutaneous; i.c. = intracutaneous

rather than 20°C (Martin et al. 1996), but others described no benefit of warming *or* buffering except when lidocaine was warmed *and* buffered (Mader et al. 1994). To add further to the confusion, saline solutions of lidocaine with a pH of 4.2 and 5.3 evoked less pain than buffered lidocaine with a pH of 8.4 (Lugo-Janer et al. 1993). In the latter study, however, only solutions with epinephrine were used, and its possible pain-evoking (or increasing) properties may have contributed to the confusion.

The reason for the painful injections is not easy to determine. None of the pain-reducing methods described before is able to make the injections painless. Although intra- and subcutaneous injections cause some pain mechanically by distracting the tissue (which may explain the pain occurring even with buffered local anesthetics), it remains unclear whether or not the substances themselves cause pain. Controlled studies using a placebo (i.e., pain testing with dermal injections of pure buffered diluent versus buffered diluent with local anesthetic) have not been performed with two exceptions:

1. Lugo-Janer and colleagues (1993) tested bacteriostatic saline solution with epinephrine 1:300,000, which was found to be significantly less painful on intradermal infiltration than lidocaine with epinephrine 1:100,000 with sodium bicarbonate 80 meq/mL. Unfortunately, two different amounts of epinephrine were used, thus decreasing the amount of information on lidocaine's intrinsic pain-evoking properties.

2. In contrast, Farley and associates (1994) found more discomfort with the injection of normal saline than with lidocaine in normal saline, which goes against its pain-evoking properties. Unfortunately, their preparation of normal saline had an acid pH of 4.8 versus a more normal pH of 6.5 with lidocaine in saline. Therefore, the acid pH of the preparations, not the local anesthetics, seem to evoke the pain with dermal injections.

Thus, pain on intra- and subcutaneous injections of local anesthetics is common, is incompatible with the idea of local anesthetics, depends in all likelihood on acid pH values, and thus can be avoided by buffering the drug solutions, which apparently does not affect the numbing activity.

Severe local reactions like skin necrosis, however, are rare. Allergic reactions, especially with local anesthetics of the esther type did occur. The systemic immediate type reactions can be serious and require immediate treatment. Local reactions were transient and usually did not cause lesions. Vasoactive additives like epinephrine may cause tissue damage, especially when applied in ear lobes or digits. The cause for necrosis is a long-lasting vasoconstriction and, therefore, is most likely due to ischemia. This type of necrosis is not related to local anesthetics but to alpha-adrenergic actions of vasoconstrictors. It may also happen following accidental application of such drugs, and serious sequelae can be prevented by immediate treatment with alpha-adrenergic blocking agents like phentolamine (Hardy and Agostini 1995).

Intramuscular Injections

IM injections were widely used for more than a century and—compared to IV administration—were thought to be less harmful and equally reliable in effect. The development of methods to measure drug concentrations in blood, however, revealed interindividual as well as interdrug differences in bioavailability (Koch-Weser 1974a, b). Since this time, and paralleled by the development of better materials and techniques of IV application, IM injections may not be used as often clinically. Nevertheless, many drugs are still injected intramuscularly, e.g., analgesics and antibiotics, and some problems do occur with this route of application. Due to the blood flow through skeletal muscle, injection concentration in the tissue decreases more quickly than in subcutaneous fat, with poor blood supply. But duration of contact of the concentrated injection to the tissue is long, when compared to IV injections with rapid dilution by blood.

Although skeletal muscle is poorly innervated nociceptively, *pain* is frequent with intramuscular injections, and the reasons for this have been studied for years (Travell 1955; Taggart 1972). Research has shown that solutions with pH levels far above the physiologically tolerable range, and with high or very low osmolality give rise to pain on injection. The volume of the injection relates to pain intensity, so that, in addition to chemical activation, muscular nociceptors obviously respond to tissue distention. The size and cut of the needle used also contribute to pain on intramuscular injection. The nerve fibers stimulated by the needle, however, seem to be located in the skin and in subcutaneous connective tissue, since this type of pain can be reduced by local cooling. Adding local anesthetics to the injection has been recommended for pain relief, but are not used very often. Digital pressure applied to the region immediately before intramuscular injection reduced pain intensity by 37 percent (Barnhill et al. 1996).

Damage to muscle cells seems to occur with each intramuscular injection, leading to measurable elevations in serum creatine kinase (CK) concentrations. Numerous studies reported this nuisance in the diagnostic use of the enzyme in patients after intramuscular injections. Direct muscle toxicity of drugs, the distention trauma, the effects of certain drugs on cell membrane permeability, and other mechanisms were all accused of being responsible for enzyme release.

One ingenious study related the dimension of muscle damage to the physicochemical data of the injection (Sidell et al. 1974):

- With injection of constant volumes, CK response depends on the concentration of the drug and the osmolality of the solvents.

Injections of saline above an osmolality of 1.6 osmol/L increased CK activity in a concentration dependant manner up to 160 mU/mL with 3.2 osmol/L.

- Some drugs/solvents may have their own muscle toxicity, since osmolality/effect curves differ between substances and vehicles, e.g., pralidoxime chloride with an osmolality below 2.0 osmol/L increased CK activity to the same level as an equal volume of saline with an osmolality of 3.2 osmol/L.

- With the injection of constant concentrations, CK response was related to the injected volume, i.e., the total dose.

- Muscle activity after an IM injection increased the CK response.

This local cellular damage ("needle myopathy") seems to be unspecific, and the muscle usually regains normal function and histological appearance within several weeks. The reasons for this seem to be the same as those for pain and for cellular damage, i.e., injection volume, osmolality, and pH. Thus, common mechanisms may be responsible for the occurrence of both and pain on IM injection may be a predictor of damage, but studies relating pain incidence or intensity to CK response do not exist.

More permanent damage with muscle fibrosis, indurations, and even development of contractures has been reported with repeated injections of antibiotics, especially in children. More *specific muscular sequelae* (myotonia, necrosing myopathy, muscle lipidosis) due to drug interaction with skeletal muscle tissue have also been described (for a review, see Mastaglia [1982]). This was due not to the injection site but to muscle binding properties of the drugs.

Inattentive intravascular injections are a great problem in deep IM injections. A blood aspiration test is requested, but it does not guarantee its safety (see Figure 2.2).

Most of the disastrous IM injections leading to severe sequelae and extended tissue loss were probably administered intra-arterially. With intragluteal injections, thrombosis of the gluteal artery with necrosis of the gluteus maximus muscle has been described (Tokodi and Huber 1995). Such situations are especially serious in children, who are disproportionally affected by arterial injuries with IM injections (Weir 1988).

Local infections and abscess formations are also known sequelae of intramuscular injections. They are probably supported by the local tissue damage. Infections may be more serious, and tissue necrosis with necrotizing fasciitis has been found in six patients with intramuscular injections of a nonsteroidal anti-inflammatory drug. These conditions were also associated with septic complications and lethal outcomes in two of the patients (Pillans and O'Connor 1995).

Nerve damage with IM injections is not rare when incorrect techniques are used. With intragluteal injections, injury of the sciatic nerve was

Figure 2.2. Possible reasons for inattentive intravascular application with IM injections.

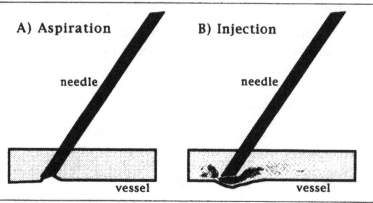

A) Aspiration   **B) Injection**

needle   needle

vessel   vessel

Although the needle tip was located intravascularly, aspiration test (A) is negative due to suction of the vessel wall into the needle lumen. The following injection (B) is completely intravascular.

reported, but nerve injury may also occur with other injection locations. Intraneural and intra-arterial injections cause immediate pain extending from the site of injection to the area supplied by the injured nerve or artery. The occurrence of such pain should force an immediate stop of the injection.

Thus, pain, irritation, infection, and nerve and tissue damage may occur with IM injections. Pain and local cellular damage are related to volume, osmolality, and pH of the injection, but some drugs may have an intrinsic potential for causing muscle damage (see also Chapter 3).

Intra-arterial Injections

Intra-arterial injections were performed either in order to get a local effect in the tissues supplied by the artery (e.g., intracoronarily) or inattentively when an IV or IM injection was intentional. Damage with arterial injections is frequent because of poor dilution of the injection (see Figure 2.3).

With IV injections, vessel diameter increases with blood flow direction, and the blood from all side branches dilutes the injection more and more, so that maximum concentration is present only at the tip of the IV needle. With intra-arterial injections, in contrast, vessel diameter decreases in the direction of the bloodstream. Initial dilution at the site of injection depends on the relation between local blood flow and injection speed. Rapid injection into a small artery let the bolus stream nearly undiluted into the small branches and into the microcirculation. The walls of arterioles and

Figure 2.3. Schematic figure of different dilution with intra-arterial and IV injections.

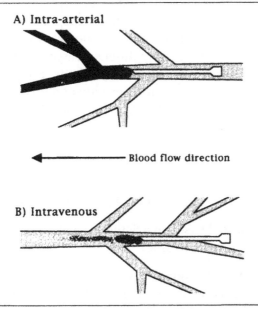

A) Intra-arterial

◄——————————— Blood flow direction

B) Intravenous

While with IV injection, the vessel diameter increases with the blood flow direction and injectate is diluted more and more by blood from side branches (B), intra-arterial bolus injection results in an immediate dilution only at the needle tip (A). This initially diluted bolus maintains its concentration while diverging into the small branches and into microcirculation.

capillaries are in contact with the bolus concentration as long as the injection lasts.

Another possibility is retrograde intra-arterial injection. Whenever injection speed exceeds the blood flow and microcirculation overload occurs, the injection may cause retrograde arterial flow and thus reach other, unintended, blood supply regions. In the past few years, invasive arterial catheter techniques have been developed for the diagnosis and selective treatment of arteriovenous malformations or cancer. With inattentive retrograde flow, chemotherapeutics or sclerosing agents may find the wrong regions with disastrous consequences. (For a review of potential complications with embolization therapy of brain arteriovenous malformations, see Frizzel and Fisher [1995]).

Even the intra-arterial use of vasodilators for treatment of acute vasospasm during catheter procedures may cause problems. Due to the different diluting properties of veins and arteries, IV formulations may cause problems when given intra-arterially, as described using a preparation of glyceryl trinitrate in the treatment of coronary vasospasm (Webb et al. 1983).

Most of the reports concerning damage after intra-arterial injections, however, refer to accidental and inattentive applications. Intra-arterial injection of irritants is accompanied by an immediate excruciating pain from the artery's region of blood supply. Intense vasoconstriction occurs with loss of peripheral pulses and blanching of the extremity, followed by cyanosis and, possibly, gangrene and permanent damage. The mechanisms remain unclear, but the following possibilities have been advocated to contribute to the damage:

- Precipitation of drug crystals in capillaries (e.g., with penicillin, barbiturates, diazepam)

- Hemolysis and aggregation of platelets occluding end-arterioles

- Local release of vasoconstrictive mediators (e.g., norepinephrine, endothelin, thromboxane)

Since both pain and vasoconstriction usually occur immediately, the latter mechanism seems to be the most likely candidate. Nitric oxide and endothelin, functional opponents in the control of vascular tone, were able to evoke pain and influence platelet function. Platelets release thromboxane, a vasoconstrictive mediator of inflammation. This close relationship between mediators of pain, vasotonus, and platelet function indicates common pathways in the involved mechanisms leading to irritation, ischemia, and thus damage with arterial injections.

In the case of propofol, an induction agent of anesthesia with well-known pain-evoking properties (see "What Causes Pain on IV Injection?"), another mechanism may be responsible for pain on injection, since intra-arterial injections will cause pain without damage (Holley and Cuthrell 1990; Brimacombe et al. 1994).

Due to contributing factors, therapy for accidental arterial injection of irritants includes immediate dilution, vasodilators, heparin, thrombolytic agents, and sympathetic blockade (Berger et al. 1988; Vangerven et al. 1989; Crawford and Terranova 1990; Treiman et al. 1990). The use of inhibitors of inflammatory mediation, like thromboxane (Zachary et al. 1987) was also proclaimed, and hyperbaric oxygen therapy may help to improve the result of therapy (Adir et al. 1991).

Nevertheless, despite all rapid, invasive, and aggressive treatment, permanent damage can still occur following accidental intra-arterial injection of irritants.

Intravenous Injections

The IV route for drug and fluid administration is widely used. It offers advantages like rapid onset of action if desired (e.g., drugs in emergency cases or for anesthesia induction), and therefore easy control by modulating the injection or infusion speed. Rapid dilution and buffering in the presence of blood (Figure 2.3) allows use of drug formulations with potential tissue damage potency that cannot be injected subcutaneously or intramuscularly without damage. Nevertheless, complications with IV application can occur. They include pain on injection, thrombophlebitis, as well as severe tissue damage.

The Nociceptive System of Veins

Although pain and discomfort on IV injections have been reported since the technique was established, nothing was known about the mediating nociceptors. That veins are innervated afferently has been known since 1926 (Woolard 1926), when light microscopy revealed thinly myelinated fibers ending in the paravascular tissue but also penetrating into the wall of peripheral veins. These fibers did not degenerate after sympathectomy and, therefore, were judged to form an afferent system. In neurophysiological experiments in animals, cooling (Minut-Sorokhtina and Glebova 1976) and stretching (Davenport and Thompson 1987) vein walls increased the spike traffic in afferent fibers, while in humans, injecting cold saline was found to be painful (Fruhstorfer and Lindblom 1983).

These observations, together with the clinical reports of pain on injection, led to the systematic exploration of the nociceptive system of veins some years ago. The technique of vascularly isolated vein segments was used, which were cannulated from both sides and separated from systemic circulation by external occluders (see Figure 2.4). Through both cannulas, probes for electrical, mechanical, and thermal stimulation could be placed in the vein, and relationships between the power of stimulation and the intensity of the evoked pain could be derived.

Sometimes, nonpainful cosensations occur with IV stimulation, i.e., coldness during cooling or mechanical sensations during wall stretch or electrostimulation. Therefore, blocking strategies were developed to locate the involved receptors including paravenous block (venous nociceptors blocked, but receptors of the overlaying skin intact), and transdermal block with benzocaine ointment (skin numbed, but venous nociceptors intact).

Electrostimulation, stretching, cooling, and heating of the venous wall all evoke pain of a similar quality and with equal intensity functions, therefore indicating the existence of a polymodal venous nociceptor (Arndt and Klement 1991). The physiological function of these nociceptors seems to be the mediation of strong cold pain when cold nociceptors of the skin were numbed by low temperatures (Klement and Arndt 1992).

The described experimental setup, moreover, is perfectly suited for perfusion of the isolated vein segment. Thus, the venous wall can be brought in contact with definite and constant concentrations of any substance in any vehicle. Since polymodal nociceptors should also be sensitive

Figure 2.4. Experimental setup for stimulating venous nociceptors in humans.

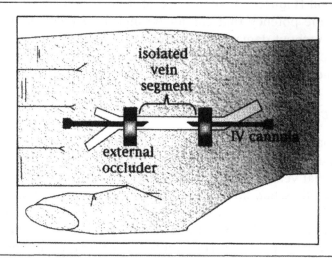

A vein segment free of side branches is cannulated from both sides. The vein is compressed by external occluders to isolate the segment vascularly. The cannulas can be used to perfuse the vein segment with various substances in known concentrations, or for the insertion of probes for electrical, mechanical, or thermal stimulation.

to chemical stimuli, and in order to explore possible reasons for pain on injections, the pain occurring with the injection and perfusion of high osmolalities (saline 1.0 to 6.0 osmol/L) was studied, as well as injections of acid or basic solutions (saline with added hydrochloric acid or sodium hydroxide, respectively, osmolality constant 0.3 osmol/L). Hyperosmolality and unphysiological pH evoked pain (see Figure 2.5) and venous sequelae (Klement and Arndt 1991a).

Injections with acid and basic solutions evoked pain with a pH below 4 and above 11, reaching the individual tolerance maximum (visual analogue scale = 100 percent) at 2 and 13, respectively. One needs to keep in mind that these experiments were done as injections into a running infusion. We do not know the effective pH at the venous wall. Perfusion experiments with long-lasting contact of the solutions with the endothelium were not performed, because even with single injections, serious venous sequelae could be observed (see "Pain and Possibly Serious Sequelae"). Similar to the experiments with hyperosmolality, perfusion with acid and basic pH can be expected to evoke pain with lower acidity or basicity than with injections diluted by an infusion.

From our experiments, the following conclusions can be derived:

Figure 2.5. Mean pain intensities with injections and constant perfusions of hyperosmolar solution in human vascularly isolated vein segments (data from Klement and Arndt 1991a).

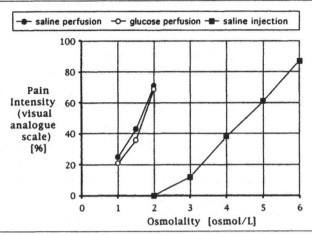

Injections (1 mL within 1 sec) were done into a running infusion (3 mL per minute) to imitate the clinical situation. Therefore, pain started and rose with higher osmolalities than in the perfusion experiments (constant perfusion 15 mL in 10 min). Pain was caused by osmolality and not by ionic strength, since saline and glucose evoked equal pain intensities.

- Cutaneous veins of humans are afferently innervated with a system of polymodal nociceptors that also respond to chemical stimuli.

- Solutions with unphysiologic osmolalities and acid or basic pH evoke pain.

- The intensity of pain depends on the osmolality and pH of the injection.

- Dilution and buffering by infusions and blood decrease the evoked pain.

What Causes Pain on IV Injections?

The experiments described above give rise to the presumption that drugs with formulations of osmolality above 2 osmol/L or of pH below 4 and above 11 can evoke pain due to the physicochemical properties of the solvents rather than the algogenity of the drug itself. If so, the osmolality and pH of drug formulations usually said to evoke pain should be within the range found to be painful in our study. Furthermore, whenever formulations of a drug have been changed or a drug is available in other and more physiologic formulations, these should evoke less or no pain.

Some vagueness exists in interpretation of the painful range of the pH level. Firstly, the effective pH at the vein wall was not known in our experiments. Secondly, in the clinical situation, a drug is injected into a running infusion which, in its turn, enters a vein with an unknown bloodstream velocity. This is not only a situation of diluting a certain injection volume of known pH with unknown volumes of infusion (often with an unknown pH level) and blood, but also a situation of reciprocal buffering of different buffer systems with various buffer capacities. Thus, the resulting pH of such a situation can only be estimated. For example, the immediate mixture of a 2.5 percent solution of thiopental (pH 10.8) with the five-fold volume of venous blood (pH 7.35) resulted in a pH of 9.1 (our measurement), thus indicating a higher buffer capacity for thiopental than for blood. During injection of thiopental in a peripheral vein, it would be difficult to achieve an injection velocity that would be able to induce anesthesia with the injection diluted by the five-fold volume of blood.

Concerning osmolality, things are easier. Changes in osmolality mainly reflect the dilution of the injection with blood and are, therefore, a function of injection velocity and blood flow in the vessel. It is not surprising that the former hyperosmolar ionic X-ray contrast media evoke pain when injected rapidly in large volumes intravasally for phlebography or arteriography. The new nonionic contrast agents were formulated in iso-osmolar solutions, evoke local reactions with only low incidences, and have low systemic and organ-specific toxicity (Dawson 1996).

Figures 2.6 and 2.7 show osmolality and pH, respectively, for some anesthesia-related drug formulations known to evoke pain on injection. Some alternative formulations are included. The preparations of etomidate and diazepam have osmolalities far beyond the physiologic range. Pain on injection with these formulations is due to their 17- and 27-fold osmolality compared to that of blood.

Remember, maximum pain was found with the injection of 1 mL of solution with 6,000 mosmol/L, which is exceeded by a normal injection volume of 1 to 2 mL of Valium® with an osmolality of 7,775 mosmol/L. Hypnomidate® has a somewhat lower osmolality of 5,000 mosmol/L, but it is injected in higher volumes, and, moreover, it has a pH of 5. If indeed pain is caused by the osmolality and there are no algogenic properties of etomidate and diazepam, the alternative iso-osmolar preparations of these substances in fat emulsions should fail to evoke pain.

Barbiturates are suspected to evoke pain through their basic pH of 10.5 and 11.2, which at first glance seems to be moderate compared to the pH of 12.5 to 13.0 needed to evoke maximal pain. Barbiturates, however, have been injected at high volumes of up to 20 mL, and they have a high buffer capacity (see above). Muscle relaxants, in contrast, were acidic but have been normally injected after the induction agent of general anesthesia. Thus, no studies were performed on their pain-evoking properties, despite patients frequently withdrawing the arm in which vecuronium was

Figure 2.6. Osmolality of some drugs known to cause pain on injection.

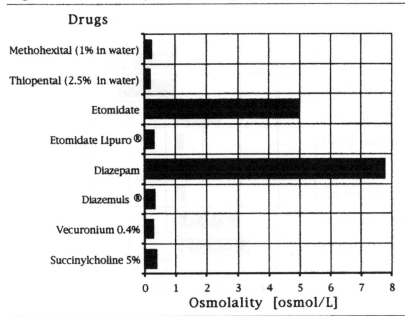

In diazepam (Valium®) and etomidate (Hypnomidate®), osmolality exceeds 17-fold and 27-fold, respectively, the osmolality of blood. This may explain the pain on injection. Change of the formulation into fat emulsion (Diazemuls®, Etomidate Lipuro®) significantly reduced the incidence and intensity of pain on injection. Data are based on our own measurements and from Trissel (1992). Values may differ between manufacturers and the use of various diluents.

injected, although they had received their induction agents and had fallen asleep.

Table 2.2 shows the results of representative, but not complete, studies dealing with pain on injection of the drug solutions mentioned above. Please note that in most of the studies no data were given about the drug preparations and their actual osmolality and pH. Furthermore, the studies were hardly comparable for several reasons. The studies differed in their vein puncture site; use of spontaneous pain complaint versus complaint sought; scales for pain and/or discomfort; injection velocity; and onset of central-nervous action of the drugs. Astonishingly, the data in Table 2.2 are, by and large, comparable. Taken together with the information from Figure 2.5, the data from pH stimulation, and the data from Figures 2.6 and 2.7, the results of the clinical studies of pain on injection can be interpreted as follows:

- Barbiturates cause pain on injection because of their basic pH level. That methohexital evokes higher incidences of pain than thiopental seems confusing, but it may have a higher buffer

Figure 2.7. The pH levels of some drugs known to cause pain on injection.

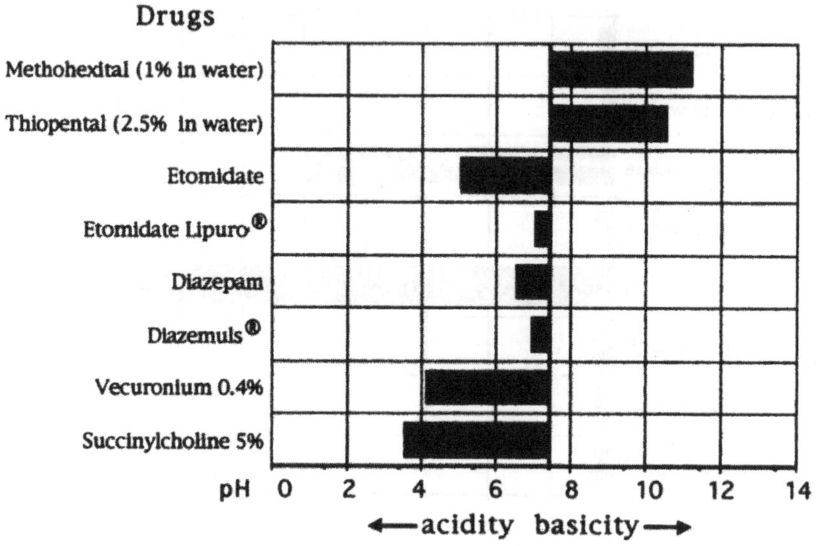

For the basic barbituates (methohexital and thiopental) and the acid muscle relaxants (vecuronium and succinylcholine), the pH explains the occurrence of pain on injection. Data were based on the author's own measurements and from Trissel (1992). Values may differ between manufacturers and the use of various diluents.

capacity and a pH difference of 0.7 reflects a five-fold higher concentration of hydroxyl ions. In our study, the injection of 0.5 more basic pH evoked a two- to threefold higher pain intensity.

- The formulations of diazepam and etomidate evoke pain by their hyperosmolality. Lipid formulations (i.e., emulsions or mixed micelles) have normal osmolalities and evoke pain on injection with a negligible incidence.

- The emulsion formulation of propofol, in contrast, does evoke pain although osmolality and pH are near the physiologic range (303 mosmol/L and pH 8.0, respectively).

Propofol, an IV anesthetic and a phenolic derivate, was available in the United Kingdom in a 2 percent solution in Cremophor EL and other vehicles with high osmolality. The first descriptions reported high incidences and intensities of pain. The formulation was changed, and today propofol is available worldwide with a 1 percent emulsion. Surprisingly, the new formulation continued to evoke pain. Since this did not fit our hypothesis,

Table 2.2. Pain Incidences with IV Injections of Some Anesthesia-Related Substances

Reference	Drug and Solution/Vehicles						
	Methohexital in water or saline	Thiopental in water or saline	Diazepam in Valium®, propylene glycol, ethanol	Diazepam in fat soybean oil or micelles	Etomidate in Hypnomidate®, propylene glycol	Etomidate in fat, in fat, Intralipid®	Propofol in in fat, Intralipid®
Kawar and Dundee (1982)	12%	9%	37%	0%			
Van Dardel et al. (1983)				0.4%			
Martin and Tweedle (1983)			34%	21%			
Galletly et al. (1985)			90%				
Gran et al. (1983)	33%				68%	2%	
Giese et al. (1985)		5%			44%		
Hynynen et al. (1985)	80%	0%					100%
McCulloch and Lees (1985)							37.5%
Simpson et al. (1989)	49%						
Rühmann and Maier (1990)					57%		
Westrin et al. (1992)	83%						
Raphael and Bexton (1994)	67%						
Nathanson et al. (1996)							67%

propofol was perfused in various dilutions through isolated vein segments and we found the pain intensities to depend on the solvent used (see Figure 2.8).

When diluted with one aliquot of Intralipid®, which doubles the fat/propofol ratio, pain was markedly reduced. When a glucose level of 5 percent was used for dilution, the fat/propofol ratio was kept constant, and the pain intensity was slightly attenuated. Since the fat/propofol ratio should determine propofol's free aqueous concentration and thus the concentration in contact with the vein wall, propofol was inferred to have intrinsic pain-evoking properties and that pain intensity depends on its free concentration in the aqueous phase. Recently, this assumption was confirmed by relating pain intensities to measurements of aqueous concentrations with fat diluents (Doenicke et al. 1996).

Thus, drug formulations with unphysiologic osmolality and pH were able to evoke pain. The example of propofol, however, reminds us that drugs or vehicles may exist that have an algogenic potency of their own and may hurt in the absence of aggressive physicochemical properties.

Alleviation of Pain on IV Injection

There are many possibilities for manufacturers to develop less painful and irritating injectables in the future. But there are some hints from the data

Figure 2.8. Effect of diluting propofol with either fat emulsion or glucose on mean pain score during perfusion of vascularly isolated vein segments (data from Klement and Arndt 1991b).

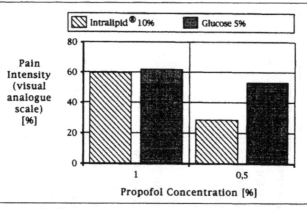

Undiluted propofol (1 percent) evoked a pain intensity of 60 percent of the scale. Concentration was decreased by half, diluting the original emulsion with equal volumes of Intralipid® or glucose. Dilution with lipids was more effective in reducing pain, which supports intrinsic algogenic properties of propofol, since dilution with lipids enhances the fat/propofol ratio, thus reducing the free aqueous concentration of propofol.

described above as to what clinicians can do with available drugs to minimize pain on injection. Therefore the following are some guidelines based on the author's experiments and clinical experience, and on a critical survey of the numerous studies dealing with the prevention of pain on injection.

Dilution and Buffering. *Hyperosmolar* injections can be diluted in water without solution stability problems, which has been tested with etomidate (Rühmann and Maier 1990). It may be that 20 mL with an osmolality of about 2,500 mosmol/L, due to longer contact time with the vessel wall evokes pain similar to 10 mL with an osmolality of 5,000 mosmol/L. Therefore, dilution with water seems to be a promising method for only small volumes of injection (e.g., Valium®), which can be diluted with multiples of the volume. It may also be advantageous with drugs where rapid onset is not desired, i.e., when the injection speed does not matter and administration of higher volumes over a longer time period is possible (e.g., with chemotherapeutics with high osmolalities).

Acid or basic injections cannot be neutralized because this could affect the stability of the solutions. Often, reactions like immediate precipitation take place, which is a common event to any anesthesiologist who has watched the precipitate of barbiturates with an acid muscle relaxant when injected together into an infusion line. Dilution with water has little effect on pH, but increases the volume of the injection. The dilution with blood drawn back into the syringe is possible and will also lead to buffering, but from most of the peripheral infusion lines, blood cannot be drawn back. Dilution with fat emulsions has been tested in the case of methohexital, and pain on injection was almost eliminated (Westrin et al. 1992) while ED 50 was not influenced. This was promising, but it remains to be tested for each individual dilution of such drugs.

Algogenes (e.g., propofol) may be dilutable without problems for stability, but higher injection volumes and slower onset of action will be the price. In the case of the emulsion form of propofol, dilution with fat emulsion is promising as is obvious from our experiments (Klement and Arndt 1991b) and does not affect bioavailability (Doenicke et al. 1996).

Site and Speed of Injection. It is obvious that veins differ in diameter and blood flow velocity. Under normal conditions, peripheral veins at the dorsum of the hand have blood flow velocities of approximately a few mL per min. Injecting 10 to 20 mL of a basic barbiturate within 15 sec is standard clinical procedure, resulting in a barbiturate flow that can be estimated to exceed by 20-fold the blood flow within the first few centimeters of this vein. This is a strict limitation for immediate dilution and buffering of the drug solution at this site of injection.

Whenever possible, the injection speed of potential irritants should be low, and the solution should be injected into a running infusion or should be administered as a slow infusion. Keep in mind that veins contract when irritated, i.e., especially small veins constrict around the infusion cannula and minimize remaining blood flow between the vein wall and cannula. Do not count on dilution by blood at the tip of your cannula, there may be none.

With anesthesia-inducting agents, the decrease of injection speed results in a later onset of action and the potential need for a higher dosage. With propofol, slow injections lead to higher incidences and intensities of pain (Scott et al. 1988), perhaps due to the later onset of anesthesia. When a rapid injection of solution is desired, a larger vein on the forearm with higher blood flow should be chosen. With the injection of propofol, a 37.5 percent incidence of pain occured with injections in hand veins, with only a 2.5 percent incidence with injections into large forearm veins (McCulloch and Lees 1985). Single injections into veins of the cubital fossa should be avoided, especially with irritants, since a high risk for paravascular or intra-arterial injection is reported at this site.

Local Anesthetics. *Preinjection of local anesthetics* should be able to block the venous nociceptors so that no pain on injection can occur. Since Bier described his regional IV anesthesia (Bier's block) in 1907, we know that intravenously applied local anesthetics to a limb with a tourniquet causes an almost complete block of the whole limb. Lower volumes of local anesthetics, given in the infusion line immediately before injecting a potential irritant, should be able to minimize pain on injection.

Various methods and dosages had been described. Twenty mg of lidocaine had little effect on pain on injection of propofol (Lee et al. 1994), while 40 mg decreased the incidence and intensity of venous discomfort following propofol injection (Haugen et al. 1995). The best prophylaxis for pain with propofol injection was 100 mg lidocaine, which reduced mean pain intensity from 75 mm of a 100 mm visual analogue scale in the placebo group to 21 mm. When lidocaine was administered during cuff inflation at the upper arm, applied for 1 min after gravity drainage of venous blood, pain was negligible (Mangar and Holak 1992). Similar results were obtained with the same technique, but with a dose of 20 mg lidocaine prior to etomidate injection (Rühmann and Maier 1990). Digital venous occlusion during preinjection of 20 and 40 mg of lidocaine reduced pain incidence from 73 percent in the placebo group to 23 and 5 percent, respectively (Johnson et al. 1990).

All of the studies using local anesthetics in the prevention of injection pain differ in time course and dose of local anesthetic application, tourniquet time, and time between applying the local anesthetic and the injection of the irritant. Since blocking concentrations and time course of action of local anesthetics at the vein wall were not known, vascularly isolated vein segments were exposed to increasing concentrations of procaine and bupivacaine during painful electrostimulation until no pain was felt. In this way, for each of the 6 subjects, individual minimal blocking concentrations were determined to be 15×10^{-3} M for procaine and 1.5×10^{-3} M for bupivacaine. In a second experiment, the veins were perfused with these blocking concentrations during continuous electrostimulation to register the time course of blocking (see Figure 2.9).

From the data collected for procaine and bupivacaine (blocking concentration and time course), which did not differ in onset of blockade although they differ extremely in lipophilicity (oil-water partitition coefficients 0.02 for procaine and 27.5 for bupivacaine) and pK_a (8.9 and 8.1), one can infer that lidocaine should block with concentrations above 0.2 percent within 1 to 1.5 min.

Thus, local anesthetics, intravenously applied using appropriate techniques prior to the injection of an irritant, are able to prevent pain on injection.

In many studies since 1988, propofol was *mixed with lidocaine* in doses of 5 to 40 mg in 20 mL propofol, a method at least as effective for the prevention of pain on injection as preinjection of lidocaine (see Table 2.3). This is unlikely to be only a matter of blocking the venous afferents with lidocaine, since pain with propofol injection mostly occurs within 30 sec, and onset of complete lidocaine block should last 1 min or more. Pain, therefore, is likely to be alleviated by another mechanism, which is not known. Or it may be that more hydrophil in a local anesthetic decreases the free aqueous concentration of propofol by displacing it into the lipid phase. It may be that local anesthetics bind to the propofol molecule and thus affect its pain-evoking properties in a reversible manner or without affecting its anesthetic effect.

Figure 2.9. Mean time course of blockade of the venous nociceptors during perfusion with procaine and rinsing (unpublished data from 6 subjects).

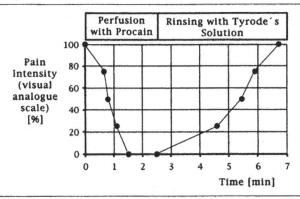

Procaine was perfused with the individual minimal blocking concentration (mean 15×10^{-3} M) during continuous painful electrostimulation until no pain was felt by the subjects. One min later, rinsing started until pain intensity regained control level.

Table 2.3. List of Studies Reflecting Efforts to Minimize Pain on Injection with Propofol Over the Last 10 Years (results are indicated as ∅ = no effect (or worsens), ↓ = reduced pain, and ↓↓ = markedly reduced pain)

Reference	Method	Dilution	Local Anesth.	Analgesics	Other Drugs	Miscellaneous
Fletcher et al. (1996)	W		L, pre, ↓			37°C, ↓
Lyons et al. (1996)						
Doenicke et al. (1996)		lipids, ↓				
Nathanson et al. (1996)	W		L, mix, ↓↓	A, 1, pre, ↓↓		
Haugen et al. (1995)			L, pre, ↓		T, 50, pre, ↓	
Tham and Khoo (1995)			L, pre, Df, ↓↓			
Eriksson (1995)	W		L, mix, ↓↓ / Pi, mix, ↓↓	K, 30, IM, ∅		
Mecklem (1994)			L, mix, ↓		M', 10, mix, ↓	
Lee et al. (1994)			L, pre, ↓		T, 100, pre, ↓↓	
Lin et al. (1994)			L, pre & mix, ↓			
Fletcher et al. (1994)	W			A, 1, pre, ↓↓		4°C, ∅
Wilkinson et al. (1993)					N, skin, ↓↓	
Ganta and Fee (1992)			L, pre, ↓↓			
Hiller and Saarnivaara (1992)	C		L, mix, ↓↓	A, Df, pre, ↓	M', 10, pre, ↓↓	
Cameron et al. (1992)	C		L, mix, Df, ↓			
Mangar and Holak (1992)			L, pre, +T, ↓↓			
Barker et al. (1991)			L, pre, ↓			4°C saline pre and 4°C ↓↓

Reference	Method	Dilution	Local Anesth.	Analgesics	Other Drugs	Miscellaneous
Gehan et al. (1991)			L, pre, Df, ↓↓			
Klement and Arndt (1991b)		lipics, ↓ glucose, ∅				
Nicol et al. (1991)			L, pre, ↓ P, pre, ↓			
McCrirrick and Hunter (1990)						4°C, ↓
Johnson et al. (1990)			L, pre, vo, ↓↓ L, mix, ↓↓			
Stokes et al. (1989)		glucose, ↓↓	L, mix, ↓↓			
Helbo-Hansen et al. (1988)			L, mix, ↓↓			
Scott et al. (1988)			L, pre, ↓ L, mix, ↓↓			antecub. fossa, ↓↓ slow injection, ∅

Legend: W = study with women only; C = study with children only; pre = IV projection of; mix = injectate mixed with; Df = dose finding study; L = lidocaine; P = procaine; Pi = prilocaine; +T = tourniquet; vo = venous occlusion; A = alfentanil; M = meperidine; K = keterolac; numbers represent doses in mg; T = thiopental; M' = metoclopramide; N = nitroglycerin ointment; X°C = injectate temperature.

Thus, in the case of propofol (no other drug has been tested), the addition of local anesthetics to the injectable markedly decreases pain on injection, whereas its efficacy as an induction agent remains unaltered.

Miscellaneous. From Table 2.3, it is obvious that pain on injection is a real nuisance for both the physician and the patient. Listed are the papers of the last 10 years that deal with methods to decrease pain on injection with 1 drug formulation only (propofol), thus demonstrating the dimensions of the problem and the efforts to solve it.

The first two columns were discussed previously. The preinjection of *analgesics* for the prevention of pain is reasonable. Opioids like fentanyl or so-called "peripheral analgesics" like aspirin have been tested. They showed no effect with the injections of Valium®, and only a moderate decrease in the incidence of severe pain with propofol (Bahar et al. 1982). The preinjection of 1 mg of the opioid alfentanil seemed to reduce pain on injection with propofol in adults, with an approximate 60 percent decrease of pain incidence when compared to placebo (Nathanson et al. 1996; Fletcher et al. 1996). In children, a dose equal to or higher than 0.15 µg/kg reduced the pain incidence 16 to 20 percent, but the mixture with lidocaine reduced pain incidence to 4 percent (Hiller and Saarnivaara 1992). The preinjection of the opioid meperidine (25 mg) was also able to reduce pain on injection with propofol, but it was more effective in women, while lidocaine preinjection was more effective in men (Lyons et al. 1996). This sex difference hampers interpretation of the effectiveness of methods for the alleviation of pain on propofol injection, as do age differences. Patients above age 65 years show only one-fifth the pain incidence of patients between 25 and 40 years (Scheepstra et al. 1989). Children have the highest pain incidence and need double the lidocaine concentration of adults (Cameron et al. 1992).

Nevertheless, comparing overall effectiveness, *opioids* as potent analgesics seem to reduce pain incidence and intensity occurring with the injection of propofol, but they are not as effective as preinjections or mixtures with local anesthetics.

The potency of nonsteroidal anti-inflammatory drugs *(NSAIDs)* like acetylsalicylic acid to decrease pain of injection has not been tested often. While pain incidence and intensity on Valium® injections did not decrease with aspirin preinjection, the incidence of severe pain due to propofol injections was only one-third but with unaltered overall pain incidence (Bahar et al. 1982). Keterolac injected intramuscularly 45 to 60 min prior to the injection of propofol had no effect (Eriksson 1995). Thus, NSAIDs seem to be ineffective in the prevention of injection pain.

That high doses (50 and 100 mg) of thiopental could reduce pain on injection is also reasonable (Haugen et al. 1995; Lee et al. 1994). However, the concept—to alleviate pain on injections of one anesthesia induction agent by preinjection of another—seems confusing to me.

Metoclopramide preinjections and mixtures with propofol also seem to be effective (Mecklem 1994; Ganta and Fee 1992), perhaps due to the weak local anesthetic properties of this structural analogue of procainamide.

Nitroglycerin ointment onto the skin above the venous line also reduces pain on injection, which might be a matter of increased blood flow and thus increased dilution with blood, since after transdermal nitroglycerin application, subcutaneous veins increase about 50 percent in diameter (Wilkinson 1993).

Warming (37°C) and *cooling* (4°C) of the injection, as well as preinjection of cold saline, was said to be effective in reducing pain on propofol injection (Fletcher et al. 1996; Barker et al. 1991). Especially in terms of cooling, these findings disagree with previous data from experiments showing pain was evoked by different methods of cooling the wall of veins (Arndt and Klement 1991; Klement and Arndt 1992). Despite the method used, pain started when the normal wall temperature of peripheral veins (about 35°C) was decreased by 5 to 10°C and reached its maximum at wall temperatures between 15 to 10°C (i.e., temperatures close to the borderline of numbing by coldness which occurs in myelinated fibers just below 10°C, Franz [1968]). Thus, an injection temperature of 4°C should evoke pain despite the chemical properties of the solution by cooling the vein wall. During cooling, transient but intense pain should be evoked as long as nociceptors and their axons are in the temperature range mentioned above. Nevertheless, if the vein wall is cooled below 10°C by the injection, pain on injection may no longer occur.

In conclusion, there are methods to prevent or at least decrease pain on injection when we know the problems with formulations and how to deal with them. Choosing the optimal site of injection, appropriate injection velocity, dilutions, and preinjections, e.g., with local anesthetics, are promising methods.

Pain and Possible Serious Sequelae

During most of our experiments with various painful stimulations of vein segments, minor venous sequelae like flush, transient perivenous edema, or indurations of small segments occurred. The latter normally needed 1 to 4 weeks to regain normal appearance and function. However, when the preliminary phase of a new series of experiments was entered, we used to test new methods and modifications in our setup on ourselves. These experiments normally exceeded our usual experimentation periods of 2 to 3 h by far. Regardless of the methods used, these long-acting, painful stimulations caused more serious sequelae with thrombosis or thrombophlebitis for weeks, which sometimes were not limited to the venous segment that was under stimulation, but spread over the whole back of the hand or parts of the forearm. Especially in the cases of long-acting osmotic stimuli or, as described above, following the acid or basic injections, such sequelae could be seen. This led us to the presumption that intensity and duration of pain may be related to the venous sequelae.

If so, there should exist hints on comparable relationships between the clinical situation with injectables and our artificial situation. In particular, high incidences of venous sequelae should be reported with injectables causing intense pain. It is well known that even with today's materials, indwelling venous catheters cause thrombotic complications related to the time period they were in position. This is said to be a consequence of mechanical stress of the inner vein wall, i.e., the endothelium. Formulations known to cause pain as well as thrombotic complications are recommended to be injected or infused into central vein catheters.

Little attention, however, was paid to possible thrombotic complications with single injections. Thrombophlebitis during infusions, in contrast, is extensively reported in terms of its relation to catheter materials and infused solutions. After a lot of contradictory reports, the first experimental study with the patients being their own control was performed with bilateral infusions of 10 percent invert sugar solutions with a pH between 3.5 and 4.5 versus a pH of 6.8 (Elfving and Saikku 1966). After one infusion of 500 mL, the more acidic sugar solution caused thrombophlebitis in 18 percent of the patients, while the buffered solution caused it in only 5 poercent. Probably due to slow infusion velocity (500 mL in 3 h, or approximately 3 mL per min), no pain was reported. With even lower infusion velocities, acid pH may cause venous sequelae without evoking pain. In our institution, the opioid, piritramide, was used for postoperative pain relief via a patient-controlled analgesia device. The dilution of the drug in saline (1.5 mg/mL) had a pH of 3.96 and an osmolality of 242 mosmol/L. Despite a low basal infusion rate of 0.5 ml/min and a bolus volume of 2 mL (maximum bolus administration 1 per 15 min), phlebitis and thrombophlebitis developed rapidly (usually within 6 h). All patients had the analgesia device at a peripheral vein without additional infusion, as revealed eventually by evaluation of therapy controls (Zucker and Flesche 1993). Since, with this low infusion velocity, small amounts of blood would have buffered the drug solution, this observation also supports the presumption that irritated veins constrict around the infusion needle and thus minimize blood flow at the tip.

In addition, high osmolar drugs, infusions, and X-ray contrast media are known to cause marked incidences of venous sequelae. Therefore, the question arises as to whether or not the same stimuli causing pain on injection (i.e., pH, osmolality) cause thrombosis via the same mechanisms.

Activated nociceptors produce and release increased amounts of mediators like substance P or calcitonin gene-related peptide, which, minimally, contribute to the inflammation of tissue following trauma (Lotz et al. 1988). This well-known phenomenon of cutaneous nociceptors is not studied with vascular nociceptors. Following some hints from the literature about inflammation-reducing properties of analgesia, evidence of a direct link between pain and inflammation was found recently during hyperosmolar stimulation of vein segments (Holthusen 1997).

Perivenous edema, measured as changes in skin altitude by infrared reflection, developed to a thickness of 2.0 to 3.2 mm during 30 min of painful perfusions with hyperosmolar saline. The venous nociceptors and the receptors of the overlying skin were alternately blocked with local anesthetics by a perivenous block (vein but not skin blocked), a distal ulnar nerve block (skin but not vein blocked), and a proximal ulnar nerve block (both vein and skin blocked). Marked perivenous edema only developed with intact innervation of venous nociceptors. The pain-free perfusion with irritant hyperosmolar saline during perivenous and proximal ulnar nerve block did not cause substantial edema. Thus, intact nociceptive innervation is a prerequisite for formation of inflammed paravenous edema.

Moreover, endogenous mediators of inflammation like bradykinin are able to evoke pain not only from cutaneous nociceptors, but also from paravascular and venous nociceptors at equal concentrations (Kindgen-Milles et al. 1994). Bradykinin is able to cause the release of nitric oxide from endothelial cells, which acts vasodilating (Ignarro 1989), and also evokes pain from veins and paravascular tissue (Holthusen and Arndt 1995). Neither bradykinin nor hyperosmolar solutions evoke pain from veins that have been exposed to the NO-synthase inhibitor, N^G-mono-methyl-L-arginine, indicating nitric oxide is a major mediator of vascular pain (Kindgen-Milles and Arndt 1996), at least in case of chemical stimulation (Holthusen 1997). Taken together, the nociception of veins and paravascular tissue have more than one link to the development of inflammation and damage, and the endothelium seems to be the common site of action.

These findings indicate that with IV injections, it may be possible to relate pain on injection to inflammation and tissue damage that follow. Table 2.4 lists a number of studies in which pain on injection as well as venous sequelae were observed.

Although the studies differ considerably in methods and definitions, there seems to be a relation between pain and sequelae. The clinical signs of venous sequelae are redness, tenderness, thickening, and indurations that can be painless or painful on touch. Some studies relate the incidence of sequelae to those signs, others to diagnoses. Furthermore, incidences were sometimes given for one of the possible sequelae or for overall venous morbidity. Although these incompatibilities hamper interstudy comparability, Figure 2.10 presents a correlation of the data from Table 2.4.

Nevertheless, lipid formulations, which are found at the bottom left in the plot, hardly cause pain *and* thrombophlebitis, while aqueous hyperosmotic etomidate and diazepam formulations cause pain in 50 percent or more of the patients and also cause venous sequelae in 20 to 50 percent. Overestimating the method and neglecting missing statistical significance, the regression line of the plot ($y = 4.4 + 0.4x$) could be

Table 2.4. List of Studies with Incidences of Pain on Injection as Well as Venous Sequelae

Reference	Drug Formulations or Methods	Pain Incidence (%)	Sequelae Incidence (%)
Doenicke (1990)	Etomidate, aqueous	36	22
	Etomidate, in lipids	0	0
Rühmann and Maier (1990)	Etomidate, aqueous	57	18
	Etomidate + local anesthetics	3	7
Schou-Olesen et al. (1984)	Etomidate, aqueous	24	24
	Thiopental	0	4
Martin and Tweedle (1983)	Diazepam, aqueous	34	42
	Diazepam, in lipids	21	7
Gran et al. (1983)	Etomidate, aqueous	68	20
	Etomidate, vs. in lipids	2	3
Zacharias et al. (1978, 1979)	Etomidate, aqueous, slow injection	50	9
	Etomidate, aqueous, fast injection	40	12
	Etomidate, polyethylene glycol, slow	30	8
	Etomidate, polyethylene glycol, fast	24	8
	Etomidate, propylene glycol, slow	35	21
	Etomidate, propylene glycol, fast	25	26
Schou-Olesen and Hüttel (1980)	Diazepam, Cremophor EL	38	9
	Diazepam, propylene glycol	78	48
	Diazepam, in lipids	1	6
Kawar and Dundee (1982)	Saline	0	2
	Thiopental	9	4
	Methohexital	12	10
	Propofol	4	10
	Diazepam, propylene glycol	37	40
	Diazepam, in lipids	0	2

Venous sequelae were phlebitis, thrombosis, and thrombophlebitis. Technique and volume of drug application, definitions of sequelae, and observation periods differ between authors. Note, by and large, increase in pain incidence is accompanied by an increase in sequelae.

interpreted as follows: Venous sequelae occur without injection in 4 percent of the patients with a venous infusion line, which is congruent with clinical experience. With injection of irritants, 4 out of 10 patients who report pain on injection will suffer from venous sequelae.

Back to what is known with certainty: The authors who looked at the individuals found no relationship between the experience of pain on injection and later development of venous sequelae, i.e., thrombophlebitis

Figure 2.10. Linear regression between incidences of pain on injection and of venous sequelae (data from Table 2.4).

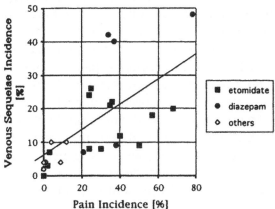

Since the comparability of studies is hampered by methodological differences, there is only a weak correlation (regression coefficient $r^2 = 0.46$). No differences between the drugs were obvious.

occurred in patients without any pain on injection and vice versa. Thus, with IV injections, only the *potential* to cause pain and that to cause sequelae seem to be related.

Can we prevent venous sequelae following IV injections and thus get hints at the mechanism? As diazepam started to be used worldwide as a promising sedative during diagnostic and therapeutic procedures, some people wondered that neither physicians nor patients paid attention to the occurrence of thrombophlebitis (Langdon et al. 1973). Injections of heparin or hydrocortisone following diazepam administration, surprisingly, were found to be useless in the prevention of thrombophlebitis, while an infusion of 150 to 250 mL saline decreased the incidence from 7 to 2.2 percent (Langdon 1973). The problems of pain and thrombophlebitis with this drug solution lead to numerous publications in the following years, most of them promoting postinjectional flushing of the vein or preinjection of (or mixing with) local anesthetics. Still, even more serious problems have occurred, such as loss of a limb following IV diazepam, but the authors could not exclude an at least partially intra-arterial injection as the cause (Schneider and Mace 1974).

Looking at the histologic level following diazepam injections into the saphenous veins of rats, the drug solution as well as the pure diluents evoked similar inflammatory response in a dose dependent manner within 48 h (i.e., vascular dilation, interstitial edema, polymorphonuclear-leukocyte infiltration, and vascular destruction and/or thrombotic organization) (Graham et al. 1977). Two results of the study go against a direct link between the origin of pain on injection and the development of venous sequelae: (1) A 100-fold dilution of the drug solution is well known to cause no pain, but caused interstitial edema and pronounced leukocyte infiltration; and (2) the addition of lidocaine to the solution, often described as pain reducing, failed to prevent inflammatory response.

Since preinjection of lidocaine, especially when combined with venous congestion, is more effective in reducing pain on injection, this procedure might also be effective in preventing thrombophlebitis. Indeed, in case of pain on injection with etomidate, preinjection of lidocaine or dilution with water decreased pain incidence by 49 and 69 percent, but thrombophlebitis still occurred with an incidence of 18 percent, independent of the mode of pain alleviation. When venous congestion was performed during lidocaine preinjection, pain incidence was decreased by 94 percent and thrombophlebitis occurred in only 7.4 percent of patients (Rühmann and Maier 1990).

Unfortunately, there is a lack of such studies on prevention of pain on injection *and* venous sequelae. This would be of great interest, because the question of whether or not pain is a prerequisite of vascular damage is still open to debate. The answer, however, relates to the basic mechanisms of pain and thrombophlebitis and is of clinical interest. If we find pain on injection to be a prerequisite (and thus a predictor) of vascular damage, we will be able to develop methods to prevent both. Preinjection of local anesthetics with venous congestion might be a promising tool whenever a new nonirritant formulation of the drug is not possible. But only preservative-free solutions of local anesthetics should be used since local anesthetic solutions containing preservatives cause phlebitic complications themselves, which can be reduced in incidence by adding heparin and/or hydrocortisone (Bassan and Sheikh Hamad 1983).

Although pain and venous sequelae evoking properties seem to be related somehow, there is room for exceptions: Propofol, which causes pain on injection although formulated in lipids, is known to cause thrombotic and phlebitic complications but with negligible incidences only.

Thus, irritant formulations known to cause pain on injection usually (but not always) cause morphologic venous sequelae. Change of the formulation (e.g., emulsions) decreased the incidence of pain and of venous sequelae, at least when the solved drug has no pain-evoking properties of its own. Injection into larger veins (e.g., cubital) and preinjection of preservative-free local anesthetics during venous congestion, are the only promising methods in reducing high incidences of venous damage with irritant injectables.

Is IV Injection Really IV Injection?

This last section of the IV route is dedicated to increasing the awareness of potential complications during IV injections. It is well known that paravascular injections occur with use of the wrong needle position. It is believed that high intraluminal pressure can cause venous wall rupture with concomitant extravasate. There are no accounts of paravascular administrations with venous catheters in clearly correct positions and with intact vessel walls. Is there a possibility of paravenous administration with proper IV injection?

In clinical practice, there are a lot of patients with so-called "bad venous state" (i.e., usually patients with chronic vessel disease or patients after numerous venous punctures and/or repeated or long-lasting irritating infusions, often requiring central venous port systems for further therapy). In such patients, a phenomenon of discolored areas of the forearm is common during moderately forced injections and sometimes during gravity-forced infusions into peripheral veins. The only explanation is a retrograde flow of the injection into the microcirculation, thus displacing the blood. Retrograde flow, however, can occur only in the absence or functional insufficiency of venous flaps. Venous flaps can lose function by injury, repeated phlebitis and repair, or by overstretching of the venous wall. When irritating injections are used in such patients, pain on injection is long-lasting and intractable. The reason for the increase in intensity of pain is not only the prolonged contact of concentrated injection with the venous wall, but also contact with paravascular tissue.

The latter happened to be found during our experiments with capsaicin, a potent algogenic agent, which failed to evoke pain with IV perfusion in concentrations 100-fold above those that evoke marked pain with intracutaneous injection. At the end of such a painless perfusion experiment, the IV capsaicin was washed out by saline injection when the outflow was unfortunately closed. To our surprise, unbearable pain occurred requiring pain-relieving treatment. Scrutiny of this phenomenon revealed easy access to the paravascular tissue with injection into occluded veins, and we used injections into such occluded finger veins for the investigation of paravascular nociceptors (Arndt et al. 1993). As apparent from Figure 2.11, methylene blue injected in the described fashion spread out from the occluded finger vein to the paravascular tissue and was visible in the cutis above the finger vein.

Thus, with poor flow conditions in peripheral veins, it is possible to inject or infuse at least part of the solutions into the paravascular tissue, even when correct position of the venous line has been verified. In the case of pressure infusion, this can cause compartment syndrome (Tobias et al. 1991). The view of accepting the possibility of retrograde flow into microcirculation and tissue is uncommon, so the authors held rupture of fragile veins under pressure infusion as responsible for the compartment syndrome, although they described no visible signs of venous rupture, such as hematoma. In an unpublished case of compartment syndrome with pressure infusion, the infusion catheter was in the correct position as revealed by gravity infusion and outflow of pure blood with light gravity suction,

Figure 2.11. Series of pictures with retrograde injections of methylene blue into occluded finger veins.

A

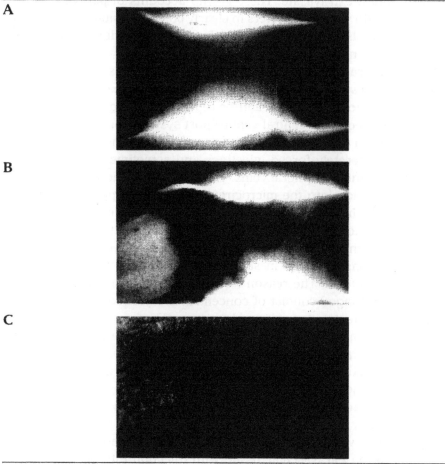

B

C

(A) Slow injection with free flow conditions. Only the vessels were made slightly visible by finger transillumination. (B) Injection into occluded finger veins obviously caused a spread of methylene blue into surrounding tissues, leading to (C) visible coloring of the skin (10 min after injection).

although the arm was swollen, mottled, and tense, and blood pressure measurement or withdrawal of blood from the radial artery cannula was not possible.

Vigilance and caution are needed whenever high injection or infusion pressure is used, or the beginning of injection or infusion reveals signs of bad flow conditions in the vein used. Irritants and hypertonic solutions may cause severe damage, and the feeling of safety with an obvious correct position of the venous catheter may be deceptive.

CONCLUSIONS AND PERSPECTIVES

Parenteral drug administration has a number of specific risks:

- *Pain* occurs with all routes of injection. Although in part caused by mechanical stress, most of the pain on injection depends on chemical activation of nociceptors. Since many drugs are poorly soluble in water, vehicles must be used for drug stability. Often, stabilizers are added to available drug formulations. Some drugs are stable only in an unphysiologic range of pH. Thus, in most cases, the osmolality and pH of these formulations are responsible for the pain on various routes of injection. Pain is usually transient and causes no serious and persistent sequelae, but pain is a warning sense, and it should recommend caution since pain and damage-evoking properties of formulations are somehow related.

- *Irritation and inflammation* of the tissue following the injection of irritant solutions reflect the reaction of the tissue to noxious stimuli. Activation of nociceptors and cellular damage cause release of mediators of the inflammation cascade. Redness, increased blood flow, edema, and hyperexcitability of nociception with spontaneous pain and/or pain with normal movements or touch occur in the irritated region. The process of repair lasts days or weeks, and the region will usually regain normal appearance and function.

Severe *damage or loss of tissue* is rare following injections, but the sequelae are horrible. (Never forget, that the patient desires help, not harm!) Different routes of parenteral drug application have different specific risks for tissue damage. Due to rapid dilution with blood during IV injection, serious sequelae are rare and in most cases caused by inattentive paravascular or intra-arterial injection. IM injections have a potential risk for loss of skeletal muscle mass. Cellular damage is frequent, usually local and transient, but severe and persistent damage has been described. Furthermore, accidental intraneural and intra-arterial injections happen with intramuscular injections causing irretrievable loss of neural function or tissue mass. Intra- and subcutaneous injections were used for slow resorption and thus longer action of the drugs applied. The resulting long duration of injection contact with the tissue may cause problems and skin necrosis can occur. Intra-arterial injections of irritants represent the worst case. Immediate pain, vasoconstriction, thrombus formations, and ischemia were caused, and tissue necrosis often occurred, despite aggressive treatment.

Since some of the worst sequelae of injections relate to inattentive and accidental injections into the wrong vessel or tissue, and since in most cases the physicochemical data of the drug vehicles are responsible for pain and tissue damage, there is a strong need for *nonirritant and safe formulations*. The progress of the last decades (e.g., development of stable lipid formulations) illustrates a step in the right direction. Sections C and D of this book deal with possible progress from today's point of view and future developments.

The user, i.e., the physician, nevertheless, should not only rely on the manufacturers. It may be that some problems are not solvable with today's techniques, and a drug cannot be made nonirritable. Furthermore, in some cases, the drug itself may be the reason for pain, irritation, and damage. Thus, physicians should pay attention to some rules with parenteral drug administration:

- Be sure that the planned route of application is the best choice for the drug effect and minimize the possibility of damage.

- Be aware of the specific tissue problems with this drug/formulation.

- Try to use methods for alleviation of pain on injection—maybe you can decrease the incidence of irritation and damage.

- Use proper injection technique. Stop injection immediately if unexpected reactions occur.

As is obvious from the data described above, a lot of problems are unsolved, and some relationships are still open to debate. Despite the numerous case reports dealing with sequelae of injections, there are fewer reports of systematic clinical and basic studies on their underlying mechanisms. The phenomenon of pain on injection is well documented, but the relationship to damage and possible common pathways in the development of pain, irritation, and damage should be the object of further studies.

ACKNOWLEDGEMENTS

I gratefully acknowledge the support of a grant from the Deutsche Forschungsgemeinschaft (Ar 64/7; Ar 64/8) for our studies on the nociceptive system of veins in humans.

REFERENCES

Adir, Y., P. Halpern, Z. Nachum, and H. Bittermann. 1991. Hyperbaric oxygen therapy for ischaemia of the hand due to intra-arterial injection of methadon and flunitrazepam. *Eur. J. Vasc. Surg.* 5:677–679.

Armstrong, P., J. Watters, and A. Whitfield. 1990. Alkalinisation of prilocaine for intravenous regional anaesthesia. Suitability for clinical use. *Anaesthesia* 45: 935–937.

Arndt, J. O., and W. Klement. 1991. Pain evoked by polymodal stimulation of hand veins in humans. *J. Physiol.* 440:467–478.

Arndt, J. O., D. Kindgen-Milles, and W. Klement. 1993. Capsaicin did not evoke pain from human hand vein segments but did so after injections into the paravascular tissue. *J. Physiol.* 463:491–499.

Bahar, M., E. McAteer, J. W. Dundee, and L. P. Briggs. 1982. Aspirin in the prevention of painful intravenous injection of di-isopropofol (ICI 35 868) and diazepam (valium). *Anaesthesia* 37:847–848.

Barker, P., J. A. Langton, P. Murphy, and D. J. Rowbotham. 1991. Effect of prior administration of cold saline on pain during propofol injection. A comparison with cold propofol and propofol with lignocaine. *Anaesthesia* 46:1069–1070.

Barnhill, B. J., M. D. Holbert, N. M. Jackson, and R. S. Erickson. 1996. Using pressure to decrease the pain of intramuscular injection. *J. Pain Symptom. Manage.* 12:52–58.

Bartfield, J. M., D. T. Ford, and P. J. Homer. 1993. Buffered versus plain lidocaine for digital nerve blocks. *Ann. Emerg. Med.* 22:216–219.

Bassan, M. M., and D. Sheikh Hamad. 1983. Prevention of lidocaine-infusion phlebitis by heparin and hydrocortisone. *Chest* 84:439–441.

Berger, J. L., M. Nimier, and J. M. Desmonts. 1988. Continuous axillary plexus block in the treatment of accidental intraarterial injection of cocaine. *N. Engl. J. Med.* 318:930.

Brimacombe, J., D. Gandini, and L. Bashford. 1994. Transient decrease in arm blood flow following accidental intra-arterial injection of propofol into the left brachial artery. *Anaesth. Intensive Care* 22:291–292.

Brogan Jr., G. X., E. Giarrusso, J. E. Hollander, G. Cassara, M. C. Maranga, and H. C. Thode. 1995. Comparison of plain, warmed, and buffered lidocaine for anesthesia of traumatic wounds. *Ann. Emerg. Med.* 26:121–125.

Cameron, E., G. Johnston, S. Crofts, and N. S. Morton. 1992. The minimum effective dose of lignocaine to prevent injection pain due to propofol in children. *Anaesthesia* 47:604–606.

Christiaens, G. C., and H. K. Nieuwenhuis. 1996. Images in clinical medicine. Heparin-induced skin necrosis. *N. Engl. J. Med.* 335:715.

Christoph, R. A., L. Buchanan, K. Begalla, and S. Schwartz. 1988. Pain reduction in local anesthetic administration through pH buffering. *Ann. Emerg. Med.* 17:117–120.

Crawford, C. R., and W. A. Terranova. 1990. The role of intraarterial vasodilators in the treatment of inadvertent intraarterial injection injuries. *Ann. Plast. Surg.* 25:279–282.

Dalton, A. M., A. Sharma, M. Redwood, J. Wadsworth, and R. Touquet. 1989. Does the warming of local anaesthetic reduce the pain of its injection? *Arch. Emerg. Med.* 6:247–250.

Davenport, P. W., and F. J. Thompson. 1987. Mechanosensitive afferents of femoral-saphenous vein. *Am. J. Physiol.* 252:R367–R370.

Davidson, J. A., and S. J. Boom. 1992. Warming lignocaine to reduce pain associated with injection. *Br. Med. J.* 305:617–618.

Dawson, P. 1996. The non-ionic isotonic contrast agents. Perspectives and controversies. *Eur. Radiol.* 6 (Suppl. 2):S20–S24.

Doenicke, A., A. Kugler, N. Vollmann, H. Suttmann, and K. Taeger. 1990. Etomidat mit einem neuen Lösungsvermittler. Klinisch-experimentelle Untersuchungen zur Venenvertraglichkeit und Bioverfügbarkeit. *Anaesthesist* 39:475–480.

Doenicke, A. W., M. F. Roizen, J. Rau, W. Kellermann, and J. Babl. 1996. Reducing pain during propofol injection: the role of the solvent. *Anesth. Analg.* 82:472–474.

Elfving, G., and K. Saikku. 1966. Effect of pH on the incidence of infusion thrombophlebitis. *Lancet* i:953.

Eriksson, M. 1995. Prilocaine reduces injection pain caused by propofol. *Acta Anaesthesiol. Scand.* 39:210–213.

Farley, J. S., R. F. Hustead, and K. E. Becker Jr. 1994. Diluting lidocaine and mepivacaine in balanced salt solution reduces the pain of intradermal injection. *Reg. Anesth.* 19:48–51.

Fletcher, G. C., J. A. Gillespie, and J. A. Davidson. 1996. The effect of temperature upon pain during injection of propofol. *Anaesthesia* 51:498–499.

Fletcher, J. E., C. R. Seavell, and D. J. Bowen. 1994. Pretreatment with alfentanil reduces pain caused by propofol. *Br. J. Anaesth.* 72:342–344.

Franz, D. N., and A. Iggo. 1968. Conduction failure in myelinated and non-myelinated axons at low temperatures. *J. Physiol.* 199:319–345.

Frizzel, R. T., and W. S. Fisher. 1995. Cure, morbidity and mortality associated with embolization of brain arteriovenous malformations: A review of 1246 patients in 32 series over a 35-year period. *Neurosurgery* 37:1039–1040.

Fruhstorfer, H., and U. Lindblom. 1983. Vascular participation in deep cold pain. *Pain* 17:235–241.

Galletly, D. C., L. F. Wilson, B. C. Treuren, and B. P. Boon. 1985. Diazepam mixed micelle-comparison with diazepam in propylene glycol and midazolam. *Anaesth. Intensive Care* 13:352–354.

Ganta, R., and J. P. Fee. 1992. Pain on injection of propofol: comparison of lignocaine with metoclopramide. *Br. J. Anaesth.* 69:316–317.

Gehan, G., P. Karoubi, F. Quinet, A. Leroy, C. Rathat, and J. L. Pourriat. 1991. Optimal dose of lignocaine for preventing pain on injection of propofol. *Br. J. Anaesth.* 66:324–326.

Giese, J. L., R. J. Stockham, T. H. Stanley, N. L. Pace, and R. H. Nelissen. 1985. Etomidate versus thiopental for induction of anesthesia. *Anesth. Analg.* 64:871–876.

Goldfine, A. B., and C. R. Kahn. 1994. Insulin allergy and insulin resistance. *Curr. Ther. Endocrinol. Metab.* 5:461–464.

Graham, C. W., R. P. Pagano, and R. L. Katz. 1977. Thrombophlebitis after intravenous diazepam—Can it be prevented? *Anesth. Analg.* 56:409–413.

Gran, L., H. Bleie, R. Jeppson, and H. Maartmann-Moe. 1983. Etomidat mit intralipid. *Anaesthesist* 32:475–477.

Hardy, S. J., and D. E. Agostini. 1995. Accidental epinephrine auto-injector-induced digital ischemia reversed by phentolamine digital block. *J. Am. Osteopath. Assoc.* 95:377–378.

Haugen, R. D., H. Vaghadia, T. Waters, and P. M. Merrick. 1995. Thiopentone pretreatment for propofol injection pain in ambulatory patients. *Can. J. Anaesth.* 42:1108–1112.

Helbo-Hansen, S., V. Westergaard, B. L. Krogh, and H. P. Svendsen. 1988. The reduction of pain on injection of propofol: The effect of addition of lignocaine. *Acta Anaesthesiol Scand.* 32:502–504.

Hiller, A., and L. Saarnivaara. 1992. Injection pain, cardiovascular changes and recovery following induction of anaesthesia with propofol in combination with alfentanil or lignocaine in children. *Acta Anaesthesiol. Scand.* 36:564–568.

Holley, H. S., and L. Cuthrell. 1990. Intraarterial injection of propofol. *Anesthesiology* 73:183–184.

Holthusen, H. 1997. Involvement of the NO/cyclic GMP pathway in bradykinin-evoked pain from veins in humans. *Pain* 69:87–92.

Holthusen, H., and J. O. Arndt. 1995. Nitric oxide evokes pain at noci-ceptors of the paravascular tissue and veins in humans. *J. Physiol.* 487:253–258.

Holthusen, H., and J. O. Arndt. 1996. The role of pain from veins for the formation of perivenous edema in humans. *Pain* 68:395–400.

Hynynen, M., K. Korttila, and T. Tammisto. 1985. Pain on i.v. injection of propofol (ICI 35868) in emulsion formulation. *Acta. Anaesth. Scand.* 29:651–652.

Ignarro, L. J. 1989. Biological actions and properties of endothelium-derived nitric oxide formed and released from artery and vein. *Circ. Res.* 65:1–21.

Johnson, R. A., N. J. Harper, S. Chadwick, and A. Vohra. 1990. Pain on injection of propofol. Methods of alleviation. *Anaesthesia* 45:439–442.

Kawar, P., and J. W. Dundee. 1982. Frequency of pain on injection and venous sequelae following the i.v. administration of certain anaesthetics and sedatives. *Br. J. Anaesth.* 54:935–939.

Kindgen-Milles, D., and J. O. Arndt. 1996. Nitric oxide as a chemical link in the generation of pain from veins in humans. *Pain* 64:139–142.

Kindgen-Milles, D., W. Klement, and J. O. Arndt. 1994. The nociceptive systems of skin, paravascular tissue and hand veins of humans and their sensitivity to bradykinin. *Neurosci. Lett.* 181:39–42.

Klement, W., and J. O. Arndt. 1991a. Pain on i.v. injections of some anaesthetic agents is evoked by the unphysiological osmolality or pH of their formulations. *Br. J. Anaesth.* 66:185–195.

Klement, W., and J. O. Arndt. 1991b. Pain on injection of propofol: Effects of concentration and diluent. *Br. J. Anaesth.* 67:281–284.

Klement, W., and J. O. Arndt. 1992. The role of nociceptors of cutaneous veins in the mediation of cold pain in man. *J. Physiol.* 449:73–83.

Koch-Weser, J. 1974a. Bioavailability of drugs. *N. Engl. J. Med.* 291:233–237.

Koch-Weser, J. 1974b. Bioavailability of drugs. *N. Engl. J. Med.* 291:503–506.

Kumar, O., L. Miller, and S. Mehtalia. 1977. Use of dexamethasone in treatment of insulin lipatrophy. *Diabetes* 26:296–299.

Langdon, C. D. E. 1973. Thrombophlebitis following diazepam. *JAMA* 225:1389.

Langdon, C. D. E., J. R. Harlan, and R. L. Bailey. 1973. Thrombophlebitis with diazepam used intravenously. *JAMA* 223:184–185.

Lee, T. W., A. E. Loewenthal, J. A. Strachan, and B. D. Todd. 1994. Pain during injection of propofol. The effect of prior administration of thiopentone. *Anaesthesia* 49:817–818.

Lin, S. S., G. T. Chen, J. C. Lin, T. Y. Chen, and M. H. Hwang. 1994. Pain on injection of propofol. *Acta Anaesthesiol. Sin.* 32:73–76.

Lotz, M., J. H. Vaughan, and D. A. Carson. 1988. Effect of neuropeptides on production of inflammatory cytokines by human monocytes. *Science* 241: 1218–1221.

Lugo-Janer, G., M. Padial, and J. L. Sanchez. 1993. Less painful alternatives for local anesthesia. *J. Dermatol. Surg. Oncol.* 19:237–240.

Lyons, B., D. Lohan, C. Flynn, and M. McCarroll. 1996. Modification of pain on injection of propofol. A comparison of pethidine and lignocaine. *Anaesthesia* 51:394–395.

Mader, T. J., S. J. Playe, and J. L. Garb. 1994. Reducing the pain of local anesthetic infiltration: warming and buffering have a synergistic effect. *Ann. Emerg. Med.* 23:550–554.

Mangar, D., and E. J. Holak. 1992. Tourniquet at 50 mm Hg followed by intravenous lidocaine diminishes hand pain associated with propofol injection. *Anesth Analg.* 74:250–252.

Mar, A. W., B. Dixon, K. Ibrahim, and J. D. Parkin. 1995. Skin necrosis following subcutaneous heparin injection. *Australas. J. Dermatol.* 36:201–203.

Martin, D. F., and D. E. Tweedle. 1983. Venous complications of two diazepam preparations related to size of vein. *Br. J. Anaesth.* 55:779–781.

Martin, S., J. S. Jones, and B. N. Wynn. 1996. Does warming local anesthetic reduce the pain of subcutaneous injection? *Am. J. Emerg. Med.* 14:10–12.

Mastaglia, F. L. 1982. Adverse effects of drugs on muscle. *Drugs* 24:304–321.

Matsumoto, A. H., A. C. Reifsnyder, G. D. Hartwell, J. F. Angle, J. B. Selby Jr. and C. J. Tegtmeyer. 1994. Reducing the discomfort of lidocaine administration through pH buffering. *J. Vasc. Interv. Radiol.* 5:171–175.

McCrirrick, A., and S. Hunter. 1990. Pain on injection of propofol: The effect of injectate temperature. *Anaesthesia* 45:443–444.

McCulloch, M. J., and N. W. Lees. 1985. Assessment and modification of pain on induction with propofol (Diprivan). *Anaesthesia* 40:1117–1120.

Mecklem, D. W. 1994. Propofol injection pain: Comparing the addition of lignocaine or metoclopramide. *Anaesth. Intensive Care* 22:568–570.

Minut-Sorokhtina, O. P., and N. F. Glebova. 1976. On the vascular component of the peripheral cold reception. *Prog. Brain Res.* 43:119–127.

Morgan, A. M. 1995a. Localized reactions to injected therapeutic materials. Part 1. Medical agents. *J. Cutan. Pathol.* 22:193–214.

Morgan, A. M. 1995b. Localized reactions to injected therapeutic materials. Part 2. Surgical agents. *J. Cutan. Pathol.* 22:289–303.

Nathanson, M. H., N. M. Gajraj, and J. A. Russell. 1996. Prevention of pain on injection of propofol: A comparison of lidocaine with alfentanil. *Anesth. Analg.* 82:469–471.

Nicol, M. E., J. Moriarty, J. Edwards, D. S. Robbie, and R. P. A'Hern. 1991. Modification of pain on injection of propofol—a comparison between lignocaine and procaine. *Anaesthesia* 46:67–69.

Pillans, P. I., and N. O'Connor. 1995. Tissue necrosis and necrotizing fasciitis after intramuscular administration of diclofenac. *Ann. Pharmacother.* 29:264–266.

Raphael, J. H., and M. D. Bexton. 1994. Improving the induction characteristics of methohexitone. A study of the effect of adding thiopentone to methohexitone. *Anaesthesia* 49:338–340.

Reeves, W. G., B. R. Allen, and R. B. Tattersall. 1980. Insulin-induced lipatrophy: Evidence for an immune pathogenesis. *Br. Med. J.* 280:1500–1503.

Rühmann, I., and C. Maier. 1990. Zur Beeinflussung des injektionsschmerzes und der thrombophlebitisrate nach etomidate. *Anaesth. Intensivther. Notfallmed.* 25:31–33.

Scheepstra, G. L., L. H. D. J. Booij, C. L. G. Rutten, and L. G. J. Coenen. 1989. Propofol for induction and maintenance of anaesthesia: Comparison between younger and older patients. *Br. J. Anaesth.* 62:54–60.

Schneider, S., and J. Mace. 1974. Loss of limb following intravenous diazepam. *Pediatrics* 53:112–114.

Schou Olesen, A., and M. S. Hüttel. 1980. Local reactions to i.v. diazepam in three different formulations. *Br. J. Anaesth.* 52:609–611.

Schou Olesen, A., M. S. Hüttel, and P. Hole. 1984. Venous sequelae following the injection of etomidate or thiopentone i.v. *Br. J. Anaesth.* 56:171–173.

Scott, R. P., D. A. Saunders, and J. Norman. 1988. Propofol: Clinical strategies for preventing the pain of injection. *Anaesthesia* 43:492–494.

Sidell, F. R., D. L. Culver, and A. Kaminskis. 1974. Serum creatine phosphokinase activity after intramuscular injection. The effect of dose, concentration and volume. *JAMA* 229:1894–1897.

Simpson, K. H., P. J. Halsall, C. A. Sides, and J. F. Keeler. 1989. Pain on injection of methohexitone. The use of lignocaine to modify pain on injection of methohexitone during anaesthesia for electroconvulsive therapy. *Anaesthesia* 44:688–689.

Stokes, D. N., N. Robson, and P. Hutton. 1989. Effect of diluting propofol on the incidence of pain on injection and venous sequelae. *Br. J. Anaesth.* 62:202–203.

Taggart, J. C. 1972. Pain and parenteral drug administration. *Bull. Parenter. Drug Assoc.* 26:87–90.

Tham, C. S. and S. T. Khoo. 1995. Modulating effects of lignocaine on propofol. *Anaesth. Intensive Care* 23:154–157.

Tobias, M. D., C. W. Hanson, R. B. Heppenstall. and S. J. Aukburg. 1991. Compartment syndrome after pressurized infusion. *Br. J. Anaesth.* 67:332–334.

Tokodi, G., and F. C. Huber. 1995. Massive tissue necrosis after hydroxine injection. *J. Am. Osteopath. Assoc.* 95:609–612.

Towse, A., M. O'Brien, F. J. Twarog, J. Braimon, and A. C. Moses. 1995. Local reaction secondary to insulin injection. A potential role for latex antigens in insulin vials and syringes. *Diabetes Care* 18:1195–1197.

Travell, J. .1955. Factors affecting pain on injection. *JAMA* 158:368–371.

Treiman, G. S., A. E. Yellin, F. A. Weaver, W. E. Barlow, R. L. Treiman, and M. R. Gaspar. 1990. An effective treatment protocol for intraarterial drug injection. *J. Vasc. Surg.* 12:456–466.

Trissel, L. A. 1992. *Handbook of injectable drugs.* Bethesda, Md., USA: American Society of Hospital Pharmacists.

Vangerven, M., G. Delrue, E. Brugman, and P. Cosaert. 1989. A new therapeutic approach to accidental intra-arterial injection of thiopentone. *Br. J. Anaesth.* 62:98–100.

von Dardel, O., C. Mebius, T. Mossberg, and B. Svensson. 1983. Fat emulsion as a vehicle for diazepam. A study of 9492 patients. *Br. J. Anaesth.* 55:41–47.

Waldbillig, D. K., J. V. Quinn, I. G. Stiell, and G. A. Wells. 1995. Randomized double-blind controlled trial comparing room-temperature and heated lidocaine for digital nerve block. *Ann. Emerg. Med.* 26:677–681.

Webb, S. C., R. Canepa Anson, A. F. Rickards, and P. A. Poole Wilson. 1983. High potassium concentration in a parenteral preparation of glyceryl trinitrate. Need for caution if given by intracoronary injection. *Br. Heart J.* 50:395–396.

Weir, M. R. 1988. Intravascular injuries from intramuscular penicillin. *Clin. Pediatr. Phila.* 27:85–90.

Westrin, P., C. Jonmarker, and O. Werner. 1992. Dissolving methohexital in a lipid emulsion reduces pain associated with intravenous injection. *Anesthesiology* 76:930–934.

Wilkinson, D., M. Anderson, and I. S. Gauntlett. 1993. Pain on injection of propofol: Modification by nitroglycerin. *Anesth. Analg.* 77:1139–1142.

Woolard, H. H. 1926. The innervation of blood vessels. *Heart* 13:319–336.

Zacharias, M., R. S. J. Clarke, J. W. Dundee, and S. B. Johnston. 1978. Evaluation of three preparations of etomidate. *Br. J. Anaesth.* 50:925–929.

Zacharias, M., R. S. J. Clarke, J. W. Dundee, and S. B. Johnston. 1979. Venous sequelae following etomidate. *Br. J. Anaesth.* 51:779–783.

Zachary, L. S., D. J. Smith, J. P. Heggers, M. C. Robson, J. A. Boertman, X. T. Niu, R. E. Schileru, and R. J. Sacks. 1987. The role of thromboxane in experimental inadvertent intra-arterial drug injections. *J. Hand Surg. Am.* 12: 240–245.

Zucker, T. P. and C. W. Flesche. 1993. Unerwünschte nebenwirkung: Thrombophlebitis unter kontinuierlicher piritramid-infusion. *Anästh. Intensivmed.* 34:360.

3

Mechanisms of Muscle Damage with Injectable Products

Anne McArdle
Malcolm J. Jackson

Muscle Research Centre, Department of Medicine
University of Liverpool
Liverpool, United Kingdom

ABSTRACT

Muscle damage can be a significant side effect following administration of certain pharmacological agents and/or the vehicle used to deliver the drugs. This damage is usually minor and reversible, but in rare instances it may be serious, and in extreme cases it may lead to widespread muscle breakdown, rhabdomyolosis and death.

Experimental studies of muscle damage caused by a variety of different stresses have indicated that the process ultimately involves one or more of only a few final common pathways. This review will summarise these data to indicate the potential mechanisms by which injectable products might cause muscle damage, and it will discuss techniques which may be used to evaluate these processes.

INTRODUCTION

Muscle damage can occur as a side effect of drug administration by intramuscular (IM) injection. Further, the drug itself or the carrier in which the drug is solubilised can cause muscle pain, weakness, cramps or damage.

Usually, the beneficial effects of the drug outweigh the side effects of muscle damage. However, in extreme situations, widespread muscle breakdown occurs. Skeletal muscle damage ultimately occurs through one or more of only a few final common pathways, including intracellular calcium overload, increased free radical activity or a decrease in energy supply within the muscle. This damage can be reversible or irreversible, but once irreversible, cell death occurs via necrosis, or (more controversially) apoptosis. The aim of this review is to summarise the mechanisms by which skeletal muscle may be damaged, the ways in which this damage may be assessed and the techniques which can be used to examine the mechanisms underlying damage in a specific situation.

MECHANISMS OF MUSCLE DAMAGE

The mechanisms by which muscle damage occurs will be considered separately, but it should be borne in mind that there is considerable overlap between these pathways. Thus, in extreme cases, a severe insult to muscle will lead to activation of all pathways, and cell death will be associated with loss of membrane integrity, influx of extracellular calcium (and thus activation of calcium dependent degradative processes), protein loss and aggregation, a fall in the cellular energy level and a stimulation of free radical production (McArdle and Jackson 1997).

Elevation of Intracellular Calcium Concentration

Intracellular calcium levels are strictly controlled in all cells, particularly skeletal muscle cells. A large concentration gradient exists across the skeletal muscle plasma membrane, with an extracellular concentration of 2 mM, and a free intracellular calcium concentration of less than 1 μM. Any perturbation of the plasma membrane will therefore result in an influx of calcium down this concentration gradient.

An increase in free intracellular calcium concentration has long been implicated in cell death (Schanne and Forber 1979). Many of the studies examining the effects of calcium overload on cellular damage have used the calcium ionophore, A23187, to elevate free intracellular calcium levels, and early studies using this agent demonstrated that an increase in intracellular calcium content caused structural damage to myofilaments (Duncan 1978; Publicover et al. 1978). Muscle damage induced by contractile activity was later shown to be associated with an influx of extracellular calcium (Jones et al. 1984; Anand and Emery 1980), although this influx of external calcium could not be solely attributed to calcium ingress through classical plasma membrane calcium channels (Jones et al. 1984). An increased cytosolic content of free calcium results in activation of a cascade of calcium-mediated degradative processes (which include proteases, phospholipases, lipolytic enzymes, lysosomal processes and mitochondrial overload), resulting in a reduction of cellular energy supply.

Calcium Activation of Proteases

Several cellular proteases are dependent on an elevation of intracellular calcium for activation. Two distinct calcium-dependent proteases have been described—calpain type I and calpain type II (DeMartino and Croall 1987), which are activated by micromolar and millimolar levels of calcium, respectively. Tissues also contain an activator protein and an inhibitor protein, which are thought to protect the cell against damage caused by activation of calpains during transient increases in intracellular calcium content (Mellgren 1987). The enzyme activity is dependent on the balance between inhibitor and activator proteins. The activity of calcium-dependent proteases is not specific for any protein sequence but may demonstrate some specificity due to subcellular compartmentalisation.

Calcium Activation of Lipases

It was previously suggested that an elevation in intracellular calcium causes muscle damage by activation of calcium-dependent phospholipases (Jackson et al. 1984). These lipases use membrane phospholipids as substrates, producing lysophospholipids and free fatty acids, which further disrupt the cell due to their detergent properties. Skeletal muscle contains phospholipase A_2, whose activity results in the production of prostanoids. Specific prostaglandins have been directly implicated in several features of calcium-mediated muscle damage (Rodemann et al. 1982).

Activation of Lysosomal Processes

Lysosomal enzymes are activated during calcium ionophore-induced damage to muscle, and it has been suggested that a calcium-mediated increase in PGE_2 causes a stimulation of lysosomal activity (Rodemann and Goldberg 1982; Rodemann et al. 1982). However, although an increase in intracellular calcium results in an increased activity of lysosomal proteases, experiments by Duncan et al. (1979) using lysosomal protease inhibitors showed that lysosomal protease activity was not a major factor in the muscle damage which occurred in this situation.

Mitochondrial Calcium Overload

With encroaching cellular calcium overload, muscle mitochondria accumulate calcium in an attempt to maintain calcium homeostasis. This results in precipitation of calcium phosphates within mitochondria (Gohil et al. 1988) and cellular energy production is inhibited (Wrogemann and Pena 1976). When the mitochondria are no longer able to cope with the calcium overload, they lyse and release the stored calcium into the (already compromised) cytoplasm of the cell.

Increased Free Radical Production

Drug-induced muscle damage may be associated with increased free radical production at a number of sites within the cell. Drugs may interfere with the mitochondrial electron transport chain (Boveris and Chance 1973) or with membrane-bound oxidases (Crane et al. 1985). In addition, muscle damage may result from an increased extracellular free radical activity by induction of an inflammatory or phagocytic response (Font et al. 1977) or activation of xanthine oxidase in the endothelial tissue (Karthuis et al. 1985; McCord 1985). Increased free radical activity can lead to oxidation of cellular proteins, deoxyribonucleic acid (DNA) and lipids. This subject has been reviewed comprehensively by Halliwell and Gutteridge (1989).

The structure, function and location of cellular proteins is extremely dependent on their inter- and intramolecular disulphide bonds, and oxidation of these bonds within proteins is known to occur early following oxidative stress (Thomas et al. 1994; McArdle et al. 1995). These proteins include the Na^+/K^+ adenosine triphosphatase (ATPase) of the plasma membrane and the Ca^{2+}-ATPase of the sarcoplasmic reticulum (Harris and Stahl 1980; Scherer and Deamer 1986), and oxidation of their disulphide bonds can result in loss of enzyme activity or protein aggregation. There is evidence that increased free radical production can inactivate the calcium pumps which are found on both the plasma membrane and the membranes of intracellular organelles, and hence cause a loss of cellular calcium homeostasis (Nicotera et al. 1985; Bellomo et al. 1985).

Free radical attack on DNA can result in base mutations or single and double strand breaks and so carcinogenesis or cell death may follow. Free radical damage results in the production of a wide range of DNA oxidation products. For example, both the aromatic ring structures and sugars of DNA are susceptible to attack by hydroxyl radicals, and the resulting products (including thymine dimers, 5-hydroxymethyl uracil or 8-hydroxyguanine) can be detected in tissues or urine.

An increase in free radical activity commonly results in peroxidation of cellular lipids. The peroxidation of a lipid is initiated by the abstraction of a hydrogen atom from a methylene group of the fatty acid by a free radical (such as the hydroxyl radical). The presence of double bonds in the fatty acid makes this abstraction more favourable. Molecular rearrangement results in the formation of a conjugated diene, which is then likely to form a peroxyl radical. The peroxyl radical is capable of abstracting a hydrogen atom from another lipid molecule and so the reaction is propagated. The overall result is the destruction of unsaturated fatty acids.

There is also evidence that an increase in muscle calcium content can influence free radical production. An increase in intracellular calcium results in activation of phospholipase enzymes, resulting in release of free fatty acids from membranes into the cytosol, where they are more susceptible to peroxidation (Jackson et al. 1984; McArdle et al. 1991, 1992). Free arachidonic acid is a substrate for the production of prostanoids by enzymatic reactions which involve production of free radicals. Activation of a calcium-dependent protease which can convert xanthine dehydrogenase to xanthine oxidase can also result in superoxide generation (McCord 1985). Xanthine dehydrogenase may not be present in skeletal muscle but is present in the endothelial cells, thus providing a potential site for production of free radicals within the muscle bulk.

In an attempt to delineate the role of increased free radical production from increased cellular calcium content during muscle damage, we have examined the effect of contractile activity (thought to result primarily in free radical–mediated damage) on calcium accumulation by vitamin E–deficient muscles. The absence of vitamin E, a membrane-soluble free radical scavenger, is known to increase the sensitivity of skeletal muscle to contraction-induced muscle damage (Jackson and Edwards 1988); it was therefore assumed that the primary damaging process during contraction-induced injury was the generation of free radicals which would lead to an increased influx of calcium. In vitamin E-sufficient muscles, calcium accumulation occurs significantly earlier than efflux of creatine kinase (CK) activity (McArdle et al. 1992). However, calcium accumulation by vitamin E-deficient muscles was similar to that of sufficient muscles, yet efflux of CK activity was greater. This suggests that, contrary to our expectations, vitamin E-deficient muscles have an increased susceptibility to the deleterious effects of calcium accumulation, which may be mediated by calcium activation of free radical processes (McArdle et al. 1993).

Loss of Energy Homeostasis

A fall in muscle energy content is associated with loss of cell viability since a release of cellular proteins has been shown to occur when cellular energy levels reach a critically low level (DeLeiris and Feuvray 1979). Early work suggested that the fall in energy supply within the cell leads directly to an instability of the plasma membrane and thus release of cellular proteins. (Pennington 1981; Cerny and Haralambie 1983). However, several authors have suggested that there is a significant delay between the fall in energy supply and loss of cellular viability, and that the loss of cellular energy supply initiates a separate mechanism that ultimately leads to loss of cell viability. This idea is supported by work in the heart, where it has been demonstrated that a loss of energy supply occurs early during ischaemia, but loss of plasma membrane integrity does not occur until much later (Hearse 1979).

The situation in skeletal muscle is less well understood. Resting skeletal muscle is much less prone to damage by transient ischaemic episodes. Our group has shown that ATP degradation is not evident until 3 to 4 h following initiation of ischaemia in the rat (McArdle et al. 1999), and other researchers have shown that skeletal muscle damage does not occur until this time (Klenerman et al. 1995). However, although there is substantial evidence supporting the association between a fall in energy levels and muscle damage, loss of skeletal muscle energy is not a prerequisite for muscle damage. West-Jordan et al. (1990, 1991) have shown that damage to skeletal muscle in-vitro may not be associated with a fall in energy content.

METHODS OF ASSESSING DRUG–INDUCED SKELETAL MUSCLE DAMAGE

The effect of drug administration on skeletal muscle in-vivo can be assessed in a number of ways. These methods include non-invasive muscle functional studies, analysis of serum/plasma or urine for markers of muscle damage or muscle biopsy analysis.

Microscopic Analysis of Skeletal Muscle

Histological and histochemical methods can be used to examine the structure and integrity of muscle fibres and the activity of muscle enzymes or the presence of enzyme substrates. The range of material which can be examined has been expanded greatly by the use of immunohistochemistry. This has allowed the analysis of a wide range of proteins which are important in muscle function. This subject has been reviewed by Helliwell (1997).

Muscle cell necrosis can be observed by light microscopy of frozen or paraffin fixed sections stained with hematoxylin and eosin. Lethally damaged muscle fibres initially swell, and subsequently invading cells such as macrophages and neutrophils can be observed clearing the site of damage. Satellite cells are activated, and fibre regeneration is evident within 1 to 2 days following insult. These mononuclear myoblasts fuse to form immature muscle fibres which can be seen on transverse section as small fibres with centrally located nuclei. Nuclei eventually migrate to the periphery of the fibres within several weeks or months depending on the species (Carlson 1973; Allbrook 1981). Electron microscopy can be used to examine fine structures within muscle and can detect abnormalities such as swollen mitochondria or disruptions in sarcomere structure.

Skeletal muscle death is routinely thought to occur by necrosis. However, there is some recent evidence that muscle cell death may also occur by a programmed pathway. Until recently, the only notable examples of skeletal muscle death occurring in a programmed manner were the classical changes in the tadpole and hawkmoth pupae during metamorphosis (Schwartz et al. 1990, 1993; Schwartz and Osbourne 1993). However, recently, several classical features of apoptosis (such as transferase UTP nick end-labelled [TUNEL] DNA and DNA ladders) have been observed in dystrophic mammalian skeletal muscle (Tidball et al. 1995; Sandri et al. 1995).

Muscle Function Studies

The loss of the ability of the muscle to generate force is a reliable measure of muscle damage (Faulkner et al. 1993; Faulkner and Brooks 1997).

Disruption or damage to the muscle fibre integrity and organisation of the contractile proteins results in a reduced ability of the muscle to generate force. The effect of muscle damage on the ability of that muscle to generate force has been most widely studied following damaging exercise (for reviews, see Jones and Round [1993] and Salmons [1997]), where it has been demonstrated that a period of damaging exercise results in a reduction in the maximum force which the muscle can generate.

Several models have been developed to measure the force characteristics of animal muscles both in-vivo and in-vitro, and in human studies. These include the use of isolated fibres, bundles of fibres and muscles in-vitro (Jones et al. 1983; Balnave and Allen 1995; Faulkner et al. 1982) and the measurement of force generation in muscles in-vivo in both rodent (McKully and Faulkner 1985; van der Meulen et al. 1997) and human (Newham et al. 1983, 1986, 1987) studies.

Neuronal or percutaneous stimulation of muscle to contract can provide considerable information on the status of the muscle. The force characteristics of a single electrical pulse (twitch) or tetanic stimuli provide information on the way in which the muscle fibres handle both the release of calcium from the sarcoplasmic reticulum (SR) and the uptake of calcium by the SR.

There is frequently some discrepancy between the amount of muscle damage which is assessed by microscopic techniques compared with maximum force generation of the same muscle. This is thought to be due to the structure of muscle cells and the nature in which they are damaged. A single muscle cell can be several centimetres in length. Damage to that fibre may be focal in nature. The damaged ends of the fibre are thought to quickly reseal in an attempt to minimise both damage and so the need to repair. This damage may go undetected by site-specific microscopic techniques. However, such damage would result in an impairment of the fibre to generate force (McKully and Faulkner 1985; Faulkner et al. 1993).

Leakage of Intramuscular Proteins

Muscle damage has, for a long time, been routinely assessed by leakage of muscle-derived enzymes such as CK and lactate dehydrogenase (LDH). For instance, values of 10,000 to 100,000 units of CK activity/L may be observed in the serum of boys with the muscle wasting disorder Duchenne muscular dystrophy (DMD) (Walton 1980; Brown and Lucy 1997). This is compared with normal values of 100 to 200 units/L; values for serum activity of CK can also be significantly elevated following unaccustomed exercise (Jones and Round 1997).

The mechanism by which muscle damage leads to elevated CK activities in serum is unclear. However, data from our group and others suggests that efflux of CK does not occur through non-specific leaks in the plasma membrane. Diederichs et al. (1979) demonstrated that damage to muscle fibres results in a gradual increase in muscle cell volume and that cell volume begins to fall when CK is seen to be released from the damaged muscle. These authors suggested that muscle cells attempt to maintain viability by extruding cytoplasm by an exocytotic type of mechanism and, in doing so, extrude cytosolic components, which include CK and other enzymes. We have demonstrated that release of CK can occur in several systems without a clear loss of membrane integrity or fall in cellular ATP levels (van der Meulen et al. 1995; West-Jordan et al. 1990, 1991, and unpublished observations). Conversely, we have also demonstrated that muscle damage can be observed by microscopic techniques, together with a loss of contractile force, when no increase in serum CK activity was seen (van der Meulen et al. 1997).

Care must be taken when using serum activity of CK as a sole index of muscle damage since CK has a short half-life (approximately 30 min) in the serum of rodents, and clearance rates may vary with interventions, such as exercise or drug administration. There is also some evidence that serum CK activity does not reflect the relative amount of muscle damage in some situations (Nosaka and Clarkson 1994; van der Meulen et al. 1991, 1997). An increase in serum CK activity relies on the total CK activity within the muscle, which may vary considerably. For example, serum CK activities in boys with DMD progressively decreases although muscle wasting continues. This is due to the gradual replacement of muscle by fat and connective tissue. Also, we have demonstrated that the total CK activity of regenerating muscle is reduced and that an equivalent amount of damage to regenerating muscle is reflected in a reduced release of CK activity (McArdle et al. 1994a).

Microdialysis Studies of Individual Muscles

A newly emerging tool for monitoring drug delivery to tissues is microdialysis (Benveniste and Huttemeier 1990; Kehr 1993). Microdialysis involves the positioning of a small dialysis membrane into the interstitial fluid of the tissue of interest. The membrane is perfused on the inside with an isotonic solution at a very slow flow rate. Tissue levels of an administered drug can be monitored dynamically by diffusion of the drug of interest across the membrane into the isotonic solution, which is subsequently collected for analysis. Thus, this technique provides information on the time course and concentration of systemic drug delivery to tissues.

It is now emerging that microdialysis can be used to continually monitor metabolic changes and damage to a specific muscle. We have demonstrated that microdialysis can be used to detect muscle metabolites such as the production of PGE_2, histamine and release of potassium from muscle (McArdle et al. 1999) and it may potentially be used to detect other small cytosolic peptides and proteins, although the need for custom-made microdialysis probes will limit the availability of this application.

Cellular Stress Response

All cells respond to stress by increased synthesis of a family of proteins known as stress or heat shock proteins (HSPs; see Feige et al. 1996 for a comprehensive review of the field). The stress response is known to occur in a variety of cells, including skeletal muscle (Guerriero et al. 1989; Salo et al. 1991; Bornman et al. 1995; Ornatsky et al. 1995; McArdle and Jackson 1996), following hyperthermia; ischaemia; treatment with toxins, heavy metals or oxidising agents; and viral infection (Feige et al. 1996). This stress response is activated by the presence of damaged or oxidised cellular proteins and can therefore be used as an indication that the cell has experienced a stressful event (Voellmy 1996).

The response is initiated by the activation of a heat shock transcription factor (HSF). There are several heat shock transcription factors (HSF1 to HSF4), but HSF1 is the most abundant and is thought to be responsible for the rapid stress response in human and rodent cells (Morimoto et al. 1996). Activation of HSF1 is thought to involve the formation of a homotrimer, translocation to the nucleus, binding to the heat shock element (HSE) of DNA and phosphorylation (Morimoto et al. 1996). The level of activation of the stress response depends on the severity of the stress. In general, HSF1 is activated within minutes of the stress, although activation is relatively transient. Increased transcription of heat shock protein mRNA (messenger ribonucleic acid) occurs very rapidly, and this results in increased cellular content of HSPs within several hours. The HSPs are relatively stable within the cell, and so elevated levels of HSPs can be seen in muscle for several days following stress. Detection of HSPs in cells will therefore indicate that the muscle has been subjected to non-lethal stress.

TECHNIQUES TO ASSESS
THE MECHANISMS OF MUSCLE DAMAGE

Models of Muscle Damage

A variety of models have been used to assess the effect of drugs on muscle damage. These include cultured myoblasts and myotubes, isolated single muscle fibres, bundles of fibres, intact isolated rodent muscles or damage to muscle in-situ in animals and man. Each model has its advantages and disadvantages.

The models differ in their accessibility and physiological relevance, thus, although muscle cells in culture are the least physiological of the models, they are the most accessible system and can provide information on whether a drug has potential myotoxicity as well as on the mechanisms by which the damage may occur. Conversely, in-situ models are the most relevant, but are inherently inefficient and minor or focal damage may not be readily detected.

Techniques to Show Changes in Muscle Calcium Content

A wide range of techniques can be employed in this area. These techniques measure changes in total muscle cellular calcium content, free intracellular calcium levels, the calcium content of intracellular organelles or the uptake of external calcium by muscles.

Compounds such as FURA-2, Indo-1 or Quin-2 have been developed to measure free intracellular calcium by fluorescent microscopy, where the level of emission reflects the free intracellular calcium level within the cell. Such techniques are primarily useful for measurement in isolated muscle fibres or cultured myoblasts or myotubes (Rivet-Bastide et al. 1993; Head 1993; Pressmar et al. 1994). Alternatively, increases in free intracellular calcium levels result in increased activity of calcium dependant enzymes such as the calpains and phospholipase A_2, and measurements of the activities of these enzymes or detection of their products can therefore also be used as an indirect measure of free intracellular calcium content.

Total muscle calcium content and mitochondrial calcium content are known to increase following muscle damage, and these can be measured in muscle biopsy samples or intact isolated muscles by atomic absorption spectroscopy (Jackson et al. 1985; McArdle et al. 1992; Reeve et al. 1996). Finally, in this area there is considerable evidence that in many situations the increase in muscle calcium which occurs during damage is derived from external sources. This accumulation can be followed in both isolated muscles and muscles in-vivo using the radioisotope, ^{45}Ca (McArdle et al. 1992, 1994b).

Markers of Increased Free Radical Activity

The highly reactive nature and extremely short half-life of free radicals makes their direct detection extremely difficult. The presence of free radical species in muscle has been measured directly by electron spin resonance (ESR) and by spin trapping techniques (Jackson et al. 1985), but these techniques are not widely applicable. Most studies rely on measurements of the stable products of oxidative free radical reactions with biological material. These include the products of fatty acid oxidation (such as lipid peroxides, malonaldehyde, diene conjugates or TBARS [thiobarbituric acid reactive substances]); the products of protein oxidation (such as protein carbonyls or a reduction in protein thiol groups); and the products of DNA oxidation (such as thymine dimers or 8 hydroxy-2-deoxy guanosine) (see Grootveld and Rhodes [1995] for a review). The adaptive response to an increase in free radical activity can also be seen in blood or tissue antioxidant enzyme levels or alterations in the tissue content of antioxidants, such as vitamin E (Robertson et al. 1991).

Methods of Measuring Cellular Energy Levels

A fall in cellular energy content can result in muscle damage or can occur as a consequence of damage due to an impairment in mitochondrial function. Muscle ATP levels can be measured in muscle biopsies by enzymatic techniques (Edwards et al. 1985) or non-invasively by ^{31}P-nuclear magnetic resonance spectroscopy (NMR; West-Jordan et al. 1990, 1991).

Conclusions

In summary, it appears that muscle cell death occurs via one of a few final common pathways. None of these pathways are independent, and there is considerable interaction between the systems. It is therefore difficult to assess which, if any, of the pathways have been initiated directly by the toxic agent. A wide variety of model systems exist in which to examine the mechanism by which muscle damage is initiated, but no single method to assess damage is infallible, and so the overall assessment of muscle damage should involve a range of techniques.

Acknowledgments

The authors would like to thank their many co-workers who have contributed to the work described in this chapter, in particular, Professor

Richard Edwards. Financial support from the Wellcome Trust, Linbury Trust, the Muscular Dystrophy Group of Great Britain and Northern Ireland and F. Hoffman-La Roche Ltd. is gratefully acknowledged.

REFERENCES

Allbrook, D. 1981. Skeletal muscle regeneration. *Muscle and Nerve* 4:234–245.

Anand, R.., and A. E. H. Emery. 1980. Calcium stimulated enzyme efflux from human skeletal muscle. *Res. Commun. Chem. Pathol. Pharmacol.* 28:541–550.

Balnave, C. D., and D. G. Allen. 1995. Intracellular calcium and force in single mouse fibres following repeated contractions with stretch. *J. Physiol.* 488:25–36.

Bellomo, G., P. Richelmi, F. Mirabelli, V. Marinoni, and A. Abbagano. 1985. Inhibition of liver microsomal calcium ion sequestration by oxidative stress: Role of protein sulphydryl groups. In *Calcium, oxygen radicals and cell damage,* edited by C. J. Duncan. Cambridge: Cambridge University Press, pp. 115–138.

Benveniste, H., and P. C. Huttemeier. 1990. Microdialysis—theory and application. *Prog. in Neurobiology* 35:195–215.

Bornman, L., B. S. Polla, B. P. Lotz, and G. S. Gericke. 1995. Expression of heat-shock/stress proteins in Duchenne muscular dystrophy. *Muscle and Nerve* 18:23–31.

Boveris, A., and B. Chance. 1973. The mitochondrial generation of hydrogen peroxide. *Biochem. J.* 134:707–716.

Brown, S. C., and J. A. Lucy,. eds. 1997. *Dystrophin: Gene, protein and cell biology.* Cambridge: Cambridge University Press.

Carlson, B. M. 1973. The regeneration of skeletal muscle—a review. *American Journal of Anatomy* 137:119–50.

Cerny, F. J., and G. Haralambie. 1983. Exercise-induced loss of muscle enzymes. In *Biochemistry of exercise,* edited by H. G. Knuttgen, J. A. Vogel and J. Poortmans. Champaign, Ill., USA: Human Kinetics Inc., pp. 441–446.

Crane, F. L., I. L. Sun, M. G. Clark, D. Grebing, and H. Low. 1985. Transplasma-membrane redox systems in growth and development. *Biochim. Biophys. Acta* 811:233–264.

DeLeiris, J., and D. Feuvray. 1979. Morphological correlates of myocardial enzyme leakage. In *Enzymes in cardiology,* edited by D. J. Hearse and J. De Leiris. Chichester, UK: John Wiley and Sons, pp. 445–460.

DeMartino, G. N., and D. E. Croall. 1987. Calcium-dependent proteases: A prevalent proteolytic system of uncertain function. *N.I.P.S.* 2:82–85.

Diederichs, F., K. Muhlhaus, and I. Trautschold. 1979. On the mechanism of lactate dehydrogenase release from skeletal muscle in relation to the control of cell volume. *Enzyme* 24:404–415.

Duncan, C. J. 1978. Role of intracellular calcium in promoting muscle damage: A strategy for controlling the dystrophic condition. *Experientia* 34:1531–1535.

Duncan, C. J., J. L. Smith, and H. C. Greenway. 1979. Failure to protect frog skeletal muscle from ionophore-induced damage by the use of a protease inhibitor, leupeptin. *Comp. Biochem. Physiol.* 63C:205–207.

Edwards, R. H. T., D. A. Jones, C. Maunder, and S. Batra. 1985. Needle biopsy for muscle biochemistry. *Lancet* I:736–738.

Faulkner, J. A., and S. V. Brooks. 1997. Muscle damage induced by contraction: An in situ single skeletal muscle model. In *Muscle damage,* edited by S. Salmons. Oxford: Oxford University Press, pp. 28–40.

Faulkner, J. A., S. V. Brooks, and J. A. Opiteck. 1993. Injury to skeletal muscle fibres during contractions: Conditions of occurrence and prevention. *Physical Therapy* 73:911–921.

Faulkner, J. A., D. R. Claflin, K. K. McKully, and D. A. Jones. 1982. Contractile properties of bundles of fiber segments from skeletal muscles. *Am. J. Physiol.* 243:C66–C73.

Feige, U., R. I. Morimoto, I. Yahara, and B. S. Polla, eds. 1996. *Stress-inducible cellular responses.* Berlin: Birkhauser Verlag.

Font, B., C. Vial, and D. Goldschmidt. 1977. Metabolite levels and enzyme release in the ischaemic myocardium. *J. Molecular Med.* 2:291–297.

Gohil, K., C. A. Viguie, W. C. Stanley, L. Packer, and G. A. Brooks. 1988. Blood glutathione oxidation during human exercise. *J. Appl. Physiol.* 64:115–119.

Grootveld, M., and C. J. Rhodes. 1995. Methods for the detection and measurement of reactive radical species in vivo and in vitro. In *Immunopharmacology of free radical species,* edited by D. Blake and P. G. Winyard. London: Academic Press.

Guerriero, V., D. A. Raynes, and J. A. Gutierrez. 1989. HSP70-related proteins in bovine skeletal muscle. *J. Cell. Physiol.* 140:471–477.

Halliwell, B., and J. M. C. Gutteridge. 1989. *Free radicals in biology and medicine.* Oxford: Clarendon Press.

Harris, W. E., and W. L. Stahl. 1980. Organisation of thiol groups of electric eel organ Na/K ion stimulated adenosine triphosphate, studied with bifunctional reagents. *Biochem. J.* 185:787–790.

Head, S. I. 1993. Membrane potential, resting calcium and calcium transients in isolated muscle fibres from normal and dystrophic mice. *J. Physiol.* 469:11–19.

Hearse, D. J. 1979. Cellular damage during myocardial ischaemia. Metabolic changes leading to enzyme leakage. In *Enzymes in cardiology: Diagnosis and research,* edited by D. J. Hearse and J. DeLeiris. Chichester, UK: Wiley & Sons, pp. 1–20.

Helliwell, T. R. 1997. Muscle damage induced by contraction: An in situ single skeletal muscle model. In *Muscle damage,* edited by S. Salmons. Oxford: Oxford University Press, pp. 168–214.

Jackson, M. J., and R. H. T. Edwards. 1988. Free radicals, muscle damage and muscular dystrophy. In *Reactive oxygen species in chemistry, biology and medicine,* edited by A. Quintilha. New York: Plenum, pp. 197–210.

Jackson, M. J., D. A. Jones, and E. J. Harris. 1984. Inhibition of lipid peroxidation in skeletal muscle homogenates by phospholipase A2 inhibitors. *Bioscience Reports* 4:581–587.

Jackson, M. J., R. H. T. Edwards, and M. C. R. Symons. 1985. Electron spin resonance studies of intact mammalian skeletal muscle. *Biochim. Biophys. Acta* 847:185–190.

Jones, D. A., and J. M. Round. 1993. *Skeletal muscle in health and disease.* Manchester, UK: Manchester University Press.

Jones, D. A. and J. M. Round. 1997. Muscle damage induced by contraction: An in situ single skeletal muscle model. In *Muscle damage,* edited by S. Salmons. Oxford: Oxford University Press, pp. 28–40.

Jones, D. A., M. J. Jackson, and R. H. T. Edwards. 1983. The release of intracellular enzymes from an isolated mammalian skeletal muscle preparation. *Clin. Sci.* 65:193–201.

Jones, D. A., M. J. Jackson, G. McPhail, and R. H. T. Edwards. 1984. Experimental muscle damage: The importance of external calcium. *Clin. Sci.* 66:317–322.

Karthius, R. J., D. N. Granger, M. I. Townsley, and A. R. Taylor. 1985. The role of oxygen-derived free radicals in ischaemia-induced increases in canine skeletal muscle vascular permeability. *Circ. Res.* 57:599–609.

Kehr, J. 1993. A survey on quantitative microdialysis: Theoretical models and practical implications. *J. Neurosci. Meth.* 48:251–261.

Klenerman, L., N. M. Lowe, I. Miller, P. R. Fryer, C. Green, and M. J. Jackson. 1995. Dantrolene sodium protects against experimental ischaemia and reperfusion damage to skeletal muscle. *Acta Orthop. Scand.* 66:347–351.

McArdle, A., and M. J. Jackson. 1996. Heat shock protein 70 expression in skeletal muscle. *Biochem. Soc. Trans.* 24:485S.

McArdle, A., and M. J. Jackson. 1997. Intracellular mechanisms involved in skeletal muscle damage. In *Muscle damage,* edited by S. Salmons. Oxford: Oxford University Press, pp. 90–108.

McArdle, A., R. H. T. Edwards, and M. J. Jackson. 1991. Effects of contractile activity on muscle damage in the dystrophin-deficient mdx mouse. *Clin. Sci.* 80:367–371.

McArdle, A., R. H. T. Edwards, and M. J. Jackson. 1992. Accumulation of calcium by normal and dystrophin-deficient muscle during contractile activity "in vitro." *Clin. Sci.* 82:455–459.

McArdle, A., R. H. T. Edwards, and M. J. Jackson. 1993. Calcium homeostasis during contractile activity of vitamin E deficient muscle. *Proc. Nutr. Soc.* 52:83A.

McArdle, A., R. H. T. Edwards, and M. J. Jackson. 1994a. Release of creatine kinase and prostaglandin E2 from regenerating skeletal muscle. *J. Appl. Physiol.* 76 (3):1274–1278.

McArdle, A., R. H. T. Edwards, and M. J. Jackson. 1994b. Time course of changes in plasma membrane permeability in the dystrophin-deficient mdx mouse. *Muscle and Nerve* 17:1378–1384.

McArdle, A., G. Khera, R. H. T. Edwards, and M. J. Jackson. 1999, in press. A microdialysis study of mediators of muscle pain during ischemia and reperfusion. *Muscle and Nerve.*

McArdle, A., J. H. van der Meulen, M. Catapano, M. C. R. Symons, J. A. Faulkner, and M. J. Jackson. 1995. Free radical activity during contraction-induced injury to the extensor digitorum longus muscle of rats. *J. Physiol.* 487:157–158P.

McCord, J. M. 1985. Oxygen derived free radicals in post-ischaemic tissue injury. *N. Eng. J. Med.* 312:159–163.

McKully, K. K., and J. A. Faulkner. 1985. Injury to skeletal muscle fibers of mice following lengthening contractions. *J. Appl. Physiol.* 59:119–126.

Mellgren, R. L. 1987. Calcium dependent proteases, an enzyme system active at cellular membranes. *F.A.S.E.B. J.* 1:110–115.

Morimoto, R. I., P. E. Kroeger, and J. J. Cotto. 1996. The transcriptional regulation of heat shock genes: A plethora of heat shock factors and regulatory conditions. In *Stress-inducible cellular responses,* edited by U. Feige, R. I. Morimoto, I. Yahara, and B. S. Polla. Berlin: Birkhauser Verlag, pp. 139–163.

Newham, D. J., D. A. Jones, and P. M. Clarkson. 1987. Repeated high-force eccentric exercise: Effects on muscle pain and damage. *J. Appl. Physiol.* 63:1381–1386.

Newham, D. J., D. A. Jones, S. E. J. Tolfree, and R. H. T. Edwards. 1986. Skeletal muscle damage: A study of isotope uptake, enzyme efflux and pain after stepping. *Eur. J. Appl. Physiol.* 55:106–112.

Newham, D. J., K. R. Mills, B. M. Quigley, and R. H. T. Edwards. 1983. Pain and fatigue after concentric and eccentric contractions. *Clin. Sci.* 64:55–62.

Nicotera, P. L., M. Moore, F. Mirabelli, G. Bellomo, and S. Orrenius. 1985. Inhibition of hepatocyte plasma membrane Ca^{2+} ATPase activity by menadione metabolism and its restoration by thiols. *Federation of European Biochemical Societies (FEBS) Letters* 181:149–153.

Nosaka, K., and P. M. Clarkson. 1994. Effect of eccentric exercise on plasma enzyme activities previously elevated by eccentric exercise. *Eur. J. Appl. Physiol.* 69:492–497.

Ornatsky, O. I., M. K. Connor, and D. A. Hood. 1995. Expression of stress proteins and mitochondrial chaperonins in chronically stimulated skeletal muscle. *Biochem. J.* 311:119–123.

Pennington, R. J. T. 1981. Biochemical aspects of muscle disease. In *Disorders of voluntary muscle,* 4th ed., edited by J. N. Walton. Edinburgh, UK: Churchill Livingstone, pp. 417–444.

Pressmar, J., H. Brinkmeier, M. J. Seewald, T. Naumann, and R. Rudel. 1994. Intracellular Ca^{2+} concentrations are not elevated in resting cultured muscle from Duchenne (DMD) patients and in mdx mouse muscle fibres. *Pflugers Arch-European J. Physiol.* 426:499–505.

Publicover, S. J., C. J. Duncan, and J. L. Smith. 1978. The use of A23187 to demonstrate the role of intracellular calcium in causing ultrastructural damage in mammalian muscle. *J. Neuropath. Exp. Neurol.* 37:544–557.

Reeve, J., A. McArdle, and M. J. Jackson. 1996. The role of calcium in muscle degeneration in the dystrophin-deficient mdx mouse. *Muscle and Nerve* 20:357–360.

Rivet-Bastide, M., N. Imbert, C. Cognard, G. Duport, Y. Rideau, and G. Raymond. 1993. Changes in cytosolic resting ionized calcium level and in calcium transients during in vitro development of normal and Duchenne muscular dystrophy cultured skeletal muscle measured by laser cytofluorimetry using Indo-1. *Cell Calcium* 14:563–571.

Robertson, J. D., R. J. Maughan, G. G. Duthie, and P. C. Morrice. 1991. Increased blood antioxidant systems of runners in response to training load. *Clin. Sci.* 80:611–618.

Rodemann, H. P. ,and A. L. Goldberg. 1982. Arachidonic acid, prostaglandin E_2 and F_{2a} influence rates of protein turnover in skeletal and cardiac muscle. *J. Biol. Chem.* 257:1632–1638.

Rodemann, H. P., L. Waxman, and A. L. Goldberg. 1982. The stimulation of protein degradation by Ca^{2+} is mediated by prostaglandin E_2 and does not require the calcium activated protease. *J. Biol. Chem.* 257:8716–8723.

Salmons, S., ed. 1997. *Muscle damage.* Oxford: Oxford University Press.

Salo, D. C., C. M. Donovan, and K. J. A. Davies. 1991. HSP70 and other possible heat shock or oxidative stress proteins are induced in skeletal muscle, heart and liver during exercise. *Free Rad. Biol. Med.* 11:239–246.

Sandri, M., U. Carraro, M. Podhorska-Okolov, C. Rizzi, P. Arslan, D. Monti, and C. Franceschi. 1995. Apoptosis, DNA damage and ubiquitin expression in normal and mdx muscle fibres after exercise. *FEBS Letters* 373:291–295.

Schanne, F. X., and J. C. Forber. 1979. Calcium dependence of toxic cell death: A final common pathway. *Science* 206:700–701.

Scherer, N. M., and E. W. Deamer. 1986. Oxidative stress impairs the function of sarcoplasmic reticulum by oxidation of sulphydryl groups in the Ca^{2+} ATPase. *Arch. Biochem. and Biophys.* 246:589–601.

Schwartz, L. M., and B. A. Osbourne. 1993. Programmed cell death, apoptosis and killer genes. *Immunology Today* 14:582–590.

Schwartz, L. M., L. Kosz, and B. K. Kay. 1990. Gene activation is required for developmentally programmed cell death. *P.N.A.S. USA* 87:6594–6598.

Schwartz, L. M., M. E. E. Jones, L. Kohz, and K. Kaah. 1993. Selective repression of actin and myosin heavy chain expression during the programmed death of insect skeletal muscle. *Develop. Bio.* 158:448–455.

Thomas, J. A., Y. C. Chai, and H. Jung. 1994. Protein-s thiolation and dethiolation. In *Methods in enzymology, oxygen radicals in biological systems,* vol. 233, edited by L. Packer. London: Academic Press, pp. 385–397.

Tidball, J. G., D. E. Albrecht, B. E. Lokensgard, and M. J. Spencer. 1995. Apoptosis precedes necrosis of dystrophin-deficient muscle. *J. Cell Sci.* 108:2197–2204.

van der Meulen, J. H., H. Kuipers, and J. Drukker. 1991. Relationship between exercise-induced muscle damage and enzyme release in rats. *J. Appl. Physiol.* 71:999–1004.

van der Meulen, J. H., A. McArdle, M. J. Jackson, and J. A. Faulkner. 1995. Lack of effect of vitamin E in contraction-induced injury to the extensor digitorum longus muscle of rats. *J. Physiol.* 487:158P.

van der Meulen, J. H., A. McArdle, M. J. Jackson, and J. A. Faulkner. 1997. Contraction-induced injury to the extensor digitorum longus muscle of rats: The role of vitamin E. *J. Appl. Physiol.* 83:817–823.

Voellmy, R. 1996. Sensing stress and responding to stress. In *Stress-inducible cellular responses,* edited by U. Feige, R. I. Morimoto, I. Yahara, and B. S. Polla. Berlin: Birkhauser Verlag, pp. 121–137.

Walton, J. N. 1981. *Disorders of voluntary muscle,* 4th ed. Edinburgh, UK: Churchill Livingstone.

West-Jordan, J. A., P. A. Martin, R. J. Abraham, R. H. T. Edwards, and M. J. Jackson. 1990. Energy dependence of cytosolic enzyme efflux from rat skeletal muscle. *Clin. Chim. Acta* 189:163–172.

West-Jordan, J. A., P. A. Martin, R. J. Abraham, R. H. T. Edwards, and M. J. Jackson. 1991. Energy metabolism during damaging contractile activity in isolated skeletal muscle: A ^{31}P-NMR study. *Clin. Chim. Acta* 203:119–134.

Wrogemann, K., and S. J. D. Pena. 1976. Mitochondrial calcium overload: A general mechanism for cell necrosis in muscle diseases. *Lancet* I:672–674.

Section B

Methods to Assess Pain, Irritation, and Muscle Damage Following Injections

4

In Vitro Methods for Evaluating Intravascular Hemolysis

Joseph F. Krzyzaniak

G. D. Searle
Pharmaceutical Development
Skokie, Illinois

Samuel H. Yalkowsky

College of Pharmacy, Department of Pharmaceutical Sciences,
The University of Arizona
Tucson, Arizona

Many medicinal agents are formulated as parenteral solutions for intravenous (IV) administration. It is often necessary to add excipients to these solutions to increase the solubility and/or stability of the drug. Some additives used in preparing parenteral formulations, which are generally considered safe, induce hemolysis after an IV injection. Since intravascular hemolysis has been associated with many undesirable medical conditions, as described in the following section, the toxic effects of pharmaceutical excipients must be determined before they are administered.

Several simple in vitro procedures have been developed to assess the potential of parenteral formulations to induce hemolysis. These methods can aid in the development of hemolytically safe formulations. In vitro methods have also been used to evaluate either the degree of hemolysis induced by an IV injection or the cell damage occurring after an intramuscular (IM) injection. The primary focus of this chapter is to provide information that will aid in selecting an appropriate in vitro method for testing potential formulations.

SIGNIFICANCE

Hemolysis is defined as an alteration of the erythrocyte membrane that results in the release of hemoglobin and other cellular components into the bloodstream. Symptoms commonly seen in patients with hemolysis are chills, fever, pain in the abdomen and back, shortness of breath, prostration, and shock (Berkow 1992). The severity of the symptoms produced by hemolysis is directly related to the amount of hemoglobin released into the bloodstream and the ability of the body to eliminate that hemoglobin.

When hemoglobin is released in the plasma, it binds to haptoglobin, a plasma protein, to form a soluble complex (Pintera 1971; Putnam 1975). This complex is cleared from the plasma by the reticuloendothelial cells in the liver, spleen, and bone marrow. In these cells, the heme groups are converted to bilirubin, which is then transported to the liver after binding to plasma albumin. In the liver, bilirubin is concentrated and conjugated to form bilirubin diglucuronide, which is then eliminated from the body. The conversion of heme into bilirubin diglucuronide is shown in Figure 4.1. Jaundice occurs when the amount of bilirubin exceeds the liver's ability to conjugate it. An accumulation of bilirubin in the bloodstream can cause kernicterus (a deposit of bilirubin on the basal ganglia of the brain that can lead to mental retardation, loss of hearing, or neonatal death).

Figure 4.1. The conversion of heme into bilirubin diglucuronide.

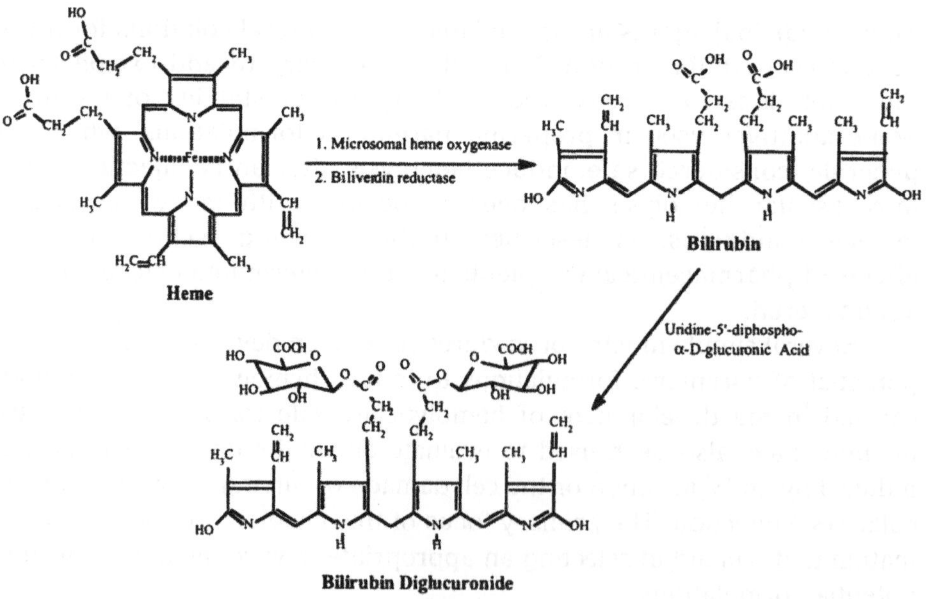

When the amount of hemoglobin released in the plasma is larger than the binding capacity of haptoglobin, unbound hemoglobin is present in the circulation. Some of the unbound hemoglobin is rapidly excreted in the urine, producing hemoglobinuria. Occasionally, intratubular hemoglobin casts are formed in the kidney. These casts obstruct the renal tubules, producing nephrosis and acute renal failure (Lucké 1946; Lalich 1955; Jaenike 1966a, b; Myers et al. 1966; Birndorf and Lopas 1970; Saitoh et al. 1993).

Unbound hemoglobin that is not excreted is either sequestered by the reticuloendothelial system or oxidized in the plasma to form methemoglobin. In the plasma, the heme groups dissociate from methemoglobin and complex with hemopexin and albumin to form heme-hemopexin and methemalbumin, respectively. These complexes are then eliminated from the plasma by the liver and metabolized in the same manner described above. The remaining globin group of methemoglobin binds to haptoglobin and is cleared from the plasma by the reticuloendothelial system.

The hemoglobin-haptoglobin complex and heme-hemopexin complex, along with fragments of the red blood cell membrane, cause the reticuloendothelial cells in the spleen to become congested. This causes splenomegaly, an increase in the size of the spleen, which produces the premature destruction of erythrocytes, i.e., hypersplenism (Berkow 1992).

It is clear from the discussion above that hemolysis can produce a wide range of undesirable medical conditions. When hemolysis is mild, these conditions are usually reversible. However, death can occur when hemolysis becomes severe. Since hemolysis can be more harmful to the patient than the condition being treated, every effort must be made to minimize its occurrence. The use of in vitro methods to evaluate the ability of a formulation to induce this condition is thus an important component of IV formulation development.

IN VITRO METHODS FOR EVALUATING HEMOLYSIS

In 1893, Hamburger developed a hemolytic method to study the permeability of red blood cells. He determined that the volume of the erythrocytes is dependent on the osmotic pressure of the surrounding fluid. Parenteral solutions that have the same osmotic pressure as the intracellular fluid of the erythrocyte were thought to be isotonic. Wokes (1936) developed a hemolytic method to evaluate the isotonicity of solutions prepared for parenteral administration. He determined that all isotonic solutions tested were nonhemolytic except solutions prepared with boric acid. Boric acid solutions induced hemolysis at all concentrations tested, i.e., 0.5 to 5 percent. Husa and Rossi (1942) outlined various calculations and experimental methods for preparing isotonic solutions. They determined that 1.8 percent boric acid should be isotonic with red blood cells, since the osmotic pressure is the same as the blood. The results of Wokes (1936) and Husa and Rossi (1942) suggest that all iso-osmotic solutions are not isotonic with red blood cells.

The fact that iso-osmotic solutions may not be isotonic was further explained in the work by Husa and Adams (1944). They showed that many iso-osmotic solutions induce hemolysis and are, therefore, not isotonic with red blood cells. This was attributed to the fact that the osmotic pressure of a solution is dependent on the total concentration of dissolved particles in it, while the tonicity of a solution depends only on the total concentration of the dissolved particles that do not pass through or alter the cell membrane. The inability of some iso-osmotic solutions to prevent hemolysis was also demonstrated by Hammarlund and Pedersen-Bjergaard (1961), who studied the degree of hemolysis induced by 161 pharmaceutical solutions. Their study showed that 71 of these iso-osmotic solutions induced varying amounts of hemolysis.

Many investigators have used in vitro methods to evaluate the hemolytic effects of solutions prepared with commonly used pharmaceutical excipients, i.e., amino acids and sugars (Husa and Adams 1944; Grosicki and Husa 1954); salts (Husa and Adams 1944; Hartman and Husa 1957, Krzyzaniak et al. 1996); cosolvents (Cadwallader 1963; Smith and Cadwallader 1967; Ku and Cadwallader 1974; Nishio et al. 1982; Reed and Yalkowsky 1985, 1986; Krzyzaniak et al. 1997); surfactants (Al-Assadi et al. 1989; Riess et al. 1991; Ohnishi and Sagitani 1993; Lowe et al. 1995; Krzyzaniak and Yalkowsky 1998); complexing agents (Rajewski et al. 1995; Shiotani et al. 1995). Note that the above is by no means a comprehensive list of the research done in this area. Some of these methods are summarized in Table 4.1. As shown by this table, each method is identified as either static or dynamic. In general, static methods determine hemolysis after incubating a predetermined volume of formulation with blood for a given period of time. The volume of formulation that is mixed with a given volume of blood is designated by the formulation:blood ratio, while the contact time determines how long the two liquids are incubated. For example, the method developed by Grosicki and Husa (1954) evaluates hemolysis after incubating 100 parts formulation with 1 part blood for 45 min. After the incubation is complete, the erythrocytes are separated by either sedimentation or centrifugation. The supernatant is then analyzed for hemoglobin.

In the case of dynamic methods, hemolysis is determined after injecting a formulation into a flow of blood and quenching the hemolytic reaction at a predetermined contact time with a large volume of normal saline. The contact time is determined by the velocity of the formulation:blood mixture and the volume of the mixing tube. After quenching, the liquid is centrifuged and the amount of free hemoglobin in the supernatant is determined. Common uses of the static and dynamic methods are described in the following sections.

Table 4.1. Summary of Various In Vitro Hemolysis Methods

In Vitro Method	Formulation: Blood Ratio	Contact Time	Type of Method
Wokes (1936)	—	30 min	static
Husa and Adams (1944)	50	30 min	static
Grosicki and Husa (1954)	100	45 min	static
Oshida et al. (1979)	10	30 min	static
Fort et al. (1984)	100	20 min	static
Reed and Yalkowsky (1985)	0.1	2 min	static
Al-Assadi et al. (1989)	100	20 min	static
Obeng and Cadwallader (1989)	—	—	dynamic
Lowe et al. (1995)	100	60 min	static
Shiotani et al. (1995)	20	30 min	static
Krzyzaniak et al. (1997)	0.1	1 sec	dynamic

— not specified

Static Methods

Static methods are commonly used in determining the hemolytic potential of excipients used in parenteral formulations. Since many formulations are known to induce hemolysis, static methods have also been used to evaluate the ability of "protecting agents" to decrease the degree of hemolysis induced by hemolytic formulations. Many studies have been conducted to decrease hemolysis by the addition of sodium chloride to these formulations (Husa and Adams 1944; Cadwallader 1963; Smith and Cadwallader 1967; Ku and Cadwallader 1974; Nishio et al. 1982; Reed and Yalkowsky 1986; Fu et al. 1987). In many cases, the hemolytic effect of the solution decreased and sometimes disappeared when sodium chloride was added.

In addition to determining the protecting effects of sodium chloride, Fu et al. (1987) evaluated the ability of sorbitol and polyethylene glycol 400 to prevent hemolysis induced by a 15 percent propylene glycol solution. They concluded that the addition of either of these substances at concentrations of approximately 20 percent gives maximum protection against hemolysis induced by the propylene glycol vehicle. The protective abilities of the additives used in their study were attributed to the increase in the tonicity of the test vehicle as well as to the potential formation of a complex between the excipients.

Static methods are also used to determine the rank order of hemolytic potentials for excipients used in formulations. The rank order determined by several workers for various cosolvents, surfactants, and complexing agents are summarized below.

- Reed and Yalkowsky (1985) evaluated the hemolytic effect of many cosolvents and determined that pure dimethyl sulfoxide is more hemolytic than pure propylene glycol, which is followed by a vehicle containing 10 percent ethanol and 40 percent propylene glycol, pure ethanol, pure polyethylene glycol 400, pure dimethyl-acetamide, and pure dimethylisosorbide.

- Ohnishi and Sagitani (1993) evaluated the hemolytic effects of nonionic surfactants and determined the following hemolytic relationship: Polyoxyethylene(20) oleyl ether is the most hemolytic followed by polyoxyethylene(40) monostearate, polyoxyethylene(20) sorbitan monooleate, and polyoxyethylene(20) hydrogenated castor oil. These surfactants are also known as Brij 97, Myrj 52, Tween 80, and Cremophor RH20, respectively.

- In the study by Rajewski et al. (1995), the following rank order was determined for various cyclodextrins. β-cyclodextrin was determined to be more hemolytic than hydroxypropyl-β-cyclodextrin, while sulfobutylether-β-cyclodextrin derivatives (SBE4-β-CD and SBE7-β-CD) were the least hemolytic.

In general, the same rank order for a given group of vehicles is obtained using different in vitro methods. With this information, excipients can be selected on the basis of their relative hemolytic safety as well as their ability to solubilize the solute. For example, polyethylene glycol 400 was shown to be less hemolytic than propylene glycol (Reed and Yalkowsky 1985; Krzyzaniak et al. 1997) and a better solubilizing agent for some medicinal agents (Rubino and Yalkowsky 1985).

Dynamic Methods

Dynamic methods are potentially very useful in evaluating the degree of hemolysis occurring after an IV injection. In developing such a method, the dynamics at the injection site must be considered. When a formulation containing components at their initial concentration is injected into a vein, as shown in Figure 4.2, the formulation is rapidly mixed with blood, resulting in a decrease in both drug and vehicle concentration. The concentration of these components in the blood immediately after the injection is dependent on their concentration in the formulation and the ratio of injection rate to the blood flow rate at the site of injection. The formulation and blood remain in contact at this ratio until the vein in which the injection occurred is joined by other veins, after which the formulation:blood ratio progressively

Figure 4.2. The interaction of a formulation with a red blood cell after an intravenous injection.

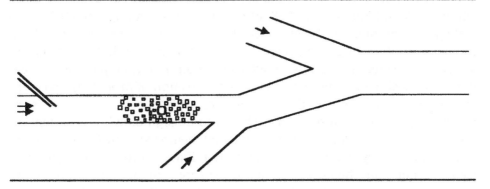

decreases as the formulation approaches the heart. All component concentrations will decrease further with continued distribution and circulation in the body.

The dynamics of an IV injection are responsible for the effect of the formulation composition and injection rate on hemolysis. Hemolysis is dependent on the hemolytic nature of both the drug and vehicle components in a formulation, as well as their concentrations as they are initially diluted with blood at the injection site. The initial dilution of the formulation by blood is described by the formulation:blood ratio. As the ratio of formulation to blood decreases with increasing dilution, the rate of hemolysis will decrease until the formulation is diluted enough that it becomes nonhemolytic and hemolysis ceases. The formulation:blood contact time is used to identify the time required for the formulation to become nonhemolytic.

In vitro methods that are intended to evaluate intravascular hemolysis should use an appropriate formulation:blood ratio and contact time to simulate the brief interaction of the initially diluted formulation with blood following an IV injection. In order to develop such a method, the effect of these parameters on in vitro hemolysis must be determined. Reed and Yalkowsky (1985), while evaluating the hemolytic effects of several cosolvents, determined that hemolysis is dependent on the formulation:blood ratio. With this information, they developed an in vitro method using a formulation:blood ratio of 0.1 that is able to mimic the initial dilution of the formulation by blood that follows an IV injection. Their method also uses a relatively short, 2-min, contact time to evaluate the hemolytic potential of pharmaceutical cosolvents. Although their method is more physiologically realistic than previous methods, a contact time of 2 min is still too long to model the fluid dynamics of an injection accurately.

Recently, Krzyzaniak et al. (1996) developed a dynamic in vitro method to evaluate the effect of contact time on hemolysis. Their experimental apparatus, which is illustrated in Figure 4.3, enabled them to determine the degree of hemolysis induced by hypotonic solutions (Krzyzaniak et al. 1996), cosolvent vehicles (Krzyzaniak et al. 1997), and surfactant vehicles (Krzyzaniak and Yalkowsky 1998) at contact times ranging from 0.5 sec to 100 min. From their results, it is clear that hemolysis is dependent on both the concentration of the excipient in the formulation and the time during which the formulation is in contact with blood. For example, the percent hemolysis is shown to increase as the concentration of propylene glycol increases above its iso-osmotic concentration of 2.1 percent. Hemolysis induced by propylene glycol is also shown to be sigmoidally dependent on the logarithm of contact time. Sigmoidal hemolysis curves have been obtained for every hemolytic vehicle tested. Each curve can be characterized by a minimum hemolysis occurring at short contact times and a maximum hemolysis occurring at long contact times. Both the minimum and maximum hemolytic potentials are shown to be dependent on both the concentration and hemolytic nature of the excipient in the formulation.

From the studies described above, it is clear that the percent hemolysis determined by in vitro methods that use a large formulation:blood ratio and a long contact time will be larger than that occurring after an IV injection. Therefore, an in vitro method that uses physiologically realistic parameters must be used to evaluate hemolysis occurring during the short period of time that the initially diluted formulation components mix with blood before further dilution occurs.

Figure 4.3. Dynamic in vitro method developed by Krzyzaniak et al. (1996).

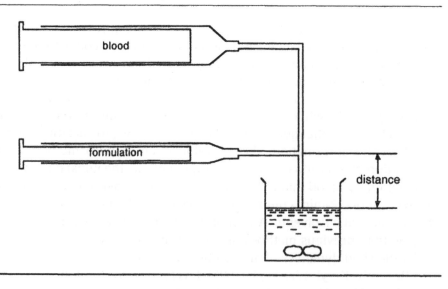

The actual in vivo formulation:blood ratio and contact time will depend on many factors, including the physical condition of the subject, blood flow at the site of injection, and the injection rate. Although no single formulation:blood ratio and contact time are appropriate for all conditions, the ratio of 0.1 with a contact time of 1 sec, which is used in the in vitro method by Krzyzaniak et al. (1997), is believed to be a reasonable approximation for the average human situation. This ratio is representative of a 1 mL formulation injected over 15 seconds into a vein with a blood flow rate of 40 mL/min. A contact time of 1 sec corresponds to the time in which the formulation becomes nonhemolytic as it is rapidly diluted with blood from intersecting veins.

COMPARISON OF IN VITRO AND IN VIVO HEMOLYSIS DATA

Although the in vitro dynamic method described above is able to simulate the dynamics of the injection site better than static methods, its ability to determine the degree of hemolysis occurring after an IV injection must be confirmed. This can be accomplished by comparing in vitro hemolysis data generated using this dynamic method to in vivo hemolysis data.

Recently, Krzyzaniak and Yalkowsky (1996) compared literature data for in vivo hemolysis to hemolysis data obtained from both their dynamic in vitro method and the static in vitro method used by Fort et al. (1984). The results of this comparison are given in Table 4.2, where "yes" indicates the formulation is hemolytic, while a "no" indicates that formulation is nonhemolytic. Note that Fort et al. (1984) suggested that a formulation is nonhemolytic if the percent hemolysis is less than 20 percent, while a hemolysis limit of 2 percent is used in the method by Krzyzaniak et al. (1997).

Hemolysis data generated using the method by Krzyzaniak et al. (1997) are clearly in better agreement with in vivo hemolysis data than that of Fort et al. (1984). This is attributed to the fact that a formulation:blood ratio of 0.1 and a contact time of 1 sec is more representative of the rapid dilution of a formulation with blood occurring after an IV injection. The unrealistically high formulation:blood ratios and/or contact times are believed to be responsible for the false-positive results obtained by static methods such as those of Fort et al. (1984). Since static hemolytic methods may give false-positive results for intravenously administered formulations, they are not recommended for the evaluation of hemolysis induced by an IV injection.

On the other hand, static methods may be useful as an indication of cell damage resulting from IM injections. This is shown in a study by Oshida et al. (1979) that evaluated the toxic effects (i.e., hemolytic potential, cytotoxic effect, and muscle lesions) of many parenteral formulations. Hemolytic effects were determined using an in vitro method with a

Table 4.2. In Vivo and In Vitro Hemolysis Data

Formulation Vehicle	In Vivo	In Vitro Method	
		Fort et al.[c]	Krzyzaniak et al.[d]
Normal saline (NS)	no[a,b,c]	no	no
10% ETOH[e] in NS	no[b]	no	no
30% ETOH in NS	no[c]	yes	no
40% PG[f] in NS	yes[b]	yes	yes
60% PG in water	yes[c]	yes	yes
10% ETOH + 20% PG in water	no[a]	yes[d]	no
10% PG + 30% ETOH in NS	no[c]	yes	no
10% ETOH + 40% PG in water	yes[a]	yes	yes
20% ETOH + 30% PEG[g] 400 in water	no[c]	yes	no

a. Banziger (1967)
b. Gentry and Black (1976)
c. Fort et al. (1984)
d. Krzyzaniak et al. (1997)

e. Ethanol
f. Propylene glycol
g. Polyethylene glycol

formulation:blood ratio of 10 and a contact time of 30 min. Muscle damage was evaluated after injecting a solution into either the rabbit's vastus lateralis or sacrospinalis muscle. From their data, a strong correlation between hemolytic potential and muscle lesions is evident. When parenteral formulations were determined to be nonhemolytic to slightly hemolytic, either no change or a slight change in muscle tissue was observed in 81 percent of the formulations. In the case where more than slight hemolysis is present, 91 percent of the solutions were shown to cause severe muscle damage. The correlation between hemolytic potential and muscle damage is supported by the study by Nishijima (1977). Nishijima also determined that muscle contractures were seen one month after injection in 70 percent of the cases in which the injection was determined to be very hemolytic.

SUMMARY OF IN VITRO METHODS

The biocompatibility of pharmaceutical excipients is an important consideration in the preparation of parenteral formulations. In vitro hemolytic methods have been developed to evaluate the potential toxicity induced by formulations after parenteral administration. These methods can be classified into two groups: (1) methods with a large formulation:blood ratio and long contact time and (2) methods with a small formulation:blood ratio and short contact time.

In vitro methods that use a large formulation:blood ratio and a long contact time are useful in determining the isotonicity of formulations as well as the cell damaging potential of IM injections. This type of method has been shown to be unable to distinguish the rank order for hemolytic cosolvent vehicles (Krzyzaniak and Yalkowsky 1996). Furthermore, they have the potential to give false-positive results when evaluating hemolysis occurring after an IV injection.

In vitro methods that use a small formulation:blood ratio and a short contact time are useful in determining the rank order for hemolytic solutions, since the percent hemolysis is much less than 100 percent. This type of method can also be used to evaluate the hemolytic effects of formulations administered intravenously. For example, the percent hemolysis determined by the dynamic method of Krzyzaniak et al. (1997) shows that the cosolvent and surfactant vehicles used in their studies are generally nonhemolytic, even though they produce nearly complete hemolysis in static tests. The low hemolytic potential determined for these excipients is consistent with the fact that they are commonly used in marketed IV formulations. Furthermore, the dynamic method does not give the false-positive results that are characteristic of static methods.

The methods described above can aid in the development of parenteral formulations for which hemolysis or muscle damage is minimized. The safety of potential formulations can accurately be evaluated for either IV or IM administration using the appropriate in vitro method.

REFERENCES

Al-Assadi, H., A. J. Baillie, and A. T. Florence. 1989. The haemolytic activity of nonionic surfactants. *Int. J. Pharm.* 53:161.

Banziger, R. 1967. Hemolysis testing in vivo of parenteral formulations. *Bull. Parent. Drug Assoc.* 21:148–151.

Berkow, R. 1992. *The Merck manual of diagnosis and therapy.* Rahway, N.J., USA: Merck Research Laboratories.

Birndorf, N. I., and H. Lopas. 1970. Effects of red cell stroma-free hemoglobin solution on renal function in monkeys. *J. Appl. Physiol.* 29:573–578.

Cadwallader, D. E. 1963. Behavior of erythrocytes in various solvent systems I: Water-glycerin and water-propylene glycol. *J. Pharm. Sci.* 52:1175–1180.

Fort, F. L., I. A. Hayman, and J. W. Kesterson. 1984. Hemolysis Study of aqueous polyethylene glycol 400, propylene glycol and ethanol combinations in vivo and in vitro. *J. Parent. Sci. Tech.* 38:82–87.

Fu, R. C-C., D. M. Lidgate, J. L. Whatley, and T. McCullough. 1987. The biocompatibility of parenteral vehicles: In vitro/in vivo screening comparison and the effect of excipients on hemolysis. *J. Parent. Sci. Tech.* 41:164–168.

Gentry, P. A., and W. D. Black. 1976. Influence of pentobarbital sodium anesthesia on hematologic values in the dog. *Am. J. Vet. Res.* 37:1349–1352.

Grosicki, T. S., and W. J. Husa. 1954. Isotonic solutions III. Amino acids and sugars. *J. Am. Pharm. Assoc., Sci. Ed.* 43:632–635.

Hamburger, H. J. 1893. Hydrops Von Mikrobiellem Ursprung. *Zieglers Beitr. allgem. Path. & Pathol. Anat.* 14:443–480.

Hammarlund, E. R., and K. Pedersen-Bjergaard. 1961. Hemolysis of erythrocytes in various iso-osmotic solutions. *J. Pharm. Sci.* 50:24–30.

Hartman, C. W., and W. J. Husa. 1957. Isotonic solutions V. The permeability of red corpuscles to various salts. *J. Am. Pharm. Assoc., Sci. Ed.* 46:430–433.

Husa, W. J., and J. R. Adams. 1944. Isotonic solutions II. The permeability of red corpuscles to various substances. *J. Am. Pharm. Assoc., Sci. Ed.* 33:329–332.

Husa, W. J., and O. A. Rossi. 1942. A study of isotonic solutions. *J. Am. Pharm. Assoc., Sci. Ed.* 31:270–277.

Jaenike, J. R. 1966a. The renal lesion associated with hemoglobinemia I. Its production and functional evolution in the rat. *J. Exp. Med.* 123:523–535.

Jaenike, J. R. 1966b. The renal lesion associated with hemoglobinemia II. Its structural characteristics in the rat. *J. Exp. Med.* 123:537–546.

Krzyzaniak, J. F., D. M. Raymond, and S. H. Yalkowsky. 1996. Lysis of human red blood cells 1: Effect of contact time on water induced hemolysis. *PDA J. Pharm. Sci. & Tech.* 50:223–226.

Krzyzaniak, J. F., D. M. Raymond, and S. H. Yalkowsky. 1997. Lysis of human red blood cells 2: Effect of contact time on cosolvent induced hemolysis. *Int. J. Pharm.* 152:193–200.

Krzyzaniak, J. F., and S. H. Yalkowsky. 1998. Lysis of human red blood cells 3: Effect of contact time on surfactant induced hemolysis. *PDA J. Pharm. Sci. & Tech.* 52:66–69.

Krzyzaniak, J. F., and S. H. Yalkowsky. 1996. A new dynamic in vitro method for evaluating lysis of human red blood cells. *Pharm. Res.* (Supplement) 13:367.

Ku, S-H., and D. E. Cadwallader. 1974. Behavior of erythrocytes in various solvent systems VI: Water-monohydric alcohols. *J. Pharm. Sci.* 63:60–64.

Lalich, J. J. 1955. The role of brown pigment in experimental hemoglobinuric nephrosis. *Arch. Pathol.* 60:387–392.

Lowe, K., B. Furmidge, and S. Thomas. 1995. Haemolytic properties of pluronic surfactants and Effects of purification. *Art. Cells. Blood Subs., and Immob. Biotech.* 23:135–139.

Lucké, B. 1946. Lower nephron nephrosis. *Mill. Surg.* 99:371–396.

Myers, J. K., D. Storrs, T. Miller, and C. B. Mueller. 1966. The Role of renal tubular flow in the pathogenesis of traumatic renal failure. *Surg. Gynecol. Obstet.* 130:1243–1251.

Nishio, T., S. Hirota, J. Yamashita, K. Kobayashi, Y. Motohashi, and Y. Kato. 1982. Erythrocyte changes in aqueous polyethylene glycol solutions containing sodium chloride. *J. Pharm. Sci.* 71:977–979.

Nishijima, Y. 1977. An experimental study of quadriceps contracture. *Centr. Jap. J. Orthop. Traumat. Surg.* 20:829–845.

Obeng, E. K., and D. E. Cadwallader. 1989. In Vitro method for evaluating the hemolytic potential of intravenous solutions. *J. Parent. Sci. Tech.* 43:167–173.

Ohnishi, M., and H. Sagitani. 1993. The effect of nonionic surfactant structure on hemolysis. *J. Am. Oil Chem. Soc.* 70:679–684.

Oshida, S., K. Degawa, Y. Takahashi, and S. Akaishi. 1979. Physico-chemical properties and local toxic effects of injectables. *Tnhoku J. exp. Med.* 127:301–316.

Pintera, J. 1971. *The biochemical, genetic, and clinicopathological aspects of haptoglobin,* edited by K. G. Jensen and S-A. Killmann. Baltimore: The Williams and Wilkins Company.

Putnam, F. W., ed. 1975. *The plasma proteins: Structure, function, and genetic control.* New York: Academic Press, Inc.

Rajewski, R. A., G. Traiger, J. Bresnahan, P. Jaberaboansari, V. J. Stella, and D. O. Thompson. 1995. Preliminary safety evaluation of parenterally administered sulfoalkyl ether β-cyclodextrin derivatives. *J. Pharm. Sci.* 84:927–932.

Reed, K. W., and S. H. Yalkowsky. 1985. Lysis of human red blood cells in the presence of various cosolvents. *J. Parent. Sci. Tech.* 39:64–68.

Reed, K. W., and S. H. Yalkowsky. 1986. Lysis of human red blood cells in the presence of various cosolvents II. The effect of differing NaCl concentrations. *J. Parent. Sci. Tech.* 40:88–94.

Riess, J. G., S. Pace, and L. Zarif. 1991. Highly effective surfactants with low hemolytic activity. *Adv. Mater.* 3:249–251.

Rubino, J. T., and S. H. Yalkowsky. 1985. Solubilization by cosolvents III: Diazepam and benzocaine in binary solvents. *J. Parent. Sci. Tech.* 39:106–111.

Saitoh, D., T. Kadota, A. Senoh, T. Takahara, Y. Okada, K. Mimura, H. Yamashita, H. Ohno, and M. Inoue. 1993. Superoxide dimutase with prolonged in vivo half-life inhibits intravascular hemolysis and renal injury in burned rats. *Am. J. Emerg. Med.* 11:355–359.

Shiotani, K., K. Uehata, T. Irie, K. Uekama, D. O. Thompson, and V. J. Stella. 1995. Differential effects of sulfate and sulfobutyl ether of β-cyclodextrin on erythrocyte membranes in vitro. *Pharm. Res.* 12:78–84.

Smith, B. L., and D. E. Cadwallader. 1967. Behavior of erythrocytes in various solvent systems III: Water-polyethylene glycols. *J. Pharm. Sci.* 56:351–355.

Wokes, F. 1936. Isotonic solutions for injection. *Quart. J. Pharm. Pharmacol.* 9:455–459.

5

Lesion and Edema Models

Steven C. Sutton

Pfizer Central Research
Groton, Connecticut

For intramuscular (IM) therapy, toleration of the injected formulation is often an issue. To aid the formulation scientist in achieving the least irritating formulation, a variety of in vivo and in vitro screening tools are now available. In 1981, Gray wrote that the relatively simple procedure for (testing) in the rabbit (had) been developed without much notice in the literature. FDA officials did not mention this type of testing in their *Appraisal of the Safety of Chemicals in Foods, Drugs and Cosmetics* that was published in 1959. Indeed, the current animal model generally accepted by the pharmaceutical industry and the FDA (Food and Drug Administration) for the prediction of muscle damage following IM administration in humans is the rabbit lesion volume model. Other commonly reported animal models are the rabbit creatine kinase (CK) models (Gray 1978; Gray 1981; Svendson 1988), rat lesion and CK models, (Surber and Sucker 1987) and the rat paw-lick model (for the assessment of pain [Comereski et al. 1986]).

In this chapter, animal models to assess lesion and edema are compared and contrasted. The utility of these models for immediate-release and extended-release formulations is also discussed.

EDEMA AND INFLAMMATION

While a comprehensive review of the process of inflammation is beyond the scope of this chapter, a brief discussion outlining the process is appropriate. Irrespective of the cause of tissue damage, substances are released by injured tissues that produce inflammation. Inflammation can include an increased local blood flow, leakage of capillaries (extravasation), clotting in interstitial fluid, migration of monocytes, and tissue swelling (Guyton 1991). Often the increased capillary permeability, which leads to increased fibrinogen and interstitial clotting, results in a "walling off" of the injured area.

The inflammatory process is often described in four stages. Regardless of whether or not the initial cause of cellular injury is chemotactic per se[1], chemotactic substances will be released from the damaged cells. Within minutes, these substances serve to attract tissue macrophages and neutrophils from nearby capillaries. Within hours, monocytes also reach the injured site, maturing and increasing in quantities, until days to weeks later, macrophages eventually become the predominate phagocytes in the inflamed region. The final phase consists of bone marrow production of granulocytes and monocytes, formation of white blood cells, and removal of the cause of inflammation. These events, which are primarily caused by tumor necrosis factor (TNF) and interleukin-1 (IL-1), take days to reach the injured site, but can continue for years if the stimulus continues. For details on mechanisms of neurologic inflammation, see Lowe et al. (1996).

Edema, the presence of excess fluid in body tissues, can occur intracellularly when either the sodium pump in the cell membrane can no longer function or there is insufficient energy to drive the pump, and is usually followed by cell death. In addition to the processes described above, substances released by damaged cells (e.g., around an inflammation) increase the membrane permeability in neighboring cells (Guyton 1991). Nearby mast cells may release a variety of mediators (e.g., histamine, serotonin, bradykinin, arachidonate metabolites, substance P), accelerating the inflammatory process (Wang et al. 1996).

LESION MODELS

If the damaged area is sufficiently large, it is generally considered a lesion. Lesion models were among the earliest models established to predict irritation from IM formulations. Perhaps this was because the damaged region was readily visible and easily described.

Rabbit

Since first described in 1949 (Nelson et al.), the rabbit lesion model has been extensively referenced (Shintani et al. 1967; Svendsen 1983; Svendsen et al. 1979; Pettipher et al. 1988; Oshida et al. 1979; Olling et al. 1995; Dness 1985), and remains the "gold standard" (Gray 1981) for predicting formulation tolerability in humans.

The model remained attractive, despite being resource and time intensive, primarily because of the large database of published correlations

---

1. There are various causes of cell injury: membrane perturbation, leakage, disruption of the sodium pump, tonicity, pH, etc.

between rabbit and human IM formulations. Furthermore, the rabbit is normally gentle, has a relatively large muscle mass (e.g., sacrospinalis), and is normally more sensitive to IM inflammation than humans. This sensitivity may result in a reduction in numbers of animals required to determine a less-irritating formulation.

Method

Our use of the model consisted of using New Zealand White rabbits (2.7–2.9 kg) of either sex (3–8 per time point, per formulation) injected approximately 0.6 cm deep into the sacrospinalis muscle with 1.0 mL of the formulation of interest, using 23-gauge sterile needles. Groups of animals were euthanatized at 1, 2, 3, 7, 11, 14 and 21 days postinjection.

Hemorrhage. In our lab, lesions were subjectively scored (Shintani et al. 1967) for hemorrhage (rabbit hemorrhage score [RbHS], reddening) as follows: 0 (no grossly detectable coloration), 1 (slightly red), 2 (mild), 3 (moderate), and 4 (black). While scoring was achieved by averaging the independent evaluation of two unblinded investigators, the preferred method would "blind" the scoring.

Lesion Volume. The size of the lesion was often reported in our laboratory as an additional parameter. The total RbLV volume of abnormal appearing tissue (necrotic, hemorrhagic, etc.) was measured as length (anterior to posterior) by width (midline to side) by depth (top to bottom of lesioned muscle) at the point of maximum involvement.

Histology. Histological evaluation can provide additional information about mechanisms, or subtle differences between formulations. Samples were fixed in 10 percent formalin; trimmed sections were dehydrated in graded alcohols, embedded in paraffin, sectioned at a thickness of 6 μm, placed on glass slides, stained with hematoxylin and eosin, and coverslipped. Microscopic changes in skeletal muscle were quantified by subjective evaluation of the following criteria, which were scored on a scale of 1 (least) to 5 (greatest): necrosis of myofibers, hemorrhage, granulocytic cell infiltration, and mononuclear cell infiltration. The score for each sample was based on the most severe changes present but did not reflect the relative size of a lesion. An example of the histological evaluation of a 60 mg/mL danofloxacin aqueous formulation is shown in Figures 5.1 and 5.2. One can conclude from Figure 5.1 that the variability in rabbit necrosis scores was small for this formulation. Figure 5.2 demonstrates the similarity in 21-day profiles of necrosis scores and histology indices.

Since histopathological scoring can be somewhat subjective, it is important that the same pathologist score all samples in a study. When this is not possible, representative samples with their assigned scores may be kept

Figure 5.1. Individual (bars) and average (line) necrosis scores in rabbits following intramuscular injection of 60 mg/mL danofloxacin formulation, showing general shape of lesion onset and repair profile, and extent of variability for this measurement (*no data).

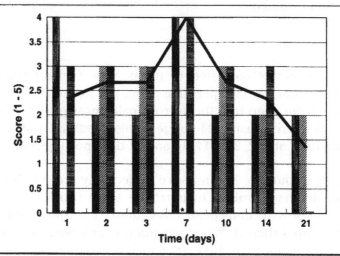

Figure 5.2. Average score following intramuscular injection of 60 mg/mL danofloxacin aqueous formulation. All indices appeared to increase 48 to 72 h after injection, with maximum scores on day 7, followed by a return toward baseline. (Note that on days 10 to 21, granulocytes were completely absent).

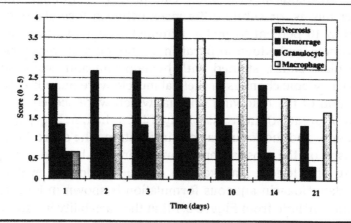

on file to help standardize the scoring between pathologists. For a number of reasons (e.g., incomplete study design, change in study personnel), a complete set of histological evaluations may not be possible for every formulation examined. When this occurred in our lab (Sutton et al. 1996), the scores were averaged across animals for each day and index and then summed across days 3, 7, 14, and 21 to give a cumulative histology score (CHS). While the CHS was shown to rank correlate with RbLV, the correlation appeared formulation dependent (Figure 5.3).

Methodological Concerns

While rare, an aggressive rabbit was occasionally encountered. One possible explanation is an animal's poor health or insufficient/inadequate training of either animal or investigator. Standard Operating Procedures (e.g., injection volume, needle depth) are important to minimize "noise" in the data. Needle depth can be standardized though the use of an adapter that fits snugly over the needle. All formulations should be rendered sterile.

Even with extreme care, persistent variability, subjectivity, and inconsistency may require a large number of animals (*n*). We have found that an *n* = 3 is inadequate for most studies. A minimum of six replicates will provide a more reliable conclusion.

Figure 5.3. Relationship of rabbit lesion volume (RbLV) and cumulative histology score (CHS) for intramuscular formulations DanoIR (immediate release danofloxacin [■]) DanoAQUEOUS (aqueous extended-release danofloxacin [●]), and DanoOIL (oily extended-release danofloxacin, [▲]). In general, as the lesion volume increased, so did CHS. Note that the two extended-release formulations appeared to demonstrate a slightly steeper relationship than the immediate-release formulation.

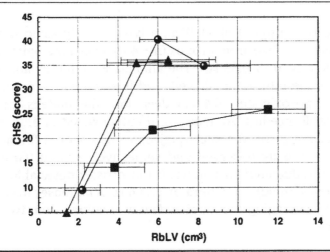

Pain on Injection. The issue of pain and its relationship to muscle damage is controversial. Comereski et al. (1986) ranked pain (measured by the rat paw-lick model) with muscle damage (gross pathology and histopathology in the rabbit lesion model) for a series of cephalosporins. However, Svendsen (1988) implied that pain resulting from injection may not be related to muscle damage. For example, faulty technique may have lead to injection into or near a nerve. In the event that an injection causes severe discomfort, the study protocol must clearly state procedure. Standard protocols should be defined (e.g., the animal is immediately pulled off the study and administered analgesics).

Mice

Direct examination of muscle damage in lesions following IM injection in mice was reported by Gutiérrez et al. 1991. In a study using groups of white mice, 50 μL of a myotoxic phospholipase A_2, bothropstoxin II (BthTX-II) ($n = 5$), or PBS (phosphate buffered saline) ($n = 3$) was injected in the gastrocnemius muscle. While lesions were not evident on gross examination, light and electron microscopy detailed muscle fiber damage. Macrophages were present at 24 h, and swollen mitochondria were evident 1 h after injection of the toxin.

Rat

In 1978, Gray dismissed the rat as an alternative to the rabbit for lack of a suitable database. However, the rat has become the most studied of all species (including human), and the rodent database has steadily grown. This is not surprising as the laboratory rat is docile, genetically well-defined, and relatively inexpensive to house.

Method

As reported by Sutton et al. (1996a), a typical study using the rat lesion models consisted of separate groups ($n = 4$ to 6 per time point) of Sprague Dawley male rats (0.25–0.35 kg). The animals were lightly anesthetized by methoxyflourane inhalation, shaved, and injected with 0.5 mL of the test formulation approximately 0.4 cm deep into the gluteus medius using 23-gauge sterile needles. Animals were euthanatized at 1, 2, 3, 4, 6, and 24 h postinjection, and the site of injection was scored for hemorrhage. Lesions were visually observed and subjectively scored (Gray 1978) for hemorrhage (reddening) as follows: 0 (no grossly detectable coloration), 1 (slightly red), 2 (mild), 3 (moderate), and 4 (black). Biases in scoring were minimized by averaging the *independent* evaluations from two unblinded investigators.

BIOCHEMICAL MODELS

The lesion models are labor and resource intensive. As mechanisms of edema and inflammation were elucidated, investigators searched for methods that were more sensitive and might detect tissue damage earlier than lesion models. The need for a less resource and labor intensive surrogate to the lesion model lead to biochemical models. Several enzyme models have been shown to correlate with muscle damage. Among the numerous biochemical markers commonly correlated with lesion models, four deserve mention: SGOT, NAβG, MyPo, and CPK. Since the enzyme action can generally be determined by published methods, this section is limited to precautions. In the case of CK, correlations will be discussed.

Serum Glutamic-Oxaloacetic Transaminase

Knirsch and Gralla (1970) reported elevated SGOT (serum glutamic-oxaloacetic transaminase) levels in humans and dogs following IM injection of carbenicillin. In humans, SGOT activity peaked at 3 h and returned to baseline 8 h postinjection. Caution must be exercised when using SGOT since elevated levels are also manifested by liver damage. The investigators reported that liver function tests were normal, and SGOT levels did not elevate following IV (intravenous) administration of carbenicillin.

N-Acetyl-β-Glucosaminidase

NAβG (N-acetyl-β-glucosaminidase) is an enzyme commonly associated with tissue inflammation, as its presence is an indication of monocyte infiltration (Pettipher et al. 1988). Sutton et al. (1996a) found no correlation between tissue NAβG activity and lesion or creatine phosphokinase (CPK) activity following IM injection of danofloxacin formulations (Figure 5.4). However, the presence of monocytes could not be confirmed by microscopic examination. Perhaps this biochemical test would be useful for those irritants that do result in monocyte infiltration.

Myeloperoxidase

MyPo (myeloperoxidase) is an enzyme found in neutrophils and monocytes (Lefkowitz et al. 1992; Miller et al. 1993). As summarized earlier, these cell types are often found in areas of advanced inflammation. We evaluated the potential use of MyPo as a predictive indicator of muscle damage following IM injection of various formulations (Sutton et al. 1996a). Compared to a saline control, MyPo activities were generally higher in tissues injected with the "positive control" digoxin; however, all values were much lower

Figure 5.4. The apparent lack of a correlation is shown between N-acetyl-β-glucosaminidase (NAβG) and rabbit lesion volume (RbLV) following intramuscular injection of danofloxacin formulations ($r^2 = 0.11$).

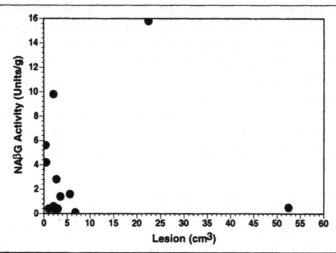

than expected (Table 5.1). Tissue histology (data not shown) on these tissues suggested a paucity of neutrophils. This may be due to the fact that all of the formulations were sterile, or that the cytotoxic nature of digoxin did not stimulate migration of neutrophils. The MyPo tissue assay, therefore, may not be a useful biochemical predictor of IM toleration caused by pharmaceutical preparations.

Creatine Kinase

The intracellular enzyme creatine kinase (CK) (a.k.a. creatine phosphokinase [CPK] or creatine phosphotransferase) is primarily located in skeletal, brain, and heart muscle. Damage to these tissues results in the release of CK into blood. Cardiac muscle injury following myocardial infarction results in a rise in serum CK activity within 18 to 30 h in humans (Sigma 1990). Muscle injury following IM injection causes an earlier increase in CK activity in humans (e.g., 2–3 h) (Knirsch and Gralla 1970). As was the case for the liver enzyme SGOT, release of CK by cardiac tissue damage can be easily ruled out by IV administration.

Assay Considerations

While by far the most commonly cited biochemical marker, the measurement of CK is not without issue (Szasz et al. 1976). Interference of formulation on the assay must first be ruled out before accurate analysis of this

Table 5.1. Summary of Tissue Myeloperoxidase Assay Activity (Units/100 mg) Following Intramuscular Injection of Saline or Digoxin

Time (postinjection)	Saline[a] (0.9%)	Digoxin[a] (0.25 mg/mL)
24 h	0.44	1.32
48 h	0.67	0.74
72 h	0.56	0.83
11 day	0.24	0.06
14 day	0.28 ± 0.28	0.46 ± 0.29
21 day	0.05 ± 0.05	0.09 ± 0.08

[a]Mean of tissues from two animals, or mean ± SD of tissues from three animals.

enzyme can be made (Attar and Mata 1971; Meltzer 1971; Meltzer et al. 1970; Andersen and Damsgaard 1976; Brazeau and Fung 1989). Additionally, any muscle damage caused by the agent(s) that is not related to the initial IM injection should be determined though an oral and/or IV administration of the agent(s). We used a commercially available kit (47-UV, Sigma, St. Louis, Mo.), to determine plasma CK concentrations. The assay was linear over a range of 5 to 50 units/L. Samples were stable at room temperature for 24 h, but were always assayed on the day of the experiment. The test compound was directly added to the CK standards in concentrations expected in vivo, and compared to the CK standard alone. If an effect of the test compound on the CK standard was observed, a baseline correction was made.

Methodology Considerations

If surgery or animal handling is involved, sufficient time for recovery is required (see "Rabbit" section below). This allows CK levels to return to baseline before the study is begun. If the test procedure is relatively stressful, a training period should be implemented. Finally, a sham study, where sterile normal saline is injected, should be included as a control for the handling and injection procedures.

CK activity has been measured in a variety of species. Table 5.2 summarizes the CK activity in several species following IM injection of an irritating substance. The data are intended for a qualitative comparison among the species mentioned here. Specie selection may be made based on customer endpoint (e.g., husbandry, companion animals), ease of use, and/or cost.

Table 5.2. CK Activity in Species Following IM Injection of an Irritating Substance[1]

Species	CK C_{max} (units/L)	CK T_{max} (units/L)	Time CK Activity Returned to Baseline (h)
Mice	700	1 to 3	24
Rat	1,000	1 to 3	24
Rabbit	3,000	8	72
Dog	3,000	24	96
Mini pig	70	8	—
Cattle	1,800	8	> 72
Human	1,300	6	> 72

[1]See specific sections for references.

Mice. In the study by Gutiérrez et al. (1991) cited earlier, blood was collected at 1, 3, 6, and 24 h by cutting the tip of the tail, and plasma CK activity was determined. Average CK activity increased sharply in the toxin group, reaching a maximum of around 700 units/mL at 1 to 3 h postinjection, then falling to 200 units/mL at 6 h, and returning to baseline ($\approx$ 25 units/L) by 24 h. This profile of CK release closely paralleled the muscle damage observed by light and electron microscopy.

Rat. In our hands, a typical study using the rat CK models consisted of separate groups (n = 4 to 6 per time point) of Sprague Dawley male rats (0.25–0.35 kg) briefly anesthetized with methoxyflourane, shaved, and injected with 0.5 mL of the test formulation approximately 0.4 cm deep into the gluteus medius using 23-gauge sterile needles. Blood was collected from animals by cardiac puncture at 1, 2, 3, 4, 6, and 24 h postinjection, centrifuged, and plasma separated for immediate CK determination. To establish whether cardiac puncture resulted in an uncontrolled release of CK, studies completed in our lab revealed that 2 h after a saline injection, CK activity in samples obtained by cardiac puncture (158 $\pm$ 76.7 units/L) were similar to samples obtained via retro-orbital vein plexus under ether narcosis (115 $\pm$ 38.1 units/L) (Surber and Sucker 1987).

Rabbit. In our lab, rabbits were surgically cannulated at the jugular vein with a vascular access port (Model SLA, Access Technologies, Skokie, Ill.). Ports were flushed with heparinized saline (500 units/mL) weekly, and CK activity was determined. Usually within 1 week following aseptic surgery,

CK activity was back to baseline values. For each study, 4 to 6 cannulated rabbits were injected approximately 0.6 cm deep into the sacrospinalis muscle with 1.0 mL of the formulation of interest, using 23-gauge sterile needles. Blood was collected from the ports just before, and 2, 4, 6, 24, 48, and 72 h after IM injection of the test formulation, centrifuged, and plasma CK activity immediately determined (Sutton et al. 1996a).

Dog. Gray (1978) reported single and multiple dose studies in the dog. Baseline measurements were collected at least twice before the start of treatment. Injection volume was 1.5 mL per site. CK levels peaked (3,000 units/L) at 24 h following IM injection of U-21, 251F (a "moderately irritating antibiotic"), and returned to baseline by 96 h.

Mini-pig. A few reports of studies using the pig have appeared in the literature (Steiness et al. 1978; Gray 1978; Steiness et al. 1974). Pigs weighing 20 to 30 kg each were intramuscularly injected in the back with 2 mL of the formulation. Compared to a saline control, lidocaine produced only a twofold increase in CK activity ($\approx$ 300 and 725 units/L, respectively) at 8 h.

Cattle. Pyörälä et al. (1994) reported the effect of IM administration of several commercially available formulations on CK activity in cattle. Baseline serum CK activity was approximately 125 units/L. Following IM injection, CK activity increased to a maximum at 8 h, followed by a steady decrease over the next 3 days. For some formulations, CK activity was elevated for days before declining. The most irritating formulations produced a peak CK activity of $\approx$ 1800 units/L.

Comparison of Parameters

Several different parameters describing CK activity have appeared in the literature (see references in the following sections). These include the enzyme activity at a specified time following the IM injection (e.g., C_{2h}), the maximum enzyme activity (C_{max}), the time of maximum activity (T_{max}), and the area under the activity versus time curve, over a specified interval (e.g., AUC_{0-24h}). The correlation of these parameters to the rabbit lesion model are compared in this section.

Rabbit. As reported in earlier work, rabbit CK (RbCK) C_{max} and CK AUC_{0-72} were both about equal in their ability to predict muscle damage (see below, "Correlation of Models"). We determined how robust the parameters were by examining which parameter could best distinguish subtle differences between eight formulations (Sutton et al. 1996a). Differences in the parameter following IM injection of the eight formulations were determined by analysis of variance (ANOVA) using SAS statistical software (SAS

Institute Inc., Cary, N.C.). Differences were considered significant ($p < 0.05$) using the GLM[2] procedure. Robustness (ρ) was defined as the total number of statistically significant differences determined among the eight formulations. As detailed in Table 5.3, and summarized in Table 5.4, the parameters RbCK C_{max} and RbCK AUC_{0-72} had a similar number of significant differences between formulations ($\rho = 21$, Table 5.4). This suggested that a shorter sampling schedule (defining C_{max} and not the entire CK activity profile) may be sufficient to describe the relationship between CK activity and lesion.

Johnston and Miller (1985) also showed an excellent correlation for gross tissue morphology and CK both after single and multiple dosing. Using the rabbit, they reported CK profiles after injection of poloxamers 238 and 407 that were similar in shape to that of peanut oil and saline, while poloxamers 335 and 403 caused much greater and prolonged CK levels. CK was not elevated beyond 72 h in any of the above studies. Thus it appeared that RbCK correlated well with muscle damage observed within a few days of IM injection.

Rat. Early studies (Paget and Scott 1957) suggested the rat CK (RtCK) model may be predictive of muscle damage. Surber and Sucker (1987) reported "very severe" macroscopic damage in the rat after IM imipramine and navaminsulfon-Na. Of the formulations tested, only these two produced 2 h RtCK activities in the 1,000 units/L range.

Our studies supported those of Surber and Sucker (1987) and confirmed the predictive value of RtCK. In our examination of the rat CK model, we also determined how robust (ρ) a 2 h CK level (RtCK$_{2h}$) was compared to a 4 h level, or the cumulative CK levels over the time course of the study (RtCK$_{0-24h}$) (Sutton et al. 1996a). As shown in Table 5.3 and summarized in Table 5.4, the parameters RtCK$_{4h}$ and RtCK$_{0-24h}$ detected a greater number of significant differences between formulations ($\rho = 19$ and 20, respectively) than did the parameter RtCK$_{2h}$ ($\rho = 15$, Table 5.4). Since RtCK C_{max} was usually the larger of RtCK$_{2h}$ and RtCK$_{4h}$, the C_{max} parameter detected more differences in this comparison than either the 2 h or 4 h parameters ($\rho = 21$).

Summary of CK Model. As shown in Figure 5.5 for digoxin, CK is more rapidly cleared from the rat than from the rabbit. Therefore, characterization of the CK C_{max} in the rat requires frequent sampling during the first few hours postinjection. Additionally, the muscle damage caused by the formulations need not be instantaneous. For some formulations, CK T_{max} will occur at 2 h, for others, at 4h. While the best parameter is probably a time-averaged one (e.g., AUC), its determination required numerous CK sampling times to profile the entire CK curve. While rat CK C_{max} was as

---

2. General linear models post hoc means comparison test.

Table 5.3. Comparison of Parameters: Ability to Determine Statistically Significant Differences Among Eight Formulations

The table presents a series of pairwise comparison matrices (formulations 1–8) for the following parameters:

- RbLV Days 1-3
- RbHS Days 1-3
- RbCK C_{max}
- RbAUC
- RtCK C_{max}
- RtCK$_{4h}$
- RtCK$_{0-24h}$
- RtCK$_{2h}$
- RtHS$_{4h}$
- RtHS$_{0-24h}$
- RtHS$_{24h}$
- RFE

Each matrix uses the symbols: * = significant ($p < 0.05$), o = not significant, nd = not done, − = self comparison.

One-way ANOVA (SAS) comparisons for each model were completed against the eight formulations, using the GLM procedure to determine statistical significance (*$p < 0.05$). Formulations were identified as follows:

1 = saline, 2 = digoxin, 3 = digoxin vehicle, 4 = azithomycin, 5 = azithomycin vehicle, 6 = danofloxacin vehicle, 7 = danofloxacin 25 mg/mL, and 8 = danofloxacin 60 mg/mL. (o = not significant; nd = not done; see text for details).

Table 5.4. Summary Table Comparing the Total Number of Significant Differences from Table 5.3 (ρ)

Model	Parameter	# Differences (ρ)
RtHS	Cumulative 0–24 h	22
RbCK	AUC	21
RbCK	Cmax	21
RtCK	Cmax	21
RbLV	Cumulative days 1–3	20a
RtCK	Cumulative 0–24 h	20
RtCK	4 h	19
RFE	—	18
RtHS	24 h	16
RtCK	2 h	15
RtHS	4 h	15
RbHS	Cumulative days 1–3	8a

[a]Scaled to equate the 28-way comparisons of other parameters.

Figure 5.5. Comparison of average CK levels after intramuscular administration of digoxin to rats and rabbits. Note that compared to the rabbit, the profile in the rat appears condensed.

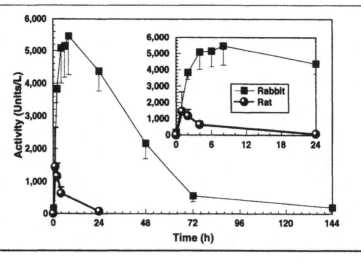

discriminating as rat CK AUC, $RtCK_{4h}$ was found to be an adequate labor and resource sparing alternative.

EDEMA MODELS

Edema models developed in parallel with the lesion models. In combination with various biochemical tests, they provided a rapid readout on experimental therapies and hypothesis testing.

Inducing Edema

In most of the aforementioned models, a formulation consisting of some compound of medicinal value was injected. In the edema literature, however, these compounds are used to elucidate edema mechanisms. The most common agents used to induce edema in those studies were carrageenin, kaolin, and glass (Riesterer et al. 1971). Such material is inert, having no pharmacological action per se. Recently, the use of pharmacologically active agents (e.g., polymyxin B and serotonin) in these models has also been reported (Wang et al. 1996). In pharmaceutical research, the irritant also has intrinsic pharmacological activity. The challenge is to separate the effects of formulation actives and excipients.

Exudative Models of Inflammation

Otterness and Bliven (1985) described a model that allows for the collection of exudate from an object/formulation that causes an inflammation. A sterilized sponge impregnated with the compound of interest was surgically implanted subcutaneously in an anesthetized rat. Animals were sacrificed at specified times from 6 to 24 h after implantation, depending on which marker information was desired (e.g., neutrophils, mononuclear, PGE_2, TxB_2, LTB_4). The sponge was then removed, the exudate collected and examined. This model has been useful to determine the effects of specific agents and mechanisms of inflammation.

Vascular Permeability Models

A major cause of edema is an increased vascular permeability, leading to excess fluid in the affected area. Vascular permeability can be determined by IV injection of a substance normally restricted to the vascular space (e.g., Evans blue dye, ^{67}Ga).

^{67}Ga-Citrate

The ^{67}Ga-citrate vascular permeability model consists of injecting the radioisotope into the rat tail vein, and determining the extent of extravasation in the rat footpad. Gallium forms a complex with transferrin once it enters the circulation. At various times following subcutaneous injection of the test substance into the subplantar area of the hind paw, the radioactivity of ^{67}Ga in each hind paw is measured using a sodium iodide (NaI) scintillation detector. The radioactivity in the paw generally follows a profile similar to edema measured by the water displacement method. A reasonable correlation between accumulation of ^{67}Ga and edema was reported. This method may hold some advantages over the water displacement method (see "Footpad Edema Models"), since continuous monitoring of acute inflammation may be possible (Kohno et al. 1987).

Mouse Ear Model

In the mouse ear model, extravasation of intravenously injected Evans blue is measured in the treated ear, with a correction from the control ear (Wang et al. [1986] and references therein). Five min after the dye is intravenously injected, the test substance is subcutaneously injected into one ear (saline is injected into the other ear). Animals were killed at specified times after the induction of edema, and an ear punch from both ears is obtained. Exuded blue dye in the tissue sample is extracted and quantitated by absorbance. The intensity of the inflammatory response is determined by the difference in the plasma leakage (using a standard curve for absorbance change vs. plasma volume) between the two tissue samples from each animal.

Rat Footpad Exudative Model

In the rat footpad exudative model, Evans blue is intravenously injected prior to subcutaneous administration of the test substance into the footpad, and dye extracted from the tissue is spectrophotometrically determined (Reisterer and Jaques 1967).

Footpad Edema Models

In these models, the ability of a test formulation to swell the footpad with edema (thereby increasing the volume or weight) often was shown to be correlated with a formulation's local irritancy.

Rat

The rat footpad edema model has been heavily cited in the literature (Reisterer and Jaques 1967), due to the relative ease of handling and wide database accumulated on this common laboratory animal (Ando et al. 1991). In one variation of this model, the animal was physically restrained, the right hind footpad of each rat was injected with 0.1 mL of the formulation, and the left footpad served as a control. The control consisted of "no injection" or saline (preferred). The animals were euthanatized 24 h later, the hind feet were amputated and weighed (Sutton et al. 1996a; Gilligan et al. 1994). A variation of this model used serial volume measurements determined with a plethysmometer (Prelon et al. 1994).

Mouse

The mouse is a scaled-down version of the rat foot edema model. In this model, 5 μL of the test substance or sterile saline was injected just under the footpad of the right and left hindpaw, respectively. The volumes of both hind paws were measured with a plethysmometer just before, and at specified times after administration of the test substance. Hind paw swelling (compared to control hind paw) was calculated at a specific endpoint (e.g., 24 h), or the area under the time–paw swelling curve (AUC) was used for a time-averaged indication of edema (Wang et al. 1996).

CORRELATION OF MODELS

While one might conclude from the previous section that the edema models generally predict inflammation and tissue damage, the ability of these models to discriminate among formulations was only recently reported. In this section, the ability of the various models to predict tissue damage and discriminate among a variety of formulations (e.g., aqueous vs. oil base) will be presented.

Rabbit Lesion Versus Rabbit Hemorrhage Score Model

In addition to rabbit lesion volumes, Sutton and coworkers evaluated hemorrhage (reddening) after IM administration of these IR (immediate-release) formulations (Sutton et al. 1996a). The cumulative hemorrhage scores for days 1 though 3 ($RbHS_{1-3day}$) and for days 7 though 21 ($RbHS_{7-21day}$) were compared (by ANOVA) for each formulation. Note the similar scores for saline and digoxin injections for the first two days (Figure 5.6). There were only a few statistically significant differences among the formulations tested for the parameter $RbHS_{1-3day}$. While the

Figure 5.6. Hemorrhage scores in rabbits following intramuscular injection of saline or digoxin. Note the large standard deviation associated with each score.

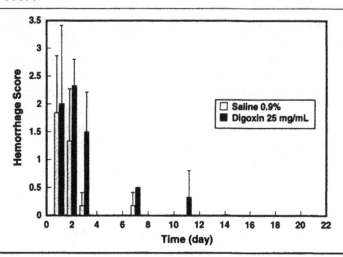

rabbit lesion volume model accumulated 20 significant comparisons ($\rho = 20$, Tables 5.2, 5.3), the rabbit hemorrhage score model accumulated only 6 significant comparisons ($\rho = 6$). Perhaps the injection technique contributed to the variability associated with the day 1 and 2 hemorrhage scores. Because of this and the subjective nature of the evaluation, we did not see any advantage in this model.

Rabbit Lesion Versus Rabbit CK Model

As shown in Tables 5.2 and 5.3, ρ for the RbCK measurements RbCK AUC ($\rho = 21$) and C_{max} ($\rho = 21$) was similar to that for RbLV model ($\rho = 20$). Furthermore, since the CK assay was rather precise, the CK models were less prone to the inconsistencies associated with the characterization of the lesion. In studies with an undiluted IV formulation of the macrolide azithomycin and its vehicle (2 mM citric acid), the importance of secondary tests became clear. In an initial evaluation, RbLV showed similar, marked muscle damage for azithomycin ($n = 9$) and azithomycin vehicle ($n = 3$) on day 3 (Figure 5.7). However, the vehicle did not produce an increase in RbCK levels consistent with significant muscle damage. In this case, a follow-up lesion study ($n = 11$) confirmed the apparent lack of muscle damage suggested by the low RbCK levels. In conclusion, either a large n must be used for the lesion model (e.g., $n = 6$), or supportive tests must be run in parallel.

Figure 5.7. Daily lesion volumes and CK levels in rabbits following intramuscular injection of digoxin or azithomycin formulations. Note that when an appropriately sized *n* was used for RbLV, the two models were in agreement.

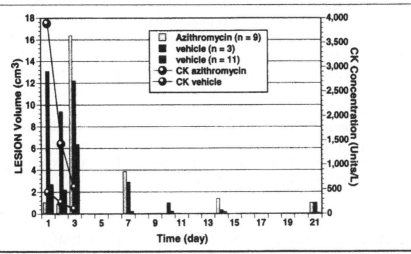

Rabbit Lesion Versus Rat Footpad Edema Model

As part of our systematic evaluation of IM models, the rat footpad edema (RFE) model was compared to the rabbit lesion model (Sutton et al. 1996a). The ability of RFE to discriminate among immediate-release formulations in general was good ($\rho = 18$, Table 5.4). This was unexpected, since the mechanism of action for edema following a subcutaneous injection may be different from that of muscle damage following IM injection of some formulations (see above discussion "Edema and Inflammation"). RFE was less predictive of muscle damage for extended-release IM formulations (Sutton et al. 1996b). Since the prediction of muscle damage appeared unreliable, caution should be excercised when evaluating RFE model predictions of muscle damage following IM injection of extended-release formulations.

Rabbit Lesion Versus Rat CK Model

As shown in Tables 5.3 and 5.4, ρ for RtCK C_{max} ($\rho = 21$), RtCK C_{4h} ($\rho = 19$), and RtCK CK_{0-24h} ($\rho = 20$) was similar to the value for RbLV ($\rho = 20$). This suggested that like the RbCK model, the RtCK model was about as sensitive as the rabbit lesion volume model (Sutton et al. 1996a).

Rat and Human

Following IM injection in humans, an experimental diazepam formulation containing half the amount of propylene glycol as in the commercial formulation, and the rest of the solvent as polyethylene glycol, resulted in similar pharmacokinetic profiles but less pain on injection than the proprietor's formulation (Korttila et al. 1976). While CK activities were similar during the 3 h study, there was a trend toward less CK at 3 h for the less painful formulation. The experimental formulation also had a lower propensity to precipitate with common IV diluents than the commercial formulation.

Following IM injection in rats, the experimental formulation resulted in histological observations that were similar to saline (Kortilla et al. 1976). Thus the formulation that apparently resulted in less muscle damage in rats was less painful on injection in humans.

MODELS FOR EXTENDED-RELEASE FORMULATIONS

Reports evaluating the tissue response to prolonged or extended-release formulations are few. Johnston and Miller (1985) evaluated the use of Cremophor EL, peanut oil, and poloxamer vehicles for IM use in the rabbit. Svendsen and Aaes-Jørgensen (1979) studied the muscle damage following IM injection of vegetable oil in rats, rabbits, and dogs. Gupta et al. (1993) reported the effect of IM injection of poly(lactic acid) microspheres in dogs.

Sutton and coworkers (1996b) examined the effect of IM injection of vehicle (aqueous vs. sesame oil) and the dissolution of an active compound in numerous models. In that study, the rat lesion, CK, and RFE models were evaluated as resource sparing alternatives to the rabbit lesion model for assessing injection site tolerance in extended-release formulation screening (Sutton et al. 1996b). Whereas for immediate-release formulations, attention was usually focused on *acute* muscle damage (e.g., 1–3 days postinjection), for extended-release formulations, equally important was the prediction of chronic muscle damage. Formulations that delayed the release of the active compound were screened in the alternative models and compared to the rabbit lesion model.

None of the short-term models (CK, RFE, or $RbLV_{days1-3}$) predicted the chronic effects of the extended-release formulations, since these models apparently reflected only the acute muscle damage of such components of the extended-release formulation that were immediately available to surrounding tissue at the time of injection. As was the case for immediate-release formulations, the RtCK model could screen those extended-release formulations with unacceptable acute damage due to immediately available components. However, to evaluate potential *delayed* effects from extended-release formulations, the long-term model RbLV was still recommended (Sutton et al. 1996b).

Predicting Muscle Damage from Extended-Release Formulations

Muscle damage is probably a function of both local tissue concentration and contact time of drug and/or formulation components. A poorly tolerated immediate-release formulation may be typified by the immediate-release of muscle damaging components that exceed a critical level (C_{crit}, Figure 5.8). Once C_{crit} is reached, cell lysis occurs, and released CK is detected (Curve A). However, an extended-release formulation may release muscle damaging components at a slower rate than immediate-release formulations. When released at slow rates, dilution and lymphatic clearance of these damaging components, as well as cellular repair, may lessen muscle damage (Curve D). On the other hand, an extended-release formulation that releases too many of these components soon after injection would

Figure 5.8. Hypothetical relationship between component concentration and exposure time on muscle damage. Curve A: an immediate-release formulation, which would cause acute muscle damage (predicted by CK models); curves B–D: extended-release formulations; B: acute and sustained muscle damage (probably predicted by CK models); C: delayed muscle damage (not predicted by CK models described here), D: ideal extended-release formulation, no muscle damage (probably predicted by CPK models).

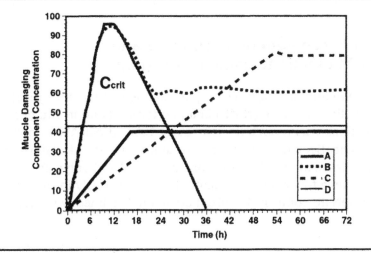

have acute muscle damage predicted by the CK models. If C_{crit} continued to be exceeded, repair might be hampered, resulting in chronic muscle damage (Curve B). Finally, if C_{crit} was not initially achieved but achieved 48 to 72 h later, then the CK models (as presented here) may not have predicted either the acute or chronic muscle damage from the delayed C_{crit} (Curve C).

FUTURE DIRECTIONS

Muscle Damage and CK

Although CK release is commonly thought of as an all-or-nothing phenomenon, the sequelae of events is likely more complicated. Gray (1978) suggested that certain lesions may release more CK than others. Brazeau and coworkers (Brazeau and Fung 1990; Brazeau et al. 1992) have reported that for organic cosolvents, the relationship between muscle damage and CK release may in some cases involve intracellular calcium mobilization. Additional studies are needed to further understand the relationship between CK and muscle lesions following IM injection of formulations. Perhaps more studies with immediate- and extended-release formulations are needed to determine whether the apparent inconsistencies are attributable to formulation or animal model.

Gamma Scintigraphy

Research from Davis' group in Nottingham (Mills et al. 1981) suggests that gamma scintigraphy may be useful to evaluate the in vivo release of IM formulations. Such studies may improve our understanding of the relationship between component C_{crit} and muscle damage.

Electron Paramagnetic Resonance and Nuclear Magnetic Resonance Imaging

While the potential use of electron paramagnetic resonance (EPR) and nuclear magnetic resonance (NMR) imaging for studying in situ performance of formulations was reported in the early 1980s (Beall 1984), only recently has their utility been detailed in the literature. Mader et al. (1997) examined the in situ release of PCA (a spin probe molecule) and polymer erosion from a biodegradable formulation implanted subcutaneously in the neck of rats. With appropriate controls, localized edema may someday be quantitated.

Effect of Edema and Lesion on Bioavailability

Effect of Lesion/Tissue Capsule

A few studies examining the relationship between edema, muscle damage, and pharmacokinetics have appeared in the literature. In one such study, stainless steel cages were implanted in several species, and the pharmacokinetics of compounds injected into the cage followed as capsules formed around the cages (Leppert et al. 1994). While lesions formed around the cages did not decrease systemic availability to cefoxitin or ivermectin in cattle and sheep, plasma levels of both drugs following administrations to the tissue cages in rats and dogs were significantly lower than those following subcutaneous injection. This group further reported the successful use of lesions generated by silastic disks in rats for the in vitro evaluation of their barrier properties on selected drugs (Wood et al. 1995).

Models to Assess Drug Absorption from Intramuscular Injection

The use of isolated rat muscle (Brazeau and Fung 1990) and perfused rabbit leg models (Nara et al. 1990) as tools to obtain information on the muscular absorption of drugs has also been reported in the literature. Although difficult, these models may help unravel the complexities of formulation effects on muscle damage and drug pharmacokinetics.

Formulation

Support Matrix

While it is generally known that solid particles cause more irritation than a semisolid, a carefully designed comparison of substances in solution versus in an eroding matrix versus in a noneroding matrix has not been published.

Preventing Inflammation

Interestingly, cortisol prevents the development of inflammation by stabilizing cellular and lysosomal membranes. By reducing the amounts of proteolytic (lysosomal) enzymes and other substances normally released by damaged cells, cortisol reduces or minimizes the inflammation process (Guyton 1991). Developmental research specifically addressing the use of such agents in IM formulations may lead to better tolerated products.

Conclusions

The rat CK model can be used as a reasonable alternative to the rabbit lesion model for immediate-release formulations. However, for extended-release formulations, the rabbit lesion model must still be used.

While much is known regarding the relationship between formulation components and muscle damage for immediate-release formulations, this cannot be said for extended-release formulations. More research is needed to unravel the mysteries of formulation and muscle damage. Perhaps some combination of EPR, NMR, and gamma scintigraphic imaging with the above drug absorption models will provide those answers.

References

Andersen, K. E., and T. Damsgaard. 1976. The effect of serum enzymes of intramuscular injections of digoxin, bumetanide, pentazocine and isotonic sodium chloride. *Acta Med. Scand.* 199:317–319.

Ando, Y., M. Inoue, S. Araki, and Y. Morino. 1991. Inhibition of carrageenin-induced paw edema by a superoxide dismutase derivative that circulates bound to albumin. *Biochim. Biophys. Acta* 1073:374–379.

Attar, A. M., and C. Mata. 1971. Increased levels of creatine phosphokinase after intramuscular injections. *Med. Chem DC.* 40:92–93.

Beall, P. T. 1984. Safe common agents for improved NMR contrast. *Physiolog. Chem. Phys. Med. NMR* 16 (2):129–135.

Brazeau, G., and H.-L. Fung. 1989. Interferences with assay of creatine kinase activity in vitro. *Biochem. J.* 257:619–624.

Brazeau, G. A, and H.-L. Fung. 1990. Effect of organic cosolvent-induced skeletal muscle damage on the bioavailability of intramuscular [14C]diazepam. *J. Pharm. Sci.* 79:773–777.

Brazeau, G. A., S. S. Watts, and L. S. Mathews. 1992. Role of calcium and arachidonic acid metabolites in creatine kinase release from isolated rat skeletal muscles damaged by organic cosolvents. *J. Paren. Sci. Technol.* 46:25–30.

Comerski, C. R., P. D. Williams, C. L. Bregman, and G. H. Hottendorf. 1986. Pain on injection and muscle irritation: A comparison of animal models for assessing parenteral antibiotics. *Fund. Appl. Tox.* 6:335–338.

Dness, V. 1985. Local tissue damage after im injections in rabbits and pigs. Quantitation by determination of creatine kinase activity at injection sites. *Acta Pharmacol. et Toxicol.* 56:410–415.

Drelon, E., P. Gillet, N. Muller, B. Terlain, and P. Netter. 1994. Anti-inflammatory properties of IL-1 in carrageenan-induced paw oedema. *Agents and Actions* 41:50–52.

Gilligan, J., S. Lovato, M. Erion, and A. Jeng. 1994. Modulation of carrageenan-induced hind paw edema by substance P. *Inflammation* 18 (3):285–292.

Gray, J. E. 1978. Pathological evaluation of injection injury. In *Sustained and controlled release delivery systems,* edited by J. Robinson. New York: Marcel Dekker, pp. 351–410.

Gray, J. E. 1981. Appraisal of the intramuscular irritation test in the rabbit. *Fund. Appl. Tox.* 1:290–292.

Gupta, P. K., H. Johnson, and C. Allexon. 1993. In vitro and in vivo evaluation of clarithromycin/poly (lactic acid) microspheres for intramuscular drug delivery. *J. Controlled Rel.* 26:229–238.

Gutiérrez, J. M., J. Núnez, C. Díaz, A. C. O. Cintra, M. I. Homsi-Brandeburgo, and J. R. Giglio. 1991. Skeletal muscle degeneration and regeneration after injection of bothropstoxin-II, a phospholipase A2 isolated from the venom of the snake *Bothrops jararacussu. Exper. Molec. Path.* 55:217–229.

Guyton, A. 1991. Resistance of the body to infection: 1. Leukocytes, granulocytes, the monocyte-macrophage system, and inflammation. In *Textbook of Medical Physiology,* edited by A. Guyton. Philadelphia: WB Saunders Co., pp. 365–373.

Johnston, T. P., and S. C. Miller. 1985. Toxicological evaluation of poloxamer vehicles for intramuscular use. *J. Paren. Sci. Technol.* 39 (2) 83–88.

Knirsch, A. K., and E. J. Gralla. 1970. Abnormal serum transaminase levels after parenteral ampicillin and carbenicillin administration. *Med. Intell.* 282 (19): 1081–1082.

Kohno, H., et al. 1987. Utilization of 67Ga-citrate for the measurement of histamine-induced edema in anesthetized rats. *Radioisotopes* 36:261–264.

Korttila, K., A. Sothman, and P. Andersson. 1976. Polyethylene glycol as a solvent for diazepam: Bioavailability and clinical effects after intramuscular administration, comparison of oral, intramuscular and rectal administration, and precipitation from intravenous solutions. *Acta Pharmacol. et Toxicol.* 39:104–117.

Lefkowitz, D. L., K. Mills, D. Morgan, and S. S. Lefkowitz. 1992. Macrophage activation and immunomodulation by myeloperoxidase. *Proc. Soc. Exp. Biol. Med.* 2:204–210.

Leppert, P., L. Cammack, R. Cargill, L. Coffman, M. Cortese, K. Engle, C. Krupco, and J. Fix. 1994. Interspecies differences in systemic drug availability following subcutaneous pulsatile administration in cattle, sheep, dogs and rats. *J. Biomed. Mat. Res.* 28 (9):713–722.

Lowe III, J. R. Snider, and D. MacLean. 1996. Nonpeptide NK1 antagonists: From discovery to the clinic. In *Neurogenic inflammation,* edited by P. Geppetti and P. Holzer. New York: CRC Press, pp. 299–309.

Mader, K., Y. Cremmilleux, A. Domb, J. Dunn, and H. Swartz. 1997. In vitro/in vivo comparison of drug release and polymer erosion from biodegradable P(FAD-SA) polyanhydrides—A noninvasive approach by the combined use of electron paramagnetic resonance spectroscopy and nuclear magnetic resonance imaging. *Pharm. Res.* 14 (6):820–826.

Meltzer, H. 1971. Chlorpromazine-induced hypothermia and increased plasma creatine phosphokinase activity. *Biochem. Pharm.* 20:1739–1748.

Meltzer, H. Y., S. Mrozak, and M. Boyer. 1970. Effect of intramuscular injections on serum creatine phosphokinase activity. *Am. J. Med. Sci.* 259:42–48.

Miller, M. J. S., H. Sadowska-Krowicka, S. Chotinaruemol, J. L. Kakkis, and D. A. Clark. 1993. Amelioration of chronic ileitis by nitric oxide synthase inhibition. *J. Pharm. Exper. Therap.* 261:11–16.

Mills, S. N., S. S. David, J. G. Hardy, C. G. Wilson, N. Thomas, and M. Frier. 1981. In vivo evaluation of colloidal dosage forms intended for intramuscular use. *J. Pharm. Pharmacol.* 33.

Nara, E., T. Hatono, M. Hashida, and H. Sezaki. 1990. A new method for assessment of drug absorption from muscle: Application of a local perfusion system. *J. Pharm. Pharmacol.* 43:272–274.

Nelson, A. A., C. W. Price, and H. Welch. 1949. Muscle irritation following the injection of various penicillin preparations in rabbits. *J. Am. Pharm. Assoc.* 38:237–239.

Olling, M., K. Van Twillert, P. Wester, A. B. T. Boink, and A. G. Rauws. 1995. Rabbit model for estimating relative bioavailability, residues and tissue tolerance of intramuscular products: Comparison of two ampicillin products. *J. Vet. Pharmacol. Therap.* 18:34–37.

Oshida, S., K. Degawa, Y. Takahashi, and S. Akaishi. 1979. Physico-chemical properties and local toxic effects of injectables. *Tnhoku J. Exp. Med.* 127:301–316.

Otterness, I., and M. Bliven. 1985. Laboratory models for testing nonsteroidal anti-inflammatory drugs. In *Nonsteroidal inflammatory drugs,* edited by J. Lombardino. New York: John Wiley & Sons, Inc., pp. 156–168.

Paget, G., and H. M. Scott. 1957. A comparison of the local effects of various intramuscular injections in the rat. *Br. J. Pharmacol.* 12:427–433.

Pettipher, E. R., B. Henderson, S. Moncada, and G. A. Higgs. 1988. Leucocyte infiltration and cartilage proteoglycan loss in immune arthritis in the rabbit. *Br. J. Pharmacol.* 95:169–176.

Pyörälä, S., L. Manner, E. Kesti, and M. Sandholm. 1994. Local tissue damage in cows after intramuscular injections of eight antimicrobial agents. *Acta Vet. Scand.* 35:107–110.

Riesterer, L., and R. Jaques. 1967. The local anti-inflammatory action of nonsteroidal compounds on the paw edema caused by kaolin in the rat. *Helv. Physiol. Pharmacol. Acta* 25:156–159.

Riesterer, L., H. Majer, and R. Jaques. 1971. On the paw edema induced by subcutaneous injection of minute glass particles in the rat. *Agents and Actions* 2 (1): 27–32.

Shintani, S., M. Yamazaki, M. Nakamura, and I. Nakayama. 1967. A new method to determine the irritation of drugs after intramuscular injection in rabbits. *Tox. Appl. Pharm.* 11:293–301.

Sigma. 1990. *Creatine kinase procedure No. 47-UV.* St. Louis: Sigma.

Steiness, E., O. Svendsen, and F. Rasmussen. 1974. Plasma digoxin after parenteral administration: Local reaction after intramuscular injection. *Clin. Pharm. Therap.* 16:430–434.

Steiness, E., F. Rasmussen, O. Svendsen, and P. Nielsen. 1978. A comparative study of serum creatine phosphokinase (CPK) activity in rabbits, pigs and humans after intramuscular injection of local damaging drugs. *Acta Pharmacol. et Toxicol.* 42:357–364.

Surber, C., and H. Sucker. 1987. Tissue tolerance of intramuscular injectables and plasma enzyme activities in rats. *Pharm. Res.* 4:490–494.

Sutton, S., L. Evans, M. Rinaldi, and K. Norton. 1996a. Predicting injection site muscle damage I: Evaluation of immediate release parenteral formulations in animal models. *Pharm. Res.* 13 (10):1507–1513.

Sutton, S., L. Evans, M. Rinaldi, and K. Norton. 1996b. Predicting injection site muscle damage II: Evaluation of extended release parenteral formulations in animal models. *Pharm. Res.* 13 (10):1514–1518.

Svendsen, O. 1983. Local muscle damage and oily vehicles: A study on local reactions in rabbits after intramuscular injection of neuroleptic drugs in aqueous or oily vehicles. *Acta Pharmacol. et Toxicol.* 52:298–304.

Svendsen, O. 1988. *Studies of tissue injuries caused by intramuscular injection of drugs and vehicles. Methods for quantitation and effects of concentration, volume, vehicle, injection speed and intralipomatous injection.*

Svendsen, O., and T. Aaes-Jørgensen. 1979. Studies on the fate of vegetable oil after intramuscular injection into experimental animals. *Acta Pharmacol. et Toxicol.* 45:352–378.

Svendsen, O., F. Rasmussen, P. Nielsen, and E. Steiness. 1979. The loss of creatine phosphokinase (CK) from intramuscular injection sites in rabbits. A predictive tool for local toxicity. *Acta Pharmacol. et Toxicol.* 44:324–328.

Szasz, G., W. Gruber, and E. Bernt. 1976. Creatine kinase in serum: 1. Determination of optimum reaction conditions. *Clin. Chem.* 22:650–656.

Wang, J., Y. Chen, and S. Kuo. 1996. Inhibition of hind-paw edema and cutaneous vascular plasma extravasation by 2-chloro-3-methoxycarbonylpropionamide-1,4-naphthoquinone (PP1D1) in mice. *Naunyn-Schmiedeberg's Archives of Pharmacology* 354:779–784.

Wood, R., E. LeCluyse, and J. Fix. 1995. Assessment of a model for measuring drug diffusion through implant-generated fibrous capsule membranes. *Biomaterials* 16 (12):957–959.

6

Rat Paw-Lick Model

Pramod K. Gupta

TAP Holdings, Inc.
Deerfield, Illinois

Parenteral formulations are often painful and irritating following injection. At times, the pain/irritation response is associated with the active drug in a formulation, e.g., macrolide antibiotics (Marlin et al. 1983; Klement and Arndt 1991). In other cases, this may be associated with the excipients used in the formulation (Ku and Cadwallder 1975; Svendsen 1983; Fort et al. 1984; Reed and Yalkowsky 1987; Fu et al. 1987; Simamora et al. 1995; Fransson and Espander-Jansson 1996), the volume of fluid for local injection (Jorgensen et al. 1996), and the size of needle used for injection (Coley et al. 1997). The use of cosolvents, surfactants, and/or pH adjustments are popular approaches often investigated to solubilize water-insoluble compounds for parenteral administration (Yalkowsky 1981). However, the use of high levels of cosolvents, and/or adjustment of pH in nonphysiological range, is also known to cause pain and irritation following local administration (Ku and Cadwallder 1975; Fort et al. 1984; Reed and Yalkowsky 1987; Gray 1981; Steiness et al. 1987; Brazeau and Fung 1989a; Brazeau and Fung 1989b; Marcek et al. 1992).

Various in vitro and in vivo models have been developed to assess pain and irritation following the injection of formulations. These tests can assist in formula optimization from the standpoint of physiologic and pathologic acceptability, particularly during the initial stage of the development program. However, some of these tests suffer from being actually performed in vitro and perhaps not mimicking the real-life situations (Fort et al. 1984; Reed and Yalkowsky 1985; Reed and Yalkowsky 1987; Brazeau and Fung 1989a). Others are too cumbersome and expensive to be applied for rapid screening of prototype formulations, e.g., the creatine kinase (CK) release test in rabbits (Gray 1981; Steiness et al. 1987).

This chapter discusses application of an alternative test, called the rat paw-lick model, for relatively rapid in vivo screening of parenteral products for pain on injection. The model is particularly useful for testing products for local injection, e.g., subcutaneous injection. However, it also provides a good estimation of potential pain upon intravenous (IV) injection. The test was first reported in 1980 (Celozzi et al.). Further reports supporting the use of this animal model in the assessment of pain and muscle irritation upon local injections appeared in 1986 (Comerski et al.) and 1990 (Chellman et al.). We have investigated the application of this model to differentiating formulations likely to cause pain upon IV injection (Gupta et al. 1991; Gupta et al. 1994; Lovell et al. 1994).

METHODOLOGY

Groups of rats (generally $n = 5$) receive a single subplantar injection of 0.1 mL test solution in the hind paw. Thereafter, the paw licks in 3 min intervals, over a total 15 min study period, are monitored. A paw-lick episode is defined as either a licking response at the injection site followed by a turning of the head away from the paw, or 5 sec of uninterrupted licking (Gupta et al. 1994). Typically, the more painful and irritating the formulation, the greater the number of paw licks (Celozzi et al. 1980; Comerski et al. 1986; Chellman et al. 1990; Gupta et al. 1994).

CORRELATION BETWEEN RAT PAW-LICK AND OTHER PAIN/IRRITATION MODELS

A rat paw-lick test for the measurement of pain upon intramuscular (IM) injection was first reported by Celozzi and coworkers (1980). This study assessed the potential for pain following subplantar injections of cefoxitin, cephalothin, cephradine, cefazolin, cephaloridine, and carbenicillin. Increases in the concentration of injected drug resulted in greater numbers of paw licks, indicating a higher potential for pain (see Table 6.1). Overall, the results obtained with this model were found to agree well with the clinical outcome. Inclusion of lidocaine was found to reduce the number of paw licks (see Table 6.2), thus indicating its effectiveness as a good local anesthetic in injected products.

In 1986, Comereski et al. compared the results from the paw-lick model with those from a rabbit muscle irritation study (see Figure 6.1). A correlation in pain/irritation response following the administration of Water for Injection (WFI), cephaloridine, and cefotoxine in the rat paw-lick model versus change in CK levels after 24 h in rabbits was made. The latter is a well-established test that monitors tissue injury and damage following local injection. A strong correlation was obtained between the CK levels and the paw licks monitored over 6, 9, and 12 min after injection ($r^2 \geq 0.970$) (Comerski et al. 1986).

Table 6.1. Application of Rat Paw-Lick Model in the Measurement of Effect of Drug Concentration on Pain Upon Subplantar Injection to Rats*

Drug	Drug Dose (mg)	N	Mean Paw Licks/Rat ± SD**		
			3 min	6 min	12 min
Cefoxitin	25	20	4.1 ± 2.2	2.7 ± 2.5	1.8 ± 2.3
	40	20	6.0 ± 2.9	5.2 ± 2.9	4.4 ± 3.6
Cefazolin	25	18	0.6 ± 0.8	0.3 ± 0.7	0.3 ± 1.0
	40	20	4.5 ± 2.6	2.3 ± 2.8	1.7 ± 2.0

*Adapted from Celozzi et al. (1980).

**All results with higher drug dose are significantly different compared to results with same drug at lower dose ($p \leq 0.05$).

Table 6.2. Application of Rat Paw-Lick Model in the Measurement of Effect of Lidocaine in Formulation on Pain on Subplantar Injection to Rats*

Drug	Drug Dose (mg)	Lidocaine (%)	N	Mean Paw Licks/Rat ± SD**		
				3 min	6 min	12 min
Water	—	—	20	0.5 ± 1.4	0.3 ± 0.4	0.4 ± 0.6
Cefoxitin	40	0	20	4.7 ± 2.6	4.5 ± 3.1	2.9 ± 3.2
	40	0.5	20	3.2 ± 2.5**	1.9 ± 1.8	0.3 ± 0.7**
Carbenicillin	25	0	10	5.0 ± 2.2	3.5 ± 2.6	2.2 ± 3.0
	25	0.5	10	1.1 ± 1.5**	1.1 ± 1.7**	1.5 ± 1.5

*Adapted from Celozzi et al. (1980).

**Results in presence of lidocaine are significantly different compared to results without lidocaine ($p \leq 0.05$).

These results supported the usefulness of the rat paw-lick model in screening parenteral antibiotics. In addition, this study led to the belief that the rat paw-lick model may not only allow assessment of injectables that elicit acute pain immediately upon injection, but it may also allow evaluation of products that cause muscle damage several hours following injection.

This hypothesis was later confirmed by Chellman and colleagues (1990), who developed a two-phase test for the assessment of pain and muscle irritation using rats. Phase one of the test was used to assess pain

Figure 6.1. Relationship between CK release and paw licks. Adapted from Comerski et al. (1986).

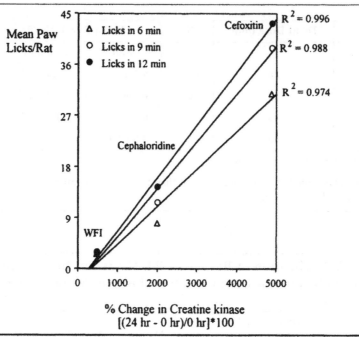

upon injection in a manner similar to that proposed by Celozzi et al. (1980) and Comereski et al. (1986). Phase two of the method was initiated after a one-week recovery period, where the same animals were intramuscularly injected with 0.2 mL of test product in the anterior thigh. Thereafter, blood samples from the orbital sinus were collected at 2, 6, and 24 h after dosing to monitor serum CK. In this study, several cephalosporin-type antibiotics (e.g., cefazoline, cephalothin, and cefoxitin) produced pain upon injection as well as irritation and muscle damage consistent with the clinical results. On the other hand, a number of nonantibiotic drugs (e.g., diazepam, digoxin, phenytoin, and lidocaine) did not produce acute pain upon injection but did produce moderate to marked muscle damage, observations again consistent with the clinical findings (Chellman et al. 1990).

The in vitro blood hemolysis test is a useful tool for screening formulations and provides an indication of their potential irritation in vivo (Fort et al. 1984; Reed and Yalkowsky 1985; Reed and Yalkowsky 1987). Injectable formulations can have a wide range of pH, e.g., between 2 and 12 (Wang and Kowal 1980; Sweetana and Akers 1996). Hence, four aqueous solutions at pH 2.3, 5.5, 8.5, and 12.0 were tested for in vitro blood hemolysis as well as rat paw licks. The results of this study are presented in Figure 6.2 and

Figure 6.2. Correlation between paw licks in rats and in vitro release of hemoglobin with aqueous solutions adjusted to pH between 2.3 and 12.0.

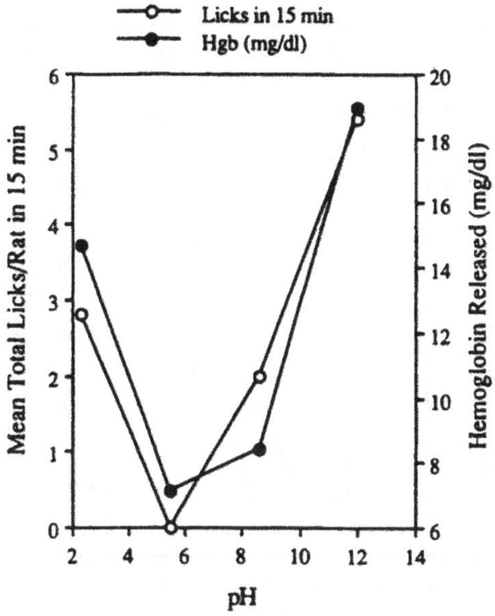

indicate that the rat paw-lick model is sensitive to changes in the pH of injected preparations.

In a separate study, 4 groups of rabbits received a single IM injection of 1 mL of aqueous solution adjusted to pH values of 2.3, 5.5, 8.5, and 12.0. Thereafter, the CK levels at 1 day after injection, which were also the maximum enzyme levels among those monitored at -1, 1, 3, and 7 days after injection, were correlated with the rat paw-lick data. A strong correlation was found between the data collected using the 2 models (see Figure 6.3). The strong correlation between the data collected using the 2 models again supports the applicability of the rat paw-lick model as a tool for in vivo estimation of pain/irritation on injection.

APPLICATION OF RAT PAW-LICK MODEL TO SCREENING COSOLVENT-BASED FORMULATIONS

Several studies were conducted using cosolvent-based solutions to assess the usefulness of the rat paw-lick model. Placebo solutions containing 0 to 25 percent v/v ethanol and/or 0 to 50 percent v/v propylene glycol in water were prepared, their pH adjusted to desired value, and freshly tested for the paw licks in rats. Figure 6.4 illustrates the effect on paw licks in rats of

Figure 6.3. Correlation between paw licks in rats and CK release in rabbits following the injection of aqueous solutions adjusted to pH between 2.3 and 12.0.

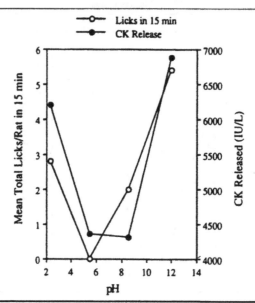

propylene glycol concentration in solutions containing either 15 or 20 percent v/v ethanol and adjusted to an apparent pH of 10.2. The increase in the propylene glycol concentration from 25 to 35 percent v/v in the presence of 15 percent v/v ethanol gradually increased the number of paw licks. A similar response was observed with solutions containing 20 to 30 percent v/v propylene glycol in the presence of 20 percent v/v ethanol. At either ethanol concentration, linear correlations were obtained between the propylene glycol concentration and the total paw licks in 15 min ($r^2 \geq 0.958$).

Table 6.3 summarizes the effects of changes in cosolvent concentration and the apparent pH of cosolvent-based solutions on the paw lick response in rats. For example, each 1 percent increase in the propylene glycol concentration from 25 to 35 percent v/v, in the presence of 15 percent v/v ethanol at pH 10.2, was found to increase the paw licks at the rate of about 0.88/rat/15 min. Similarly, with solutions containing 20 percent v/v ethanol, each 1 percent increase in the propylene glycol concentration from 20 to 30 percent v/v, increased the paw licks at the rate of about 1.38/rat/15 min (refer to Figure 6.4 for the actual data). An approximate 50 percent increase in the rate of paw licks (i.e., from 0.88 to 1.38/rat/15 min) with a 5 percent v/v increase in the ethanol concentration of the solutions (i.e., from 15 to 20 percent v/v) suggests that slight changes in the ethanol may cause appreciable changes in the pain response. In addition, it was found that each

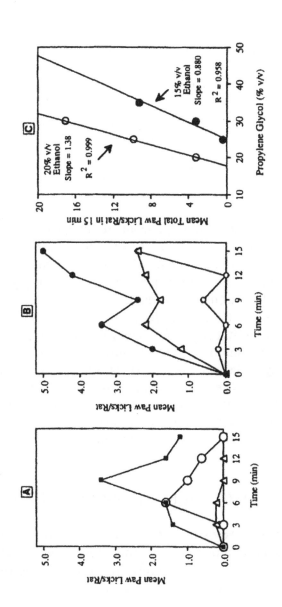

Figure 6.4. (A) Effect of propylene glycol concentration in solutions containing 15% v/v ethanol in water and adjusted to an apparent pH of 10.2, on the paw licks in rats. Key: (△) 25% v/v propylene glycol. (○) 30% v/v propylene glycol, and (■) 35% v/v propylene glycol. (B) Effect of propylene glycol concentration, in solutions containing 20% v/v ethanol in water and adjusted to an apparent pH of 10.2, on the paw licks in rats. Key: (○) 20% v/v propylene glycol, (△) 25% v/v propylene glycol, and (●) 30% v/v propylene glycol. (C) Correlation between the propylene glycol concentration and the mean total paw licks in 15 min. in rats. Key: (●) solutions containing 15% v/v ethanol and (○) solutions containing 20% v/v ethanol.

Table 6.3. The Effect of Cosolvent Concentration and Solution pH on the Rate of Increase of Pain/Irritation Response as Indicated by Paw Licks in Rats*

| Composition of Formulations | | | | |
Ethanol (%v/v)	Propylene Glycol (%v/v)	Apparent pH	Variant	Rate of Increase of Paw Licks
15	25–35	10.2	Propylene Glycol	0.88/1% increase in cosolvent
20	20–30	10.2	Propylene Glycol	1.38/1% increase in cosolvent
0	40	7–12	Apparent pH	3.14/unit increase in pH

*Adapted from Gupta et al. (1994).

unit increase in the apparent pH of solutions containing 40 percent v/v propylene glycol, from 7.2 to 12, increases the paw licks at the rate of about 3.14/rat/15 min. This type of information may be helpful in assessing pain responses with various prototype formulations during the early development of a parenteral product.

Figure 6.5 shows the paw licks in different groups of rats over the 15 min study period, following the injections of normal saline, 5 mg/mL aqueous solution of clarithromycin, 50 mg/mL aqueous solution of erythromycin lactobionate, and 200 mg/mL cosolvent-based solution of erythromycin. The results suggest that: (1) a 5 mg/mL aqueous clarithromycin is probably more painful than a 50 mg/mL aqueous erythromycin, and (2) the 200 mg/mL cosolvent-based erythromycin is probably less painful than 50 mg/mL aqueous erythromycin.

LIMITATIONS OF THE RAT PAW-LICK MODEL

Figure 6.6 shows the effect of propylene glycol concentration in solutions containing 15 percent v/v ethanol in water at pH 10.2 on the paw lick response in rats. The increase in the propylene glycol concentration from 25 to 35 percent v/v linearly increased the paw licks; however, further increase in the propylene glycol concentrations to 50 percent v/v decreased the paw licks. Figure 6.7 illustrates the effect of aqueous clarithromycin concentrations on the paw licks in rats. Whereas the increase in the clarithromycin concentrations from 0 to 5 mg/mL linearly increased the paw licks, further increase in drug concentration to 8 mg/mL did not increase the paw licks. The data displayed in Figures 6.6 and 6.7 can be explained in

Figure 6.5. Rat paw licks following the administration of normal saline (O), 5 mg/mL aqueous clarithromycin (□), 50 mg/mL aqueous erythromycin lactobionate (△), or 200 mg/mL cosolvent-based erythromycin (●).

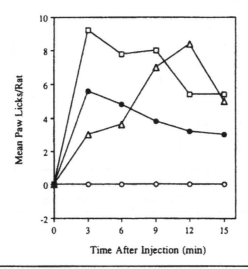

Figure 6.6. Effect of propylene glycol concentration in solutions containing 15% v/v ethanol in water and adjusted to an apparent pH of 10.2 on mean total paw licks in 15 min in rats.

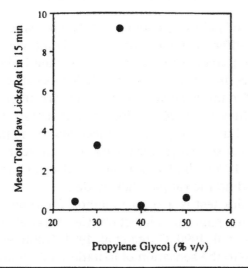

Figure 6.7. Mean paw licks following the local injection of saline and 1, 2, 5, and 8 mg/mL aqueous solution of clarithromycin lactobionate to rats.

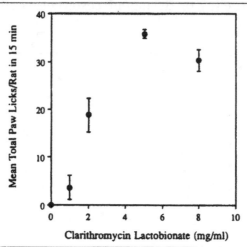

view of the fact that a "threshold" may exist between the concentration of painful component (e.g., drug or excipient) and the paw licks. Implicitly, at concentrations above the threshold, the animal does not respond to pain in a predictable manner. Therefore, for meaningful use of this model, a threshold limit should be established for each type of formulation system under evaluation.

CONCLUDING REMARKS

The measurement of pain is a complex challenge. Most in vitro methods that monitor pain offer the benefit of differentiating psychological factors contributing to the perception of pain from biochemical and pathophysiological components that may be responsible for its cause. Nonetheless, the in vivo methods for the measurement of pain are often viewed as more meaningful since they allow generation of information that perhaps more closely mimics the human response. Subjectivity in the perception of pain in humans often causes large variability in pain scores (Fransson and Espander-Jansson 1996). Similar variability is also encountered in most animal models, including the rat paw-lick model.

The rat paw-lick test is a simple method for rapid screening of formulations in vivo for pain upon injection (Celozzi et al. 1980; Comerski et al. 1986; Chellman et al. 1990; Gupta et al. 1991; Gupta et al. 1994). It measures the response to the sensation of irritation, i.e., "pain on injection." It is perhaps analogous to measurement of response following external stimuli, e.g., heat. The model has been shown to allow assessment of muscle irritation that may occur due to slow or chronic reaction between injected material and local tissue (Chellman et al. 1990). The latter aspect can also be estimated using the rabbit lesion volume and the rabbit CK models (Sutton et al. 1996a; Sutton et al. 1996b). In summary, the rat paw-lick model allows a rapid and efficient means of differentiating injectables that have the potential to cause pain upon injection from those that are relatively nonpain-producing. The model can be used for screening products for local injection (e.g., IM or subcutaneous) as well as systemic (e.g., IV) administration.

REFERENCES

Brazeau, G. A., and H.-L. Fung. 1989a. An in vitro model to evaluate muscle damage following intramuscular injections. *Pharm. Res.* 6:167–170.

Brazeau, G. A. and H.-L. Fung 1989b. Use of an in vitro model for the assessment of muscle damage from intramuscular injections: In vitro-in vivo correlation and predictability with mixed solvent systems. *Pharm. Res.* 6:766–771.

Celozzi, E., V. J. Lotti, E. O. Stapley, and A. K. Miller. 1980. An animal model for assessing pain-on-injection of antibiotics. *J. Pharmacol. Methods.* 4:285–289.

Chellman, G. J., G. F. Faurot, L. O. Lollini, and T. E. McCullough. 1990. Rat paw lick/muscle irritation model for evaluating parenteral formulations for pain-on-injection and muscle damage. *Fund. Appl. Toxicol.* 15:697–709.

Coley, R. M., C. D. Butler, B. I. Beck, and J. P. Mullane. 1987. Effect of needle size on pain and hematoma formation with subcutaneous injection of heparin sodium. *Clin. Pharm.* 6:725–727.

Comereski, C. R., P. D. Williams, C. L. Bregman, and G. H. Hottendorf. 1986. Pain on injection and muscle irritation: a comparison of animal models for assessing parenteral products. *Fund. Appl. Toxicol.* 6:335–338.

Fort, F. F., I. A. Heyman, and J. W. Keterson. 1984. Hemolysis study of aqueous polyethylene glycol 400, propylene glycol and ethanol combinations in vivo and in vitro. *J. Parent. Sci. & Tech.* 38:82–87.

Fransson, J., and A. Espander-Jansson. 1996. Local tolerance of subcutaneous injections. *J. Pharm. Pharmacol.* 48:1012–1015.

Fu, R. C. C., D. M. Lidgate, J. L. Whatley, and T. McCullough. 1987. Biocompatibility of parenteral vehicles. In vitro/in vivo screening comparison and the effet of excipients on hemolysis. *J. Parenteral Sci. Technol.* 41:164–168.

Gray, J. E. 1981. Appraisal of the intramuscular irritation test in rabbit. *Fund. Appl. Toxicol.* 1:290–292.

Gupta, P. K., J. B. Cannon, M. W. Lovell, H. Johnson, C. Allexon, and A. Riberal. 1991. Development and evaluation of a less painful IV formulation of a macrolide. II. o/w emulsion. Paper presented at the *6th Annual AAPS Meeting*, 17–21 Nov., in Washington, D.C.

Gupta, P. K., J. P. Patel, and K. R. Hahn. 1994. Evaluation of pain and irritation following local administration of parenteral formulations using the rat paw-lick model. *J. Parent. Sci. Technol.* 48:159–166.

Jorgensen, J. T., J. Romsing, M. Rasmussen, J. Moller-Sonnergaard, L. Vang, and L. Musaeus. 1996. Pain assessment of subcutaneous injections. *Ann. Pharmacotherap.* 30:729–732.

Klement, W., and J. O. Arndt. 1991. Pain on injection of propofol: Effects of concentration and diluent. *Br. J. Anesth.* 67:281–284.

Ku, S.-H., and D. E. Cadwallder. 1975. Behaviour of erythrocytes in ternary solvent systems. *J. Pharm. Sci.* 64:1818–1821.

Lovell, M. W., H. W. Johnson, H.-W. Hui, J. B. Cannon, P. K. Gupta, and C. C. Hsu. 1994. Less-painful emulsion formulations for intravenous administration of clarithromycin. *Int. J. Pharm.* 109:45–57.

Marcek, J. M., W. J. Seaman, and R. J. Weaver. 1992. A novel approach for the determination of the pain-producing potential of intravenously injected substances in the concious rat. *Pharm. Res.* 9:182–186.

Marlin, G. E. P. J. Thompson, C. R. Jenkins, K. R. Burgess, and D. A. J. LaFranier. 1983. Study of serum levels, venous irritation and gastrointestinal side-effects with intravenous erythromycin lactobionate in patients with broncopulmonary infection. *Human Toxicol.* 2:593–605.

Reed, K. W., and S. H. Yalkowsky. 1985. Lysis of human red blood cells in the presence of various cosolvents. *J. Parent. Sci. & Tech.* 39:64–68.

Reed, K. W., and S. H. Yalkowsky. 1987. Lysis of human red blood cells in the presence of various cosolvents. III. The relationship between hemolytic potential and structure. *J. Parent. Sci. & Tech.* 41:37–39.

Simamora, P., S. Pinsuwan, J. M. Alvarez, P. B. Myrdal, and S. H. Yalkowsky. 1995. Effect of pH on injection phlebitis. *J. Pharm. Sci.* 84:520–521.

Steiness, E. et al. 1987. A comparative study of serum creatine phosphokinase (CPK) activity in rabbits. *Acta Pharmacol et Toxicol.* 42:357–364.

Sutton, S. C., L. A. F. Evans, T. S. Rinaldi, and K. A. Norton. 1996a. Predicting injection site muscle damage. I. Evaluation of immediate release parenteral formulations in animal models. *Pharm. Res.* 13:1507–1513.

Sutton, S. C., L. A. F. Evans, T. S. Rinaldi, and K. A. Norton. 1996b. Predicting injection site muscle damage. II. Evaluation of extended release parenteral formulations in animal models. *Pharm. Res.* 13:1514–1518.

Svendsen, O. 1983. Local muscle damage and oily vehicles: A study on local reactions in rabbits after intramuscular injection of neuroleptic drugs in aqueous or oily vehicles. *Acta Pharmacol. Toxicol.* 52:298–304.

Sweetana, S., and M. J. Akers. 1996. Solubility principles and practices for parenteral drug dosage form development. *PDA J. Pharm. Sci. Technol.* 50:330–342.

Wang, Y. J., and R. R. Kowal. 1980. Review of excipients and pH's for parenteral products used in the United States. *J. Parent. Drug Assoc.* 34:452–462.

Yalkowsky, S. H., ed. 1981. *Techniques of solubilization of drugs.* New York: Marcel Dekker.

7

Radiopharmaceuticals for the Noninvasive Evaluation of Inflammation Following Intramuscular Injections

Agatha Feltus and Michael Jay

Division of Pharmaceutical Science
College of Pharmacy, University of Kentucky
Lexington, Kentucky

Robert M. Beihn

Scintiprox, Inc.
Indianapolis, Indiana

In this chapter, we describe how the noninvasive imaging technique known as gamma scintigraphy can be used to identify and quantify inflammatory responses to trauma, such as that which may occur following the intramuscular (IM) administration of pharmaceutical products. This technique involves the use of an external imaging device to measure the distribution of radioactive emissions following the administration of a radiopharmaceutical that accumulates at inflammatory lesion sites. We begin with a description of the imaging devices used to acquire such images and how they transform the emitted radiations into a planar or tomographic projection. We also describe how the accumulation of radioactivity at the site of interest can be quantified. This is followed by a description of the radiopharmaceuticals that are used in inflammatory lesion imaging in clinical practice, as well as some novel radioactive agents that can provide unique information on the inflammatory response. We conclude with some examples from the literature in which these techniques were used to quantify inflammatory responses in experimentally induced inflammatory lesions.

GAMMA SCINTIGRAPHY

External gamma ray scintigraphy has been utilized extensively since the early 1960s in the practice of nuclear medicine. Nuclear medicine is primarily a diagnostic discipline that involves the administration of a radiopharmaceutical designed to accumulate in an organ or tissue of interest, and the subsequent imaging of the distribution of that radiopharmaceutical in patients. There are several radiopharmaceuticals used in clinical practice for almost every organ system. Most radiopharmaceuticals are composed of a "radio" part, which possesses physical characteristics for optimum detection, as well as a "pharmaceutical" part, which directs the biodistribution of the agent. For example, a diphosphonate radiolabeled with the radionuclide ^{99m}Tc is used as a bone scanning agent because it will accumulate at sites of rapid bone growth (e.g., fractures, tumors, etc.). These diagnostic agents are designed to yield the maximum amount of information while delivering the minimal absorbed radiation doses to patients. Most nuclear medicine procedures utilize radionuclides with short half-lives and deliver the same or smaller radiation dose than the corresponding X-ray or computed tomography (CT) procedures.

These powerful and versatile nuclear imaging techniques have been exploited to evaluate pharmaceutical products. For example, controlled-release dosage forms have been radiolabeled and administered to normal, healthy volunteers under fed and fasted conditions to determine the location in the gastrointestinal tract and the time after administration when these dosage forms deliver their contents (Parr et al. 1987; Borin et al. 1990). A wide variety of other pharmaceutical products have been evaluated by gamma scintigraphy, including those administered by ophthalmic, rectal, transdermal, aerosol, and nasal routes (Ebel et al. 1993, Digenis and Sandefer 1991). Routine clinical radiopharmaceuticals have also been employed to evaluate the pharmacological responses of new drug candidates. For example, radiopharmaceuticals that measure myocardial perfusion have been used to measure the effectiveness of new drugs for the treatment of ischemic heart disease. In this chapter, we will focus on the use of radiopharmaceuticals and other radiolabeled compounds that may be useful in evaluating the inflammatory response induced by the IM injection of pharmaceuticals.

GAMMA CAMERAS

The use of a gamma ray scintillation camera was first reported in the literature in 1958. It was capable of detecting the presence of selected gamma radiation (Anger 1958), and locating the position of radiolabels in a biological system volumetric space. The modern scintillation camera with its numerous components has revolutionized the in vivo assessment of physiological function (Simmons 1988; Mettler and Guiberteau 1991; Chandra 1987).

Detectors

The radiation detector in a gamma scintillation camera is a single crystal of sodium iodide (NaI). A minuscule quantity of thallium (Tl) is present in the NaI crystal lattice to shorten the duration of the scintillation event to about 10^{-12} seconds. All NaI(Tl) scintillation detectors have the Tl to increase the capability to count high count rates (Figure 7.1). The NaI(Tl) crystal is a clear, imperfection-free solid that produces a flash of light (scintillation) when a gamma ray interacts with the crystal. To protect the crystal from

Figure 7.1. Gamma scintillation camera.

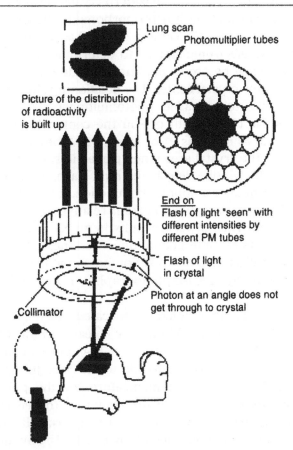

daylight and moisture from the air, the crystal is entirely covered by a thin layer of aluminum except for one top diametrical surface. The most common dimension for the right circular cylinder crystal is 15 in. in diameter by 3/8 in. in depth. Two advantages are apparent: first, this large field permits the detection of radiation from large animals, finite anatomical regions, or entire abdominal regions in a human torso. Second, the depth dimension of the crystal is nearly ideal for providing the stopping (interaction probability) power for the gamma radiation.

There are two competing processes governing gamma ray interaction in the NaI(Tl) crystal. One is the atomic number ($Z = 53$) of the iodine in the NaI. The second is the energy (E) of the gamma ray radiation from the radionuclide of the radiolabel. The probability of gamma ray interaction in the crystal is $\sigma \propto Z^3/E^3$. This relationship indicates that NaI has a Z number suitable for stopping the gamma rays, but the inverse term of E^3 indicates that lower gamma ray energies are more desirable. However, the gamma ray energies must be sufficient to escape the tissue in which they are concentrated to be detected by the detector. Radionuclides are selected for use based on their gamma ray energies, half-lives, and chemical properties.

A gamma ray interaction in the NaI(Tl) crystal results in a scintillation event. The intensity of that flash is proportional to the gamma energy deposited in the crystal. Since the camera crystal has a significant area (πr^2), multiple positioning electronic signals to determine the scintillation location in the crystal must be produced. They include +X, –X, +Y, and –Y; the origin is located at the crystal center. The positioning signals are generated using light sensitive tubes called photomultiplier (PM) tubes carefully placed in concentric circles with one in the center. Modern scintillation cameras have 37, to as many as 91 or more, PM tubes, depending on how many tubes will fit the crystal area when placed in some circular or matrix configuration. Each PM tube detects the light flash, with those nearer the event receiving the greater amount. The function of each tube is to convert the light flash intensity to a small current relative to its proximity to the light flash observed. This, in turn, results in an XY positioning pulse for each detected gamma ray interaction, one at a time. Later in the series of electronic configuration, it is this positioning signal that locates the event on an output cathode ray tube for photography, or in a computer matrix for magnetic storage.

Simultaneously, another signal is generated called a Z pulse, which is a summed output from all the PM tubes from each scintillation event. This summed pulse is subjected to amplification, then pulse magnitude analysis for selection and inclusion criteria to add to the data during the scintigraphy acquisition. The common nomenclature for the pulse selection is "energy window selection," where the center of the energy window is selected on the known specific gamma ray energy. Its width may be selected to ±5–20 percent about the energy center. The integrated detector system, including the crystal and electronics, determines the energy resolution (the separation ability of one gamma energy from another). The energy window permits only those primary photoelectric interactions to be included in the count data acquisition and discards those undesirable scatter gamma radiations from Compton interactions. With the Z pulse and the XY position, every gamma ray from a radiation source can contribute to the total data.

The number of gamma rays emanated per unit time (sec) from a radionuclide is a measure of the radioactivity in Becquerels (Bq), where one radioactive parent atom transmutation to a stable daughter is defined as one disintegration per sec (dps). One dps is equivalent to 1 Bq. For comparison, 1 microcurie (μCi) is equal to 3.7×10^4 dps. The count data recorded by the scintillation gamma camera represents some fraction of the total number of theoretical gamma emissions from the radioactivity in a location within or on the surface of a tissue or organ.

Collimators

Without directional limitation, all gamma ray emissions would be counted, yielding no spatial distributional information. After all, when a gamma emitting radioactive source is introduced into a tissue, it is clear that its location is in the volume of the biosystem, but exactly where is important to know as well. The spatial resolution has two components—the intrinsic and extrinsic. The intrinsic spatial resolution is governed by the spacing of the PM tubes and the electronic positioning of the XY location. The extrinsic spatial resolution is determined by the placement of a lead collimator between the source of the gamma rays in the tissue and the NaI(Tl) crystal. All collimators have one or more holes allowing the gamma radiation to pass unattenuated to the detector for interaction.

Gamma camera collimators have the following characteristics:

- High resolution (low energy: < 200 keV)

- High sensitivity (low energy)

- Low energy all purpose (LEAP)

- Diverging (enables larger field viewing)

- Medium energy (> 200 keV)

- Pinhole (for imaging small objects)

Pinhole collimators are conical in shape and have a single aperture with a diameter that ranges from 1 to 6 mm. The smaller the diameter, the better the spatial resolution. The overall sensitivity (the ability to record counts) increases with hole diameter, but the spatial resolution (the ability to delineate fine detail) decreases. The application of a pinhole collimator enables visualization of small anatomic regions in a biological system. This collimator will allow a ratio of x:1 in size projection on the image of the scintillation camera detector, where x is less than, equal to, or greater than 1. Thus, the recorded image can be magnified or reduced depending on the distance between the detector and the radioactive source within the tissue. With a magnified image, the apparent spatial resolution can be enhanced. A more common type of collimator for the scintillation camera is a multi-hole parallel pattern of collimation. The holes in the collimator are parallel and spaced equidistant, separated by thin lead septa. It not uncommon to use a collimator with 4,000 holes that are configured in a round or hexagonal shape. The modern scintillation camera collimator is designed to be used with gamma radiation emissions that are low, medium, or high energy (a different collimator for each energy). Most gamma rays whose energies are less than 200 keV require the use of low-energy collimators. Medium-energy collimators are for radionuclides with gamma ray energies between 200 to 400 keV, while high-energy collimators are for radionuclides with gamma ray energies above 400 keV. Low-energy collimators are further classified as high sensitivity, high resolution, or all purpose. The difference between the low-energy classifications of high sensitivity and high resolution is the thickness of the collimator. Both have identical numbers of holes and are of the same diameter. Thinner collimators require a shorter path length for the gamma rays and, thus, have higher count sensitivities. A special design called the low-energy all-purpose (LEAP) collimator represents an optimization of path length, sacrificing some resolution and count sensitivity for performance, yet yielding desirable scintigraphy images. Medium- and high-energy collimators are all-purpose in design.

There are also designs for nonparallel, multihole collimators that have unique applications. They include a converging and diverging collimator configuration where none of the holes are parallel. In the converging collimator, the holes are positioned in an arrangement such that they are focused at a theoretical point in front of the collimator. The application needed to magnify an anatomical biosystem region with increased spatial resolution would use the converging unit, whereas, if an anatomical region was greater in size than the actual scintillation camera crystal, then a diverging collimator would be used to reduce the collected image to fit the crystal surface.

Electronics and Output

All scintillation cameras have some visual display capability for observing the immediate distribution of the gamma radiation within the tissue or organ of interest. In most cases, this is an analog picture on a cathode ray tube (CRT) or television (TV) monitor. Many applications of a scintillation camera use the images generated on the CRT to create distributional information images called scintigraphs. Qualitative information can be derived from these images, but they contain little to no quantitative assessment for radiation counting. The CRT images are frequently used for correct anatomical positioning for the biosystem containing some selected gamma ray-emitting radioactivity. When the CRT image is captured on film (negative or print), a pictorial distribution may be of some value in interpreting for anatomical location.

Computers

An integral part of the modern scintillation camera is a digital computer. The computer can be used to improve the scintigraphic images by correcting for electronic imperfections in the acquired data, such as noise, crystal nonuniformity, and various other forms of distortion. The computer also permits analog-to-digital conversion for permanent or temporary storage of radiation count data (Figure 7.2), and it is also used in data processing for quantification.

Figure 7.2. Computer schematic for gamma scintillation cameras.

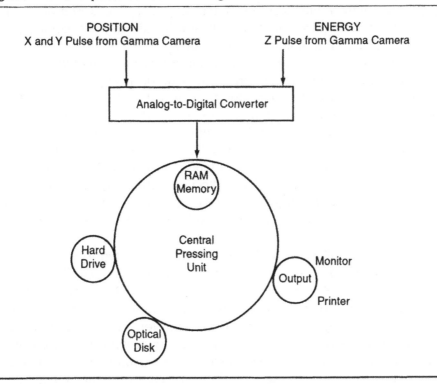

More recently, the computers used with scintillation cameras have decreased in physical size while increasing in speed of computation, volume of storage capacity, as well as display of image processing and computational results with sophisticated software. The initial interface is the analog-to-digital converter (ADC), which changes a continuously varying electronic voltage signal (analog signal) to a discrete unit voltage (digital signal). This is an assigned numerical value representing the Z pulse and the XY positioning signal. Stored count data from each scintillation event is then placed in a specific location in the computer memory depending on the XY location (a pixel in some defined X by Y matrix). Most of the storage and display matrices are 64 × 64, 128 × 128, or 256 pixels × 256 pixels. The larger the matrix, the better the resolution of the pictorial display on the output CRT screen. However, when the choice of a large matrix is selected, then the time for each acquisition should be long to decrease the statistical noise due to low counts per pixel. A common matrix size is 64 × 64.

The hardware found on scintigraphic computer systems includes random access memory (the larger the better), hard or fixed disk (high volume with disk cache desirable), floppy disk drives, and peripherals such as keyboards, CRT monitors (color, and black and white), and printers with automated image copiers. For some computers with large computational tasks, array processors are used in place of serial computations for solving mathematical algorithms. All computations are normally performed in the central processing unit (CPU). Thus, the speed of the CPU becomes critical (the quicker the better). Furthermore, since some data are stored on the hard disk drive and require retrieval and storage during the computational process, a fast access time is also necessary.

Software for any computer system interfaced to a scintillation camera allows acquisition and processing of the data for all applications involving quantification of count density for time-of-distribution experiments. Acquisition software permits numerous choices of data collection: (1) static images, where count data can be accumulated for any duration or preset total counts for an unlimited time; (2) dynamic images, where many sequential data collections are permitted with a constant time interval (e.g., 1 sec, 30 sec, 1 min, etc.); (3) count collections limited by gating using some external triggering instrument, such as a cardiac R wave EKG output; or (4) single- or dual-energy collection for single and/or dual radionuclide imaging.

Processing software can be divided into two categories: (1) image filtering (smoothing), color or black and white selection, single or multiple display of image sets, and image frame arithmetic; and (2) radiation-count curve generation from dynamic data acquisitions. The computer usually has a feature for region-of-interest (ROI) selection. This is accomplished by drawing a pixel-connected line with a cursor around a selected area in which a radionuclide has accumulated. Each computer frame can be analyzed for counts in the selected ROIs, resulting in time-activity curves.

These curves, representing the change of radioactivity, yield the most quantitative data. For example, they yield mathematical curve fittings that describe the physiological processes governing the radionuclide distributive events, including slopes and intercepts for compartmental analysis. Pharmaco-kinetic data can also be derived from the generation of curves through ROI selection.

Tomographic Imaging

All scintillation camera applications and designs previously discussed have addressed the *planar* camera, whereby only the two dimensions of an area (X and Y) are considered, even though the radiation source may emanate from the surface or depth of a tissue. The scintillation detector remains stationary throughout the data collection. A more sophisticated approach is to consider the depth dimension of the biosystem, thus producing a distributional scintigraphic image having three dimensions. This can be accomplished using the planar camera, and allowing it to rotate 360° around the biosystem. Using computer reconstruction of the acquired count data, a method of imaging has been developed called single photon emission computed tomography (SPECT). Most applications of SPECT deal with anatomical regions that are relatively large, since the general spatial resolution is limited to 2 to 4 mm. Acquisition time can also be too long for some dynamic clearance applications due to the requirement of 360° rotation of the camera head and numerous stops and acquisitions every few degrees. If the radioactivity level can be elevated, then the acquisition time can be reduced to minutes. Some modern SPECT cameras have two or three camera heads, which also reduce acquisition time. The computers necessary for the SPECT are similar to those previously discussed, except for additional software for three-dimensional reconstruction and display.

Quality Control

Scintillation camera systems must have quality control requirements for accurate, precise, and safe performance. Three parameters usually included for performance testing are detector uniformity, spatial resolution, and linearity and distortion. Additional tests may include energy resolution, count sensitivity, and collimator integrity.

Detector uniformity is usually tested daily when the scintillation cameras are used. This procedure is performed by using a flat-field radioactive source (flood source) of a similar energy level to that used in experiments. It is positioned beneath the face of the scintillation camera detector and counted for at least 10^6 counts, regardless of the time. The collimator is not present when the flood source is counted. The image is generally acquired on film or on a computer file for permanent storage for future reference.

This evaluation assesses crystal and PM tube performance. One should observe a uniform field (homogeneous image), which indicates proper functioning of the PM tubes and correct XY positioning.

The spatial resolution test defines how well close lying structures can be delineated and is also performed with the flood source, now with the addition of a bar phantom placed between the source of radiation and the detector. Bar phantoms have groups of alternating strips of lead and spaces at different distances for each group. They may be all parallel or placed at right angles in quadrants. Each group with different spacing evaluates the spatial resolution by how well the lead strips and spaces are visualized. Distortion and linearity are also evaluated using the bar phantom. This test shows the bar phantom straightness across the detector field of view. Any imperfection in spatial resolution or distortion and linearity must be corrected before reliable scintigraphic images can be obtained.

The energy resolution and count sensitivity quality control tests involve the performance of the camera electronics, which seldom fail but need to be scrutinized occasionally. Reduced count accumulation is an early clue of reduced performance of electronic instrumentation. The collimator integrity may be compromised if one or more holes are impaired, inhibiting the passing of radiation through the collimator. Evaluation of collimator performance is tested using the flood source exterior to the collimator while it is attached to the camera. Nonuniformity of the acquired image indicates damage to the collimator and repairs are required before use.

RADIONUCLIDES AND RADIATION

Not all radionuclides are suitable for external gamma ray scintigraphy. The mode of radioactive decay, or how the parent radionuclide transmutates to a stable daughter isotope, is an important consideration. The three most useful modes of decay radionuclides for scintigraphy are negatron decay (beta decay), positron decay, and electron capture (Boyd and Dalrymple 1974). It is important that the decay of radionuclides by these modes is accompanied by the emission of gamma photons. It is this gamma radiation that exits through tissues and penetrates radiation detectors for accurate assessment of its quantity and where it originated. The energy of the gamma photon must be sufficient so that it can escape the tissue and be detected by an external imaging device (gamma camera). But it must not be so great that poorly resolved images result from the penetration of the gamma rays through the septa of the collimators.

Most often, the radionuclides used for scintigraphic measurements emit relatively low-energy electromagnetic gamma radiation for detection. The low energy, and the fact that most usable radionuclides for scintigraphy have short half-lives, accounts for the low absorbed radiation doses to the tissue. This, of course, is of prime concern when performing scintigraphic studies in human volunteers or patients. A greater flexibility in the selection of radionuclides is allowed for scintigraphic studies in animals. A variety of radionuclides are employed in the clinical practice of diagnostic and therapeutic nuclear medicine as well as in the scintigraphic assessment of pharmaceutical dosage forms. Table 7.1 lists some of the more commonly employed radionuclides used in the scintigraphic assessment of inflammatory responses to muscle injury.

SCINTIGRAPHIC DETECTION OF INFLAMMATION

Several radiopharmaceuticals are known to accumulate at the sites of inflammation caused by bacteria, tumors, and tissue trauma. These include ^{67}Ga-citrate, ^{111}In- and ^{99m}Tc-labeled white blood cells, and radiolabeled antibodies. Technetium-99m, which is the most commonly employed radionuclide in the practice of nuclear medicine, decays by isomeric transition. It is essentially a pure gamma emitter. Both ^{67}Ga-citrate and ^{111}In decay by electron capture with the subsequent emission of gamma rays.

Gallium-67

Gallium-67, which decays to zinc-67 with a half-life of 78 h, was the first widely used radiopharmaceutical to identify sites of inflammation by scintigraphic imaging. It is commercially available as the weak acid citrate complex. The γ-photons emitted possess energies of 93, 185, and 300 keV, with photon yields of 37 percent, 20 percent, and 17 percent, respectively. These photons are easily detectable by a gamma camera, which can be set to record emissions at all three energies, thus optimizing the detection of ^{67}Ga.

Since smooth muscle injury due to IM drug therapy causes a coagulation necrosis that is similar to the inflammatory response caused by infections, it is also possible to detect the damage caused by the pain-inducing drug substances using these radiopharmaceuticals (Hickey et al. 1988). This

Table 7.1. Radionuclides Used in Scintigraphic Imaging

Radionuclide	Half-Life	Principal Gamma Energies (keV)
^{67}Ga	78 hours	93, 185, 300
^{111}In	2.8 days	173 , 247
^{99m}Tc	6 hours	140
^{123}I	13 hours	159

may be more sensitive and more accurate than measured levels of creatine phosphokinase (CPK) in the serum. The mechanism by which ^{67}Ga accumulates at the site of inflammation is not fully understood. Because it has a similar size and charge to the ferric ion, ^{67}Ga will form many of the same physiological complexes as iron. After intravenous injection, ^{67}Ga binds to protein, primarily to the beta globulin transferrin (Winzelberg 1984). It has been suggested that ^{67}Ga binds to the leukocytes that have already accumulated in the injection site, or possibly to migrating leukocytes. It has also been suggested that ^{67}Ga is transported into the white blood cells and is bound to the intracellular lactoferrin (Hoffer 1978). Additional studies have suggested that ferritin (another iron-binding protein) and siderophore (iron-binding molecules synthesized by bacteria) have an affinity for ^{67}Ga (Weiner et al. 1985). There is also a high background activity due to the presence of these proteins, as well as hemoglobin and other iron-binding proteins, in the blood. The best images are therefore obtained after the majority of ^{67}Ga has been cleared from noninflammed soft tissue sites. In humans, this is typically 24 to 48 h following the administration of the radioactive dose. This optimal imaging time is correspondingly shorter with smaller animals. The use of computer-assisted analytical techniques, such as pharmacokinetic imaging (Beihn and Vannier 1979), can be used to identify inflammatory lesions in a much shorter period of time, obviating the need to wait for clearance of ^{67}Ga from noninflamed soft tissue.

^{67}Ga has been shown to be useful in nuclear medicine in the detection of iatrogenic inflammatory lesions. Some of the conditions in which ^{67}Ga has proven useful in monitoring drug therapy are idiopathic pulmonary fibrosis and pseudomembranous colitis. Idiopathic pulmonary fibrosis is a potentially fatal pulmonary complication due to bleomycin toxicity. Gallium-67 scanning has proven useful for evaluating regression, as well as progression of pulmonary pathology (Richman et al. 1975). Certain patients develop pseudomembranous colitis when treated with antibiotics (Cohen et al. 1984). This drug-induced colitis has been found to result in ^{67}Ga citrate uptake in the colon. Thus, this noninvasive radiopharmaceutical technique is useful in locating inflammatory lesions (Tedesco et al. 1976). However, the literature contains conflicting reports on the value of ^{67}Ga citrate compared to other inflammatory imaging radiopharmaceuticals. One recent study showed that the use of ^{67}Ga citrate is inferior to ^{99m}Tc-labeled antibodies for imaging inflammation (Gungor et al. 1996). However, another study showed that it is an excellent alternative to ^{99m}Tc-labeled leukocytes (Bester et al. 1995). It has also been useful in detecting pericarditis (Kodama et al. 1994). The accumulation of ^{67}Ga citrate at IM injection sites can be seen clearly in Figure 7.3 (from Carter and Joo 1979).

Other groups have reported that ^{67}Ga citrate localizes in operative sites, IM injection sites, and at pressure lesions on the skin (Lentle et al. 1979). ^{67}Ga citrate was also observed to accumulate at the administration site following the injection of *Corynebacterium parvum*, which was used for immunotherapy of lymphoma (Leonard et al. 1978). Scintigraphic imaging of ^{67}Ga citrate has also been used to monitor its accumulation at inflammatory lesions following the extravasation of calcium gluconate from intravenous administration sites, as depicted in Figure 7.4 (from Sty et al. 1982).

Radiolabeled Leukocytes

Radiolabeled white blood cells have also been employed as imaging agents for inflammatory lesions. Because leukocytes migrate into sites of inflammation, radiolabeling of these cells offers a pictorial representation of the immune response. The inflammatory response involves the invasion of neutrophils into the site of inflammation within hours of the initial insult. The neutrophils will bind to endothelial cells and then squeeze through the junctions between these endothelial cells into the interstitial space. An important part of this process is the expression of three groups of adhesion molecules: integrins, selectins, and immunoglobulin supergenes. One particular integrin, leukocyte function-associated antigen (LFA-1), which is present on the surface of neutrophils, will bind to intercellular adhesion

Figure 7.3. [67]Ga scan of a patient with an abdominal wall abscess (open arrow). The intramuscular injection sites are clearly visible (closed arrows). [From Carter and Joo (1979); reprinted with permission.]	**Figure 7.4.** [67]Ga scan showing abnormal accumulation in extravasated calcium gluconate sites in lower right leg following intravenous administration. [From Sty et al. (1982); reprinted with permission.]

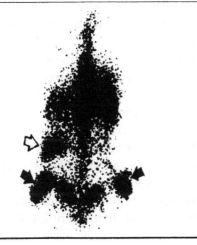

molecule-1 (ICAM-1). These ICAM-1 molecules are expressed on the surface of endothelial cells. Cytokines, chemotactic peptides, and endotoxin produced at inflammatory sites are responsible for enhancing the adhesion of white blood cells to endothelial cells by inducing the expression of ICAM-1 as well as other adhesion promoters, including vascular cellular and endothelial leukocyte adhesion molecules, and β1-integrin expression on lymphocytes (Jorgensen et al. 1995). The up-regulation of these factors promotes the overall adhesiveness of neutrophils to endothelial cells as well as transendothelial migration.

Because damage to white blood cells may affect their rate of migration and decrease their adhesion, it is very important that the radiolabeling process preserves the cellular activity for adequate imaging. Current methods involve labeling leukocytes with ^{111}In or ^{99m}Tc. Indium-111 decays by electron capture to ^{111}Cd with a half-life of 67 h. In the process, it emits photons of 171 keV and 245 keV in energy. The prevalence of these photons is 89 percent and 94 percent, respectively. In the case of ^{111}In, the trivalent ion is typically complexed by three hydrophobic chelating molecules. The most commonly employed is 8-hydroxyquinoline (also known as oxine), although tropolone (Peters 1994a), and acetylacetonate have also been used as complexing agents for ^{111}In. These complexes are lipophilic enough to freely diffuse into cells. Because indium also has a higher affinity for iron-containing proteins than for oxine, the indium binds to various intracellular components and remains in the cell. The free oxine can then diffuse out. In this case, equilibrium clearly lies on the side of indium being localized inside the cells, resulting in a high radiolabeling efficiency. In order to ensure that only white cells are labeled, blood components are typically separated before labeling. After blood from the patient is collected and anticoagulated with heparin, the red blood cells are allowed to settle out of solution. This is aided by addition of dextran, hydroxyethyl starch, or methylcellulose. The red cell layer is removed and the supernatant containing white cells and platelets is centrifuged. This results in a white-cell rich pellet, which is then incubated with ^{111}In-oxine in saline. After incubation, the white cells are again spun down and resuspended (to remove free oxine) in leukocyte-poor plasma for injection into the patient.

^{111}In-labeled white blood cells have been used to image inflammation in the urinary bladder (Swayne et al. 1995) and in passive cutaneous anaphylactic reactions (Weg et al. 1994). ^{111}In-labeled leukocytes have also been used to visualize the induction of pseudomembranous colitis induced by antibiotic therapy (Bushell 1984). Radiolabeled macrophages have also been employed to measure the inflammation induced by the injection of pristane oil into the footpad of mice. In this case, an ^{125}I-labeled compound designated at PKH95 was used to label the macrophages. This aliphatic compound binds to membrane lipids and is used for long-term in vivo cell tracking studies (Audran et al. 1995). Instead of labeling the white cells themselves, ^{111}In has also been used to image the cells actively participating in the immune response. Two somatostatin analogs, ^{111}In-pentetreotide (Dorr et al. 1993) and ^{111}In-octreotide (Vanhagen et al. 1993), have been used to target white cells, which have somatostatin receptors on their surface when active. Activated macrophages and lymphocytes are known to express somatostatin receptors (Weinstock 1992). Autoradiography with [^{125}I-Tyr]octreotide showed these binding sites in a granulatomous inflammation and was used to monitor the effect of glucocorticoid therapy.

Instead of ^{111}In, ^{99m}Tc can be used as the radiolabel for white blood cells. A recent report states that in order to optimize scanning with ^{111}In, the mixture of white cells must be purified to granulocytes, and this is more suited to imaging chronic inflammation (Frier 1994). Technetium-99m is a useful alternative and can be superior to ^{111}In for detecting inflammatory bowel disease, soft tissue sepsis, and occult fever (Peters 1994b). Technetium-99m decays by isomeric transition to technetium-99 with the emission of a 140 keV photon and a half-life of 6 h. One method of labeling white blood cells with this radionuclide depends upon the tendency of phagocytic leukocytes to engulf colloidal stannous particles, which contain [99m]Tc (Boyd et al. 1993), but this method has not proven to be as reliable as ^{111}In-oxine labeled leukocytes. The primary method for radiolabeling leukocytes with ^{99m}Tc is similar to labeling with ^{111}In, in that leukocytes are separated from other blood components, but instead of oxine, ^{99m}Tc is complexed to the lipophilic agent hexamethylpropylene amine oxine (HMPAO). The efficiency of radiolabeling is high, images are available quickly, and the radiation dose is lower than [111]In (Vorne 1994), but the complex tends to leach from the cell over time. ^{99m}Tc-labeled leukocytes have been used to visualize rheumatoid arthritis (Jorgensen et al. 1995), appendicitis (Evetts et al. 1994), and intra-abdominal abscess (Weldon et al. 1995).

Radiolabeled Antibodies

Another method of scintigraphically detecting sites of inflammation is through the use of radiolabeled antibodies. A very simple approach has been to use radiolabeled polyclonal immunoglobulin G (IgG). IgG is among the first components of the immune response to begin the inflammatory process. This radiolabeled antibody enters the inflammatory site as a result of its increased vascular permeability. The ^{111}In ion remains at the site of inflammation, presumably bound to proteins, while the free IgG diffuses out. ^{111}In-labelled IgG has been widely used in clinical applications (Buscombe 1995; Rubin and Fischman 1994; Datz et al. 1994; Corstens et al. 1993) and in animal studies, e.g., imaging of pneumonia in rats due to

Pneumocystis carinii infection (Perenboom et al. 1995). Antibodies can also be easily radiolabeled through the use of the bifunctional chelator diethyl-enetriaminepentaacetic acid (DTPA). One end of this molecule can bind to the antibody and the other can chelate the indium ion. The labeled anti-bodies are then injected, where they will circulate in the blood with a half-life of around 20 h in humans. Because of this high activity in the blood, the best images are taken between 24 and 48 h after administration to reduce background activity. At this time, a good portion of the radioactivity will still be present at inflammatory sites and the activity of the radionuclide will not be greatly reduced.

Other ^{111}In antibodies have also been used. Sasso et al. (1996) have shown that ^{111}In-labeled mouse anti-rat ICAM-1 was a useful detector of early inflammation in rats. The use of a specific radiolabeled monoclonal antibody, ^{111}In-Mab 1.2B6, which is an anti-E-selectin antibody, has been described (Keelan et al. 1994). E-selectin is a cell-specific adhesion molecule for leukocytes expressed on vascular endothelium during inflammatory response. Radiolabeled anti-E-selectin antibodies were also used to assess the inflammation induced by the IM injection of phytohaemagglutin in pigs (Jamar et al. 1995). Another ^{111}In-labeled F(ab)' antibody fragment desig-nated NCA 72, which is directed against a 95 kDa membrane protein on neutrophils, has also been used (Collet et al. 1993). A major advantage of this approach is that leukocytes could be radiolabeled in whole blood with-out having to isolate the cell population of interest. Technetium-99m has also been used for the radiolabeling of antibodies, although its shorter half-life can restrict its use in some situations. ^{99m}Tc-labeled antibodies have been used to evaluate abdominal abscess (Gungor et al. 1996) and experi-mentally induced inflammatory lesions as depicted in Figure 7.5 (from Shimpi et al. 1995).

In this latter paper, ^{99m}Tc-human polyclonal IgG was used to image the inflammatory response induced by the IM injection of turpentine oil in the hind legs of rabbits and rats. The ^{99m}Tc-IgG images were shown to be superior to those obtained with ^{99m}Tc-human serum albumin. Another paper demonstrated that both infectious lesions (induced by *Staphylococcus aureus* or *Escherichia coli*) and aseptic lesions (induced by turpentine) could be observed scintigraphically in rats using ^{99m}Tc-labeled IgG (Wong et al. 1995). Similar results were also reported in cases of acute inflammation (Jiminez-Heffernan et al. 1994).

Other antibodies and antibody fragments have been radiolabeled with [99m]Tc. A commercially available ^{99m}Tc anti-granulocyte Fab' fragment known as Leukoscan can produce adequate inflammatory lesion images within 4 h postinjection, is more convenient than preparing radiolabeled autologous leukocytes with ^{111}In-oxine or ^{99m}Tc-HMPAO, and does not in-duce a human antimouse antibody reaction (Becker et al. 1996). Inflamma-tory lesion imaging has also been accomplished using a ^{99m}Tc-labeled antigranulocyte nonspecific antibody that cross-reacts with antigen-95

Figure 7.5. Scintigraphic image demonstrating the uptake of ^{99m}Tc-Human IgG in the left thigh of a turpentine-induced inflammatory rabbit model. [From Shimpi et al. (1995); reprinted with permission.]

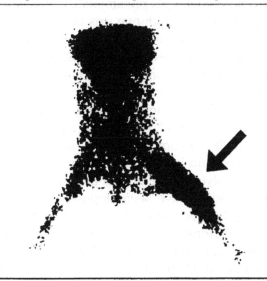

(Almers et al. 1996), and with a ^{99m}Tc- and ^{111}In-labeled antigranulocyte antibody, Mab47, which is also directed against a 95 kDa membrane protein on neutrophils (Blauenstein et al. 1995).

Other ^{99m}Tc-based radiopharmaceuticals have been used in inflammatory lesion imaging. A derivative of a chemotactic peptide was radiolabeled with ^{99m}Tc to image the region of inflammation induced by the injection of *Escherichia coli* into the thighs of rabbits (Babich et al. 1995). This peptide, formyl-methionine-leucine-phenylalanine-lysine-hydrazino nicotin-amide, was radiolabeled and administered 24 h after induction of inflammation. Images were obtained after another 16 h. The mechanism of localization was proposed to be the binding of the radiolabeled peptide to circulating and marginating leukocytes.

Other Radiopharmaceuticals

The protein avidin, which accumulates in sites of inflammation, has also been used. Preincubation with avidin, followed by administration of ^{111}In-biotin, a vitamin which binds avidin tightly and specifically, has been shown to detect inflammation associated with vascular graft infections (Chiesa et al. 1995). Technetium-99m-dextran was used for imaging inflammation following IM injection of Freund's Complete Adjuvant into rabbits (Bhatnagar et al. 1995). Well-resolved images were obtained 2 to 4 h after injection. It appeared that radiolabeled dextran was able to permeate through abnormal vascular endothelium induced by the adjuvant. Macrophages were radiolabelled with [99mTc]-labeled J001, an acylated poly-(1,3)-galactoside from the *Klebsiella pneumoniae* membrane (Miot-Noirault et al. 1996). Technetium-99m-glutathione was used to image inflammation induced by the injection of ovalbumin in rabbit knees and by the IM injection of turpentine (Ercan et al. 1994). This radiolabeled tripeptide is smaller than IgG and has better penetration into inflammatory sites. Improved image quality of [99mTc]-glutathione compared to [99mTc]-IgG may be due to the decreased diffusion of the latter agent into the circulation due to macromolecular entrapment. Oyen et al. (1996) took advantage of the lipophilic nature of the [99mTc]-HMPAO complex to label liposomes, which accumulated in sites of infection and inflammation. The same is true of the long-circulating copolymer poly(ethylene glycol)-poly-L-lysine-DTPA ([99mTc]).

Radioisotopes of iodine have been employed in inflammatory imaging. Iodine-125 decays by electron capture with a half-life of 60 days. The subsequently emitted photons have energies of 28 and 35 keV and, thus, do not provide well-resolved images. Iodine-123 also decays by electron capture, but its 13 h half-life and 159 keV photon energy make it nearly ideally suited for scintigrapic imaging. Iodine-125 has been used with success to radiolabel interleukin-8, which binds to monocytes in image peripheral inflammation (Bishayi and Samanta 1996). [125I]-labelled Substance P, which is secreted by white blood cells during the immune response, was observed to bind to spinal cord receptors following the injection of Freund's Complete Adjuvant into the paws of animals (Stucky et al. 1993). This supported the hypothesis that changes in the synaptic transmission of Substance P in the region of the spinal cord contribute to the hyperalgesia that is observed to accompany peripheral inflammation. There is also evidence that [125I]-labeled white blood cells are more stable than [111In]-white blood cells, and that they accumulate very specifically in areas of infection/inflammation (Blauenstein et al. 1995). Iodine-125-human serum albumin can also be used (Weg et al. 1994). In addition, iodine-123 has been attached to the MAb47 antibody to target granulocytes (Blauenstein et al. 1995).

SUMMARY

Gamma scintigraphy offers several advantages for the assessment of trauma as a result of the IM injection of pharmaceutical products. It is a completely noninvasive procedure that can be readily carried out in both animals and human volunteers. We have carried out a number of scintigraphic studies in humans at our institution following the approval of the Institutional Review Board, the Radioactive Drug Research Committee, and the Radiation Safety Committee. These studies generally result in low radiation absorbed doses to the subjects. The absorbed doses obtained by personnel handling radioactive animals are closely monitored and do not exceed 10 percent of the allowable Nuclear Regulatory Commission (NRC) dose. Scintigraphic measurements yield both qualitative and quantitative data, which can be obtained at any time point after the intramuscular administration of the test formulation. Tissue sampling and animal sacrifice are not required. The acquisition and analysis of scintigraphic images does, however, require specialized instrumentation and experienced personnel to carry out these measurements, as well as the infrastructure to support the regulation of radioisotopes. However, the ability to obtain a visual image of the inflammatory response and to quantify that response makes gamma scintigraphy an attractive tool for the evaluation of pharmaceuticals designed for IM administration.

REFERENCES

Almers, S., G. Granerus, L. Franzen, and M. Strom. 1996. Technetium-99m scintigraphy: More accurate assessment of ulcerative colitis with exametazime-labelled leucocytes than with antigranulocyte antibodies. *Eur. J. Nucl. Med.* 23:247–255.

Anger, H. O. 1958. Scintillation camera. *Rev. Sci. Instr.* 29:27–33.

Audran, R., B. Collet, A. Moisan, and L. Toujas. 1995. Fate of mouse macrophages radiolabelled with PKH-95 and injected intravenously. *Nucl. Med. Biol.* 22:817–821.

Babich, J. W., W. Graham, S. A. Barrow, and A. J. Fischman. 1995. Comparison of the infection imaging properties of a [99mTc] labeled chemotactic peptide with [111In] IgG. *Nucl. Med. Biol.* 22:643–648.

Becker, W., C. J. Palestro, J. Winship, T. Feld, C.M. Pinsky, F. Wolf, and D. M. Goldenberg. 1996. Rapid imaging of infections with a monoclonal antibody fragment (LeukoScan). *Clin. Orthop.* 329:263–272.

Beihn, R., and M. Vannier. 1979. Gallium pharmacokinetic imaging for early detection of tumors. *J. Nucl. Med.* 20:614.

Bester, M. J., P. D. Van Heerden, J. F. Klopper, H. J. Wasserman, S. Rubow, and F. de Klerk. 1995. Imaging infection and inflammation in an African environment: Comparison of [99mTc]-HMPAO-labelled leucocytes and [67Ga] citrate. *Nucl. Med. Commun.* 16:599–607.

Bhatnagar, A., A. K. Singh, T. Singh, and L. R. Shankar. 1995. [99mTc]-dextran: A potential inflammation-seeking radiopharmaceutical. *Nucl. Med. Commun.* 16:1058–1062.

Bishayi, B., and A. K. Samanta. 1996. Identification and characterization of specific receptor for interleukin-8 from the surface of human monocytes. *Scand. J. Immunol.* 43:531–536.

Blauenstein, P., J. T. Locher, K. Seybold, H. Koprivova, G. A. Janoki, H. R. Macke, P. Hasler, A. Ammann, I. Novak-Hofer, and A. Smith. 1995. Experience with the iodine-123 and technetium-99m labelled anti-granulaocyte antibody Mab47: A comparison of labelling methods. *Eur. J. Nucl. Med.* 22:690–698.

Borin, M. T., S. S. Khare, R. M. Beihn, and M. Jay. 1990. The effect of food on GI transit of sustained release ibuprofen tablets as evaluated by gamma scintigraphy. *Pharm. Res.* 7:304–307.

Boyd, C. M., and G. V. Dalrymple. 1974. *Basic science principles of nuclear medicine.* St. Louis: Mosby.

Boyd, S. J., R. Nour, R. J. Quinn, E. McKay, and S. P. Butler. 1993. Evaluation of white cell scintigraphy using indium-111 and technetium-99m labelled leucocytes. *Eur J. Nucl. Med.* 20:201–206.

Buscombe, J. 1995. Radiolabelled human immunoglobulins. *Nucl. Med. Commun.* 16:990–1001.

Bushell, D. L. 1984. Detection of Pseudomembranous colitis with indium-111 labelled leukocyte scintigtaphy. *Clin. Nucl. Med.* 9:294–295.

Carter, J. E., and K. G. Joo. 1979. Gallium accumulation in intramuscular injection sites. *Clin. Nucl. Med.* 4:304.

Chandra, R. 1987. *Introductory physics of nuclear medicine.* Philadelphia: Lea and Febiger.

Chiesa, R., G. Melissano, R. Castellano, C. Fernandez Zamora, D. Astore, A. Samuel, G. Paganelli, F. Fazio, and A. Grossi. 1995. Avidin and indium-111-labelled biotin scan: A new radioisotopic method for localizing vascular graft infection. *Eur. J. Endovasc. Surg.* 10:405–414.

Cohen, M. R., D. Klapp, K. B. Miller, V. L. Shaffer Jr., M. Slotfeldt, and D. E. Miller. 1984. Improving pharmacy and therapeutics committee operations. *Am. J. Hosp. Pharm.* 41:1767–1777.

Collet, B., S. Maros, A. Moisan, J. Le Cloirec, M. Moinereau, E. Aumaitre, L. Toujas, and P. Bourguet. 1993. 111-Indium-F(ab')$_2$-NCA 102 monoclonal antibody: In vitro study of a specific agent for the detection of inflammatory foci. *Nucl. Med. Biol.* 20:175–182.

Corstens, F. H., W. J. Oyen, and W. S. Becker. 1993. Radioimmunoconjugates in the detection of infection and inflammation. *Semin. Nucl. Med.* 23:148–164.

Datz, F. L., C. E. Anderson, R. Ahluwalia, J. H. Whiting, F. V. Gabor, K. A. Morton, P. E. Christian, K. Crebs, M. Neptune, and D. A. Rauh. 1994. The efficacy of indium-111-polyclonal IgG for the detection of infection and inflammation. *J. Nucl. Med.* 35:74–83.

Digenis, G. A., and E. Sandefer. 1991. Gamma scintigraphy and neutron activation techniques in the in vivo assessment of orally administered dosage forms. *Crit. Rev. Ther. Drug Carrier Sys.* 309–346.

Dorr, U., K. Frank-Raue, F. Raue, M. L. Sautter-Bihl, G. Guzman, H. J. Buhr, and H. Bihl. 1993. The potential value of somatostatin receptor scintigraphy in medullary thyroid carcinoma. *Nucl. Med. Commun.* 14:439–445.

Ebel, J. P., M. Jay, and R. M. Beihn. 1993. An in vitro/in vivo correlation for the disintegration and onset of drug release from enteric-coated pellets. *Pharm. Res.* 10:233–238.

Ercan, M. T., E. Unlenen, and A. Aktas. 1994. 99mTc-glutathione for imaging inflammatory lesions. *Nucl. Med. Commun.* 15:533–539.

Evetts, B. K., L. R. Foley, R. G. Latimer, and D. S. Rimkus. 1994. Tc-99m hexamethylpropyleneamineoxide scanning for the detection of acute appendicitis. *J. Am. Coll. Surg.* 179:197–201.

Frier, M. 1994. Leucocyte radiolabelling techniques: Practical aspects. *Scand. J. Gastroenterol. Suppl.* 203:32–35.

Gungor, F., B. Karayalcin, M. Gultekin, and N. Paksoy. 1996. Comparison of Tc-99m HIG and Ga-67 citrate in the evaluation of bacterial abscess in a rat model. *Ann. Nucl. Med.* 10:79–83.

Hickey, A. J., S. Zhou, M. Jay, S. M. Warren, M. Lord, and P. P. DeLuca. 1988. Reduced erythromycin-induced tissue trauma by incorporation in polymeric matrices prior to intramuscular injection in rabbits. *Pharm. Res.* 5:S76.

Hoffer, P. B. 1978. Mechanisms of localization. In *Gallium-67 imaging,* edited by P. B. Hoffer, C. Bekerman, and R. E. Henkin. New York: Wiley, p. 3.

Jamar, F., P. T. Chapman, A. A. Harrison, and R. M. Binns. 1995. Inflammatory arthritis: Imaging of endothelial cell activation with an indium-111-labelled F(ab')$_2$ fragment of anti-E-selectin monoclonal antibody. *Radiology* 194: 843–850.

Jimenez-Heffernan, A., J. L. Villanueva, A. Moral, and A. Rebollo. 1994. Detection of inflammation/infection with human polyclonal immunoglobulin G labelled with 99mTc. *Br. J. Radiol.* 67:770–774.

Jorgensen, C., I. Couret, C. Bologna, M. Rossi, and J. Sany. 1995. Radiolabeled lymphocyte migration in rheumatoid synovitis. *Ann. Rheum. Dis.* 54:39–44.

Keelan, E.T., A. A. Harrison, P. T. Chapman, R. M. Binns, A. M. Peters, and D. O. Haskard. 1994. Imaging vascular endothelial activation: An approach using radiolabeled monoclonal antibodies against the endothelial cell adhesion molecule E-selectin. *J. Nucl. Med.* 35:281.

Kodama, K., M. Igase, J. Funada, Y. Kazatani, K. Matsuzaki, E. Murakami, and T. Kokubu. 1994. Gallium-67 scintigraphy in idiopathic pericarditis. *Jpn. Circ. J.* 58:298–302.

Lentle, B. C., J. R. Scott, A. A. Noujaim, and F. I. Jackson. 1979. Iatrogenic alterations in radionuclide biodistributions. *Semin. Nucl. Med.* 9:131–143.

Leonard, J. C., C. B. Humphrey, and J. C. Vanhoute. 1978. Positive ^{67}Ga citrate scans in patients receiving *Corynebacterium parvum. Clin. Nucl. Med.* 3:370–371.

Mettler, F. A., and M. J. Guiberteau. 1991. *Essentials of nuclear medicine imaging.* Philadelphia: W. B. Saunders Co.

Miot-Noirault, E., F. Perin, L. Routledge, G. Normier, and A. Le Pape. 1996. Macrophage targeting with technetium-99m labelled J001 acylated polygalactoside for scintigraphy of inflammation: Optimization and assessment of imaging specificity in experimental arthritis. *Eur. J. Nucl. Med.* 23:61–68.

Oyen, W. J., O. C. Boerman, G. Storm, L. van Bloois, E. B. Koenders, R. A. Claessens, R. M. Perenboom, D. J. Crommelin, J. W. van der Meer, and F. H. Corstens. 1996. Detecting infection and iflammation with technitium-99m-labeled stealth liposomes. *J. Nucl. Med.* 37:1392–1397.

Parr, A., R. M. Beihn, R. M. Franz, G. J. Szpunar, and M. Jay. 1987. Correlation of ibuprofen bioavailability with GI transit by scintigraphic monitoring of [171]Er-labeled sustained release tablets. *Pharm. Res.* 4:487–490.

Perenboom, R. M., W. J. Oyen, A. C. van Schijndel, P. Beckers, F. H. Corstens, and J. W. van der Meer. 1995. Serial indium-111-labelled IgG biodistribution in rat pneumocystis carinii pneumonia: A tool to monitor the course and severity of the infection. *Eur. J. Nucl. Med.* 22:1129–1132.

Peters, A. M. 1994a. Development of radiolabelled white cell scanning. *Scand. J. Gastroenterol. Suppl.* 203:28–31.

Peters, A. M. 1994b. The utility of [99mTc]HMPAO-leucocytes for imaging infection. *Semin. Nucl. Med.* 24:110–127.

Richman, S. D., S. M. Levenson, P. A. Bunn, G. S. Flinn, G. S. Johnston, and V. T. De-Vita. 1975. [67]Ga accumulation in pulmonary lesions associated with bleomycin toxicity. *Cancer* 36:1966–1972.

Rubin, R. H., and A. J. Fischman. 1994. The use of radiolabeled nonspecific immunoglobulin in the detection of focal inflammation. *Semin. Nucl. Med.* 24: 169–179.

Sasso, D. E., M. A. Gionfriddo, R. S. Thrall, S. I. Syrbu, H. M. Smilowitz, and R. E. Weiner. 1996. Biodistribution of indium-111-labeled antibody directed against intercellular adhesion molecule-1. *J. Nucl. Med.* 37:656–661.

Shimpi, H. H., O. P. Noronha, and A. M. Samuel. 1995. Evaluation of [99mTc]-labelled human immunoglobulin in animal models of experimentally induced inflammatory lesions. *Nucl. Med. Commun.* 16:846–852.

Simmons, G. H. 1988. *The scintillation camera.* New York: Society of Nuclear Medicine.

Stucky, C. L., M. T. Galeazza, and V. S. Seybold. 1993. Time-dependent changes in bolton-hunter-labeled ^{125}I-substance P binding in rat spinal cord following unilateral adjuvant-induced peripheral inflammation. *Neuroscience* 57:397–409.

Sty, J. R., R. J. Starshak, and A. M. Hubbard. 1982. Gallium-67 scintigraphy-calcium gluconate extravasation. *Clin. Nucl. Med.* 7:377.

Swayne, L. C., D. Peterson, J. Collins, and C. A. Dise. 1995. Indium-111-white blood cell detection of postradiation vesicocutaneous fistulas. *J. Nucl. Med.* 36: 618–619.

Tedesco, F. J., R. E. Coleman, and B. A. Siegel. 1976. Gallium citrate (^{67}Ga) accumulation in pseudomembranous colitis. *J. Am. Med. Assoc.* 235:59–60.

Vanhagen, P. M., E. P. Krenning, J. C. Reubi, A. H. Mulder, W. H. Bakker, H. Y. Oei, B. Lowenberg, and S. W. Lamberts. 1993. Somatostatin analog scintigraphy in granulomatous diseases. *Eur. J. Nucl. Med.* 21:496–502.

Vorne, M. 1994. Imaging of abdominal inflammation using other radioisotope techniques. *Scand. J. Gastroenterol. Suppl.* 203:48–54.

Weg, V. B., M. L. Watson, L. H. Faccioli, and T. J. Williams. 1994. Investigation of the endogenous chemottractants involved in 111In-eosinophil accumulation in passive cutaneous anaphylactic reactions in the guinea pig. *Br. J. Pharmacol.* 113:35–42.

Weiner, R.E., G. J. Schreiber, P. B. Hoffer, and J. T. Bushberg. 1985. Compounds which mediate gallium-67 transfer from lactoferrin to ferritin. *J. Nucl. Med.* 26:908–910.

Weinstock, J. V. 1992. Neuropeptides and the regulation of granulatomous inflammation. *Clin. Immunol. Immunopath.* 64:17–22.

Weldon, A. J., A. E. Joseph, A. French, S. H. Saverymuttu, and J. D. Maxwell. 1995. Comparison of 99m-technetium hexamethylpropylene-amine oxime labelled leucocyte with 111-indium tropolonate labelled granulocyte scanning and ultrasound in the diagnosis of intra-abdominal abcess. *Gut.* 37:557–564.

Winzelberg, G. G. 1984. Focal gallium uptake in the liver. *Semin. Nucl. Med.* 14: 55–56.

Wong, D. W., J. I. Eisenman, and W. Wade Jr. 1995. Detection of acute infection/inflammation with Tc-99m labelled intact polyvalent human IgG. *Nucl. Med. Biol.* 22:513–519.

8

A Primer on In Vitro and In Vivo Cytosolic Enzyme Release Methods

Gayle A. Brazeau

Department of Pharmaceutics
University of Florida, College of Pharmacy
Gainesville, Florida

The extent of tissue damage or pain is a key component in formulating injectable products that must be considered in the optimization process employed by the pharmaceutical scientist (Figure 8.1). The ideal formulation for a parenteral product is one that minimizes the extent of pain and/or damage to tissues associated with the injection site (e.g., vascular epithelial cells, red blood cells, subcutaneous tissue, nerve or muscle fibers), while at the same time providing the requisite desired physicochemical (e.g., solubility, stability, injectability) and biopharmaceutical properties (e.g., extent and rate of drug release). Pharmaceutical scientists routinely characterize the physicochemical and biopharmaceutical properties of injectable products during preformulation studies. However, evaluation of the extent of pain and damage, particularly the extent of pain, remains more of a challenge to today's formulator during the drug development process.

Only in the last decade have parenteral formulators considered the importance of minimizing pain or damage during the development of parenteral products. The importance of characterizing the extent and mechanism(s) of drug- or formulation-induced pain or tissue damage is recognized by the recent work describing various evaluation methods, as discussed by other contributors to this volume. It is through the development and use of these experimental systems that pharmaceutical scientists can start to understand the mechanisms underlying the development of pain and/or tissue damage following the injection of parenteral formulations and, more importantly, to develop strategies to minimize or negate these two potential problems. The mechanisms of drug-induced pain or

Figure 8.1. Key optimization parameters in development of a parenteral formulation.

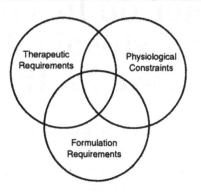

Therapeutic Requirements	Formulation Requirements	Physiological Constraints
Therapeutic indication	Solubility	Route/site of administration • Injection volume • Injection speed • Frequency of injections
Required route of administration	Stability	Local site reactions • Tissue damage • injection associated pain
Targeted patient population	Injection volume	
Desired release profile • Immediate release • Sustained release	Viscosity	
Pharmacokinetic/ pharmacodynamic profile	Incompatibilities	

tissue damage have been discussed in two recent publications (Brazeau et al. 1998; Brazeau 1998).

In our work at both the University of Houston and University of Florida, we have focused on investigating the extent of tissue damage associated with intramuscular (IM) injection using both in vitro and in vivo release of intracellular components (e.g., both structural and enzymatic proteins). The release of these intracellular components is a useful and convenient marker for the extent of drug-, excipient-, or formulation-induced tissue damage. The release of cytosolic enzymes continues to be, in basic and clinical studies, one of the simplest and most direct methods to determine whether there has been injury to a given tissue or organ. Reports in clinical and basic science literature have shown the usefulness of measuring the release of cytosolic components from isolated muscles, cells, or tissues into isolated baths or blood as a marker of damage following some type of stress or injury. The most extensively studied area utilizing the release of cellular components as a marker of cell injury has focused on evaluating the extent of myocardial damage associated with ischemic heart disease (Keffer 1996; Wu 1998).

RATIONALE FOR UTILIZING RELEASE OF CYTOSOLIC COMPONENTS AS A MARKER OF TISSUE DAMAGE

One can gain much insight into utilizing the release of cytosolic components as a marker of tissue damage by reading the literature in the area of ischemic heart disease and its clinical evaluation. Many similarities can be drawn from using this type of methodology to evaluate tissue damage associated with parenteral administration. In general, the in vitro and in vivo release of proteins, namely enzymes, measures the ability of a parenteral formulation or formulation component to cause a disruption in the tissue's outer membrane (e.g., sarcolemma in muscle) that results in the release of cytosolic enzymes into the external medium. This external medium can be either a physiological salt solution or blood. There are key assumptions and considerations a formulator must understand when utilizing these various types of experimental protocols. These are outlined in Table 8.1 and will be discussed throughout this chapter.

In our work, we have characterized the extent and/or mechanism(s) by which an injectable product can cause damage or toxicity (myotoxicity) to skeletal muscle fibers measured by the release of creatine kinase (CK). This particular enzyme is a useful marker for muscle damage. Assuming there is no other concurrent disease process, the release of this enzyme and the measurement of total CK in physiologic buffers and blood has been well correlated with the extent of tissue damage in muscle (Al-Suwayeh et al. 1996; Brazeau and Fung 1989c). This concept will be discussed in greater detail later. In the present discussion, *myotoxicity* is defined as the extent to which a formulation will cause injury to skeletal muscle fibers, and it can be assessed through the cumulative total release of CK or other cytosolic ennzymes into the incubation medium or by determining the area under the plasma or serum cytosolic enzyme curve for in vitro or in vivo studies, respectively.

The formulator who utilizes these methods must be cautioned with respect to several areas. While in vitro and in vivo systems are useful to screen test formulations for the extent of tissue irritation following parenteral administration, and have shown an excellent rank order correlation between in vitro and in vivo animal studies and clinical studies, they are not able to specifically test formulations for their pain-producing potential. However, a review of the literature and experimental findings suggests

---

Table 8.1. Assumptions or Considerations in Utilizing the Release of Intracellular Components as a Marker of Tissue Damage

---

A. General Consideration

1. Marker is specific for damage in the tissue being investigated.

2. Released protein is stable in the incubation medium or blood.

3. If enzymatic activity is being measured as the marker of tissue damage, there are no other endogenous or exogenous substances in the incubation medium or blood that interfere with the measurement of this activity by inhibiting or stimulating enzyme activity.

4. If total concentration of a protein is being quantified as the marker of tissue damage, there are no other endogenous or exogenous substances in the incubation medium or blood that shift the absorption maximum, and absorption spectroscopy can be used.

5. Appropriate controls (i.e., solvent, positive, negative) are included in the experimental design.

6. Appropriate data analysis is conducted.

B. Isolated Muscle System

1. Muscle is not damaged during the isolation procedure.

2. The injection procedure is consistent and the test solution does not leak from the site of injection.

3. The muscle is viable during the experimental time frame.

4. The possibility exists that the isolated muscle model may give false negative results.

C. Cell Culture Methods

1. The possibility exists that isolated muscle cell lines may give false negative results.

2. The cell growth curves are identical for all wells.

3. The treatment does not affect the cell number in the wells or that enzyme release is normalized to account for these differences.

4. The experimental protocol has been optimized with respect to the exposure paradigm (concentration and time) for each cell line.

5. The selection of the means to evaluate cellular toxicity is appropriate.

D. In Vivo Animal Studies

1. The experimental animal handling protocol does not increase serum enzymes.

2. The blood collection procedure does not increase serum enzyme levels.

3. The study is conducted for a time period necessary to characterize the area under the serum enzyme activity versus time curve.

4. The rate of enzyme release from the damaged tissue is faster than the rate of enzyme degradation or elimination from the blood.

---

that, in general, those formulations causing pain on injection are frequently associated with tissue damage at the injection site (Brazeau et al. 1989a; Al-Suwayeh et al. 1996). Secondly, in vitro systems are best designed to test for the acute interaction of formulation or formulation components with tissues. Therefore, these systems, particularly in vitro systems, provide the parenteral formulator with the ability to quickly and efficiently screen and select formulations with reduced tissue damage upon injection during the optimization process of formulation development.

EXPERIMENTAL MODELS

This chapter begins with a discussion of in vitro systems, including the isolated rodent muscle model and the L6 myoblast cell line. The advantages, limitations, and key assumptions and considerations required to utilize these systems will be discussed. The latter portion of this chapter will discuss the use of in vivo screening models, using rabbits and rodents, to assess parenteral formulations for their potential to cause tissue damage. While in vitro systems are useful for assessing **acute** damage by short-acting injectable formulations, in vivo systems still remain an important and critical method for testing injectable formulations. In particular, these experimental systems are beneficial for evaluating **long-term** or **repeated administration,** or when other associated cell types or tissues (not muscle) may be responsible for the pain or damage upon injection. Similarly, the advantages, limitations, and key assumptions and considerations required to utilize these in vivo methods in evaluating formulation-induced tissue damage will be discussed.

A general note prior to proceeding with this discussion: In all of these studies, we use male animals to eliminate any potential variations that may occur as a result of changes in hormonal levels. This does not mean that female animals cannot be utilized in these studies, yet caution is warranted. It has been suggested that estrogen can protect tissues (including muscle) against various forms of injury, can cause differences in the extent of CK release from isolated muscles, and can influence the levels of muscle enzymes in plasma (Amelink and Bär 1986; Amelink et al. 1990, Bär 1990).

ISOLATED RODENT SKELETAL MUSCLE MODEL

General Experimental Overview

The isolated rodent skeletal muscle system was based on the work of Dempsey and coworkers (1975). This methods provides the pharmaceutical formulator a means to quickly and directly investigate the effect of an injectable or its components to cause muscle damage using the release of CK into an isolated bath (Brazeau and Fung 1989b). There are several steps involved in utilizing this method. Initially, the rodent muscle is isolated and removed, without damaging the tissue, in a short period of time (< 5 min per muscle). It is then placed in a vial containing a physiologic isotonic buffer on ice (to help maintain viability) until being placed in the bath. This isolated muscle is then injected with the test formulation and placed into a physiologic isotonic buffer solution at a specific temperature (25°C, 30°C, or 37°C). In these studies, this buffer solution is bubbled with a mixture of 95 percent oxygen and 5 percent carbon dioxide (i.e., carbogen). The buffer solution is sampled and/or exchanged for fresh medium at specified times. The extent of tissue damage is measured by the cumulative release of CK into the medium over a selected time. We have found this total time frame in the extensor digitorum longus (EDL) muscle to be approximately 120 to 150 min.

Isolation, Extraction, and Viability of Isolated Muscles

There are several important assumptions that an investigator must realize when employing this type of screening system. To accurately assess the extent of damage caused by a given treatment upon injection, it is assumed that the muscle has not been damaged as a function of the isolation and extraction procedure and that the muscle remains viable throughout the study period. In order to not violate the isolation and extraction assumption, the muscles must be handled via tendon connections at both ends, and the body of the muscle must not be touched directly. In the rodent, the two primary muscles that can be used for in vitro studies are the EDL muscle, which is primarily composed of fast-twitch glycolytic fibers (Type II), and the soleus (SOL) muscle, which is primarily composed of slow-twitch oxidative fibers (Type I). With experience and practice, it is relatively simple to isolate and remove these two muscles in less than 5 min. These isolated muscles are then kept in the buffer solution on ice until injected.

Human muscles are mixed muscle fiber types; specifically, they are a composition of the various mixtures of slow- or fast-twitch muscle fibers. While the majority of our work has employed the EDL muscle in myotoxicity studies, investigators must understand that drug or formulation effects leading to irritation may be more prevalent in one muscle fiber type than the other fiber type. In alcoholic myopathy, basic and clinical data indicate that fast-twitch glycolytic fibers are more likely to be damaged than slow-twitch oxidative fibers (Hanid et al. 1981; Preedy and Peters 1988; Trounce et al. 1990). Estrogen deficiency appears to causes more damage to slow-twitch muscle fibers (unpublished results).

The second key assumption is that the muscle remains viable during the experimental period. The time that the muscle is viable in the incubation medium needs to be determined in preliminary experiments. Due to the lack of blood flow to the tissue after the muscle is isolated, proteolytic and degradative processes commence, and the muscle will start to develop a hypoxic core. The utilization of smaller muscles, such as the EDL or SOL muscles, is beneficial in this paradigm, since a greater fraction of muscle (versus total mass) is exposed to the medium containing carbogen. The length of time that an isolated muscle remains viable decreases as temperature increases. One can anticipate this type of finding because there would be increased enzyme activity and requirements for oxygenation with increased temperature.

Therefore, the objective for the investigator is to determine the time frame for which the release of the selected cytosolic enzyme reflects primarily the effect of the injected treatment, rather than loss of viability. A simple method to assess this would be to examine the release of the selected cytosolic enzyme from an uninjected control muscle over a 3 to 4 h period (Figure 8.2).

An examination of the cumulative release of the selected cytosolic enzyme over time is a useful index to measure muscle viability and myotoxicity. The cumulative release of a cytosolic enzyme is defined as the successive sum of the enzyme release over each short experimental period (30 to 60 min). For example, the cumulative release of a cytosolic enzyme from an uninjected control muscle is usually a biphasic curve (Figure 8.2). At some time point, a sharp increase in the slope of the curve will occur. This sharp increase in the slope most likely results from the loss of viability of the isolated muscle, leading to the increased release of cytosolic components through the dying muscle sarcolemma. Therefore, the enzyme release following this time point is the combined effect of the treatment and the loss of muscle viability. It is recommended whenever an experimental

Figure 8.2. Cumulative creatine kinase (CK) release and muscle viability. A change in the shape of the cumulative CK versus time curve is a useful indication for the loss of muscle viability.

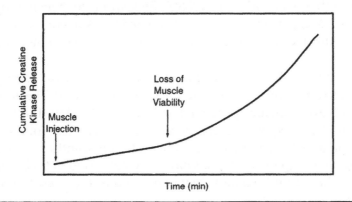

parameter has been modified that investigators determine the viability of their isolated muscle system.

A second advantage of this type of preliminary experiment using un-injected muscles is that it provides investigators with an opportunity to assess their skill in isolating the selected muscle without damaging it. If a muscle is damaged during the isolation and extraction procedure, the amount of enzyme release will be substantially higher at the beginning of the experiment. Often, a visual examination of the muscle for either nicks or tears is sufficient to make this assessment. It is the responsibility of the investigator to exclude from the analysis those muscles that were damaged during the isolation and/or extraction.

Muscle Exposure to the Test Formulation

The myotoxicity of a given treatment can be determined through the direct injection of the formulation into the muscle or by incubating the isolated muscle in buffer solution containing the test treatment. If the test formulation is to be injected into the muscle, it is imperative that the injection be standardized. It has been found that the Hamilton glass syringe with a small volume (25–100 µL) and sharp needle (those used for gas chromatographic injection) is useful for the injection. In more recent studies involving the injection of more viscous solutions, we have determined that a small gauge needle (25 G) and tuberculin syringe can also be used (unpublished data). The angle and depth of injection can be controlled by using a needle guard that is attached to the tip of the needle. A sample syringe and needle attached with the needle guard is shown in Figure 8.3.

For the EDL muscle, the injection should be made lengthwise to a depth of approximately 7 mm into the muscle body and is easily facilitated if the muscle is attached to a smooth hard surface via the tendon connections. The injection procedure often results in a pronounced welt on the muscle. Muscles that leak during the extraction procedures should be excluded from the data analysis. In the EDL muscle, an injection volume of 15 µL has been shown to be an ideal injection volume in muscles weighing 200–250 mg (Brazeau and Fung 1989b). Following the injection procedure, the muscles are placed in a Teflon®-coated basket containing holes to ensure that this tissue stays in contact with the carbongenated media (Figure 8.3).

Alternatively, the isolated muscle can be treated by adding the test compound to the buffer solution (no injection procedure). The advantage of this type of experimental paradigm is that it will allow the investigator the opportunity to expose the muscle to a given treatment for a specific period of time and to remove or add the test compound or formulation as needed by changing the buffer solution. The limitation of this experimental protocol is that the investigator must ensure that the presence of this test

Figure 8.3. Components of injection procedure for the isolated muscle study. The muscle is injected with a Hamilton 100 μL syringe and needle to which is attached a needle guard (middle). The muscles are then placed in a Teflon®-coated muscle basket to ensure the muscle stays in contact with the isotonic buffer solution.

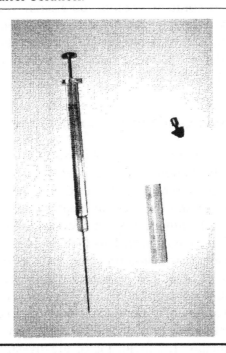

solution in the incubation medium does not interfere with (either inhibit or stimulate) the measurement of the desired cytosolic enzyme activity. If this incubation experimental procedure is to be used, it is recommended that the investigator obtain the selected enzyme in a purified form and test the extent of enzyme stimulation or inhibition caused by the proposed test formulation.

In our work, all new compounds are tested for their ability to interfere with the measurement of CK. It has been found that a number of compounds significantly inhibited CK activity (Brazeau and Fung 1989a). A second consideration occurs when the test compound is added to the buffer solution in a specific solvent. It then becomes critical to ensure that the experimental design includes appropriate solvent control and that the tonicity of the buffer solution is maintained.

Incubation Media

The incubation medium must be designed to be isotonic and contain sufficient electrolytes and nutrient sources to minimize the rate of proteolytic processes in the isolated muscle. Usually, this type of medium is a type of Ringer's solution and contains sodium, potassium, glucose, bicarbonate, and phosphate salts. Whether calcium should be added to the medium is not standardized. The presence of calcium has been shown to enhance the release of CK from the isolated EDL muscle in control and treated muscles (Brazeau and Fung 1990b).

Cytosolic Enzymes Utilized in Isolated Muscle Studies

CK (creatine kinase or creatine phosphokinase used in older literature citations) and lactate dehydrogenase (LDH) have been the cytosolic enzymes primarily utilized in isolated muscle studies due to the presence of high activity in skeletal muscle and the ease in measurement. In isolated muscle studies using untreated animals, it is not necessary to consider the various isoenzyme forms of these enzymes. This factor will be considered in more detail in the subsequent discussion on using these enzymes during in vivo studies. The activity of these two enzymes can be easily analyzed using commercially available spectrophotometric colorimetric and kinetic assays. In addition, the availability of commercial standards to calibrate assay procedures assists investigators in their ability to measure enzyme activity accurately and reproducibly. The major factor the investigator must consider in using enzymatic analyses during an isolated muscle study is the stability of the enzyme in the incubation medium. It is generally recommended that the collection periods between changes in the incubation media be kept between 30 and 60 min and that the samples be kept refrigerated until analyzed. In our work, we have found that CK activity is stable in the incubation medium for one day when the samples are stored in the refrigerator until analyzed. If one chooses other cellular components as markers of tissue damage during these isolated muscle studies, it is critical to measure the length of time that a particular one is viable in the buffer solution.

Controls and Data Analysis

The extent of the test formulation's myotoxicity can be analyzed easily by using the cumulative release of the selected cytosolic enzyme over time. It is recommended that investigators utilize positive and negative controls to calibrate their individual experimental system. Useful negative controls include uninjected control muscles, normal saline-injected muscles, or 5 percent dextrose-injected muscles, while useful positive controls are sliced muscles, phenytoin (Dilantin®), or loxapine (Loxitane®) (Al-Suwayeh et al.

1996). For example, the range of cumulative CK values from negative to positive controls is approximately 300 to 500 units/L for normal saline, 6,000 to 8,000 units/L for phenytoin, and 15,000 units/L for loxapine in our experimental systems. It is important to select negative and positive controls that have been shown through histologic analysis in basic or clinical studies to cause minimal or severe damage to muscle tissue. The enzyme release data can be normalized by wet muscle weight obtained at the beginning or end of the experiment. However, our experience indicates no significant difference in the interpretation of data that is normalized versus not normalized.

Statistical differences among the various treatments as a function of the cumulative enzyme release over time must be analyzed using repeated measures, since the values at each latter time point are dependent on the earlier values (based on the summative nature of the data). If quantifying the total cumulative release of a cytosolic enzyme at a specific time is used to assess myotoxicity, the data can be analyzed using the standard Student's t-test or analysis of variance at the specific time point. The data may be transformed logarithmically to achieve homogeneity of the variances if necessary.

Muscle Cell Culture Methods to Evaluate Muscle Injury

General Considerations

Similar to other organ systems, the utilization of isolated cells, either primary or continuous, to study formulation-induced toxicity is a useful and rapid method. While primary cell cultures are useful for other organs or tissues (e.g., neuronal), it is a more arduous task in skeletal muscle. Furthermore, the presence of commercially available clonal cell lines and their demonstration to be useful in evaluating formulation-induced toxicity has limited the interest in using primary cell culture methods. Consequently, the major continuously cultured cell lines that have been or can be employed in these studies are the L6 myoblasts or H9C2. There are other cell lines that can be purchased commercially; however, they have not been extensively studied and will not be considered in this chapter.

The advantage of using a cell line is that it enables the investigator to better control the experimental parameters and to screen a larger number of formulations simultaneously. In this respect, cell lines can be utilized to provide a rank ordering of the toxicity of selected formulations, provided there are appropriate positive and negative controls in the system. In contrast, there are limitations associated with using cell culture models. This type of system will only examine the potential toxicity of a formulation or formulation component with muscle tissue. It is very possible that the tissue toxicity associated with parenteral administration could be the result of primary effects on the associated blood vessels, nerves, and connective tissue leading to secondary muscle effects. In this situation, it is possible that utilizing such a screening system could result in a false negative. One should be cautious in interpreting the results using muscle cell lines or even isolated muscles because the possibility exists that the one could see no damage to muscle in vitro, while the in vivo experimental findings are the opposite. If this scenario occurs, it provides insight into other possible mechanisms that could be involved in causing tissue toxicity. This could include changes in blood flow to the tissue or toxicity to peripheral nerves in the muscle. Furthermore, it becomes critical for experimenters to understand the properties and characteristics associated with each cell line and to modify their experimental protocols as needed.

General Considerations in the Optimization of Experimental Cell Culture Systems

The investigator needs to determine key factors prior to utilizing a cell line to screen for formulation-induced toxicity. Factors that need to be considered include those related to the cell line itself and those related to designing the appropriate experimental design. Initially, cell growth must be optimized with respect to the selection of the medium, added medium components (such as bovine versus equine serum and other nutrients), and the environment of the incubation chamber (temperature, relative humidity). Prior to any studies, it is critical to determine the growth curve in order to obtain a sufficient number of cells per well for the study. While it is relatively easy to optimize the cell growth parameters based on research literature and commercially available information, the more difficult aspect lies in the design of the experimental protocol. There can be pronounced differences between various cell lines with respect to degree of cellular toxicity. As such, it is often necessary to optimize the experimental parameters on a case-by-case basis.

Parameters that need to be optimized include the time of exposure and the concentration of the test formulation in each well. Possible difficulties that can arise include test treatments that cause the cells to detach from the culture plate, changes in the pH of the medium, changes in the tonicity of the medium, and alterations in cellular growth rates. For example, if there is a potential for the treatment to alter the medium pH or tonicity, one needs to include in the design of the experimental protocol the appropriate control experiments to rule out pH- or tonicity-dependent effects. Equally problematic is if the test formulation causes the cells to detach from the plate. In this case, it can be difficult to compare treatments if there are differences in cell number or if one is quantifying the remaining concentration or activity of cellular components in the cells following removal of the medium (see below).

Finally, one needs to select the method to evaluate cellular toxicity. The investigator must determine whether one is quantifying cellular viability (or death), the release of cytosolic components into the medium (e.g., proteins or enzymes as discussed earlier), intracellular concentrations of selected structural proteins or enzymes or other endogenous substances, or a combination of methods. The assays that are utilized can be divided into those types that measure an immediate perturbation of membrane permeability, such as dye exclusion or enzyme release methods, or long-term survival as measured by the retention of cell growth, such as a cytotoxicity method (^{3}H-thmidine incorporation) (Freshney 1987).

In testing for formulation-induced toxicity, many studies have used the release of cytosolic enzymes into the medium followed by quantification with enzymatic activity or colorimetric assays. Like isolated muscle studies, the difficulty with this type of experimental setup is that one needs to determine the impact of the culture medium on enzyme activity or concentration. Theoretically, it is possible for one to underestimate the degree of formulation-induced cellular toxicity by measuring the release of cytosolic components if there is a change in the absorption maximum or a decrease in functional enzyme as a consequence of the presence of the specific component(s) in the culture medium. It must be considered that the decrease in intracellular levels of a cytosolic enzyme in a cell culture system will reflect not only loss from the cells but also loss due to cell necrosis or detachment from the well. In this type of release study, measurements of cellular viability and cell number should be incorporated in the experimental design.

A better approach to quantifying tissue toxicity would be to measure the concentration or activity of the remaining components in the cells following a standardized lysis and extraction protocol. This is similar to what has been suggested for red blood cells and L6 myoblast cells (Reed and Yalkowsky 1985; Williams et al. 1987; Laska et al. 1991). The results could be presented as the percentage released or retained by the cells relative to the selective positive and/or negative controls.

There are other considerations the formulator must consider when using cell lines to screen formulations for their potential to cause tissue toxicity. The characteristics of a given cell line may change as a function of the number of passages, which could lead to differences in the function and concentration of various cellular components. For example, it has been reported that CK concentration increases when there is differentiation in myotubules (Richler and Yaffe 1970). In our work with the L6 myoblast cell line, we noticed that with continuous passage of these cells, there are differences in the total concentration of CK (unpublished results). As such, it becomes critical to be consistent in using specific passage numbers if one is to make comparisons between various studies.

Another factor to be considered is the method by which one chooses to normalize the results of the study. If the investigator uses the number of cells, it becomes critical to include for every treatment a separate well intended to quantify the number of cells. The key assumption is that this well is representative of a selected treatment. Other approaches to normalize the data include total cellular protein or DNA (deoxyribonucleic acid). However, as before, it becomes critical to determine if the analysis procedure for the normalization component is unaltered by the presence of the treatment.

Selected Cell Lines in Screening for Drug-Induced Toxicity

There are a number of commercially available lines that can be used to evaluate formulation-induced tissue toxicity. However, the most extensively studied to date has been the L6 myoblast line by Williams et al. (1987), Laska (1991), and Evans et al. (1996) and the MRC-5 fibroblast line by Svendsen et al. (1985). For details on these studies, readers are referred to the work by these specific investigators. However, a general limitation with the use of myoblasts is the low levels of cellular components, either cytosolic or membrane bound. As such, this may require sensitive assay methods. A second limitation is that these cells grow extremely fast and can become confluent in a short period of time. Therefore, one must select the growth medium and design the experimental protocol to optimize the cell number and passage. Nevertheless, this model has been shown to be useful as a screen for muscle irritation of parenteral formulations as discussed Williams et al. (1987) and Laska (1991).

A cell line that might be beneficial and worth exploring is the H9C2 cell line. This clonal cell line is derived from the embryonal rat heart. Furthermore, this cell line retains the features of skeletal muscle, while also possessing features of cardiac muscle (i.e., expression of cardiac isoform of CK, L-type calcium channels, and the specific splicing protein SnM) (Mejia-Alvarez et al. 1994; Hescheler et al. 1991; Sipido and Marban 1991). As such, this line could be used to provide information on the potential effects of a formulation or drug on cardiac and/or skeletal muscle tissue. This continuous cell line can be differentiated to form multinucleated cells (unpublished data). There are two limitations with this cell line. First, the H9C2 line seems to be less sensitive to tissue injury by standard methods (unpublished results). As such, it may require higher concentrations if it is used to screen formulations. Second, the growth rate of this cell line is slow and it requires a 10 percent carbon dioxide environment to grow compared to the more conventional 5 percent carbon dioxide environment.

In Vivo Enzymatic Release Methods

General Considerations

While the in vitro methods can be used to determine the extent that short-acting formulations have on muscle tissue, these methods cannot be utilized to investigate repeated injections or long-acting formulations for their potential to cause tissue damage at an IM site. Therefore, in some circumstances, it is necessary to employ the in vivo release of cytosolic enzymes as a marker of tissue damage caused by parenteral products. The release of cytosolic enzymes as a marker of drug-induced myocardial infarction has been well established in the literature (see earlier discussion). The major advantage of this type of experimental system is that the nervous, vascular, and immune systems associated with skeletal muscle remain intact and can contribute to parenteral-induced tissue toxicity. It is theoretically possible that a given parenteral formulation does not directly damage muscle tissue; and consequently, it would not show elevated enzyme levels in the isolated muscle system. Alternatively, this formulation may result in muscle tissue damage secondary to its interaction with vascular, nervous, or immune systems. Finally, an advantage of this system is that it can be incorporated with histologic examination of tissues using light or electron microscopy.

The two species that have been primarily utilized in these types of studies are the rabbit and the rat (Brazeau and Fung 1990a; Al-Suwayeh et al. 1996; Svendsen et al. 1985; Svendsen 1983; Surber and Sucker 1987). Other larger species include the dog (Gloor et al. 1977) and the swine (Steiness et al. 1978). The use of the dog model has been problematic in that it appears there can be the potential for the presence of false positives and negatives (Aktas et al. 1994).

While there are a variety of markers that can be utilized in animal studies, CK or LDH (like the in vitro studies) are the easiest ones to use primarily due to the presence of assay methods that allow easy quantification in whole blood, serum, or plasma levels. It is also possible to measure either the total enzyme concentration or the isoenzyme fraction in these samples using electrophorectic methods. To determine the extent of muscle damage following IM injection, total CK activity can be utilized since muscle tissue is composed primarily of the MM isozyme, rather than the MB (heart) or BB (brain) isozymes. If a potential for damage to other tissues occurs, it would be better to quantify all the various isoenzymes to differentiate muscle damage from other tissue damage using standard electrophoretic methods.

Regardless of what animal species is used, it becomes critical for the investigator to collect whole blood using a sampling method that does not cause additional tissue damage and greater enzyme release. It is also important to quantify the whole blood, serum, or plasma enzyme levels prior to the injection of the test solution, and to ensure that the sampling method itself does not increase the levels in the serum. Finally, similar to the in vitro studies, it is best to include in these studies the appropriate positive and negative controls to provide a relative comparison between the various treatments and to compare between studies. Equally important is to include the appropriate solvent controls in the study design when needed, and, if repeated studies are conducted in the same animal, to randomize the injection sites. It is also recommended that the injection procedure be standardized with respect to the depth of injection, needle gauge, injection volume, and speed of injection.

Animal Models

The rabbit model has been extremely useful to evaluate formulation-induced tissue damage following IM injection because the blood samples can be taken easily via the marginal ear vein. The use of rabbits can be problematic since pronounced fluctuations in serum CK levels can occur because of the escape reaction before and during treatment (Surber and Dubach 1989; Steiness et al. 1978), and because repeated blood sampling from the ear vein can lead to increased CK levels (Olling et al. 1995). The test formulation is most often injected into the mid-lumbar muscles. The advantages of this model are that larger injection volumes (approximately 1.5 mL) can be used, larger blood volume samples can be taken over time, and more tissue is available for histologic evaluation at the conclusion of the study. It is also possible to conduct randomized crossover studies due to the large area available for injection in the mid-lumbar muscles. In addition, it has been shown that this model correlates with the results of in vitro muscle studies and clinical studies (Brazeau and Fung 1990a; Steiness et al. 1978).

The limitations of this model are primarily related to use of the rabbit. The investigator must become familiar with the animals and the animals must become familiar with the proposed experimental setup and investigator (i.e., cages, room, handling procedures, and environment) prior to the study. The use of a one-week familiarization period is recommended to avoid potential stress-induced increases in cytosolic enzyme release. The costs of acquisition and housing are higher than for the rodent. Perhaps the biggest problem is that the studies are very labor intensive and time-consuming since the experimental time frame can range from 24 to 72 h.

Based on the limitations associated with the rabbit model, we have recently started using the rodent model for in vivo studies (Al-Suwayeh et al. 1996), based on the work of Surber and Sucker (1987). Since it is necessary to cannulate these animals to obtain repeated blood samples to characterize the entire enzyme release versus time curve, the time course of CK release prior to and following the cannulation procedure was investigated. It was reported that serum CK levels following a jugular cannulation procedure peaked at approximately 2 h after completion of the surgery and returned to baseline by 12 h (Brazeau and White 1991). Thus, it would appear that the actual myotoxicity study in the rodent model could commence on the day following the cannulation procedure. The test formulation (100–300 µL) can be injected easily into the musculus rectus (thigh) or gastrocnemius muscle.

One advantage of this animal model is that peak serum enzyme levels were seen at approximately 2 h and that serum levels returned to baseline levels by 12 h for most compounds (Al-Suwayeh et al. 1996; Surber and Sucker 1987). Thus, the study in theory could be conducted within 1 day and at the most within 24 h compared to 72 h in the rabbit. However, the investigators need to be cautious in the volume and number of blood samples to prevent hematocrit depletion in the animals with repeated sampling. An ideal experimental design should include a protocol for replacement of a portion of the blood volume drawn for each sample. We have found this model useful in discriminating between various formulations and correlates with the in vitro muscle model (Al-Suwayeh et al. 1996).

Quantification of Tissue Damage

There are two key assumptions in utilizing these in vivo methods. The first assumption centers on the concept that the test formulation being investigated has damaged the sarcolemma, leading to the release of active cytosolic enzymes into the vasculature, and that this process occurs "relatively rapidly." The second assumption requires that elimination of the enzyme from the blood is slower than the release from the site so that the concentration or activity can be quantified over time. There would be minimal enzyme accumulation in the serum over the endogenous basal release if the elimination rate constant for the enzyme from the serum is larger than the release rate constant of the cytosolic enzyme from the damaged tissue. The profile of enzyme release over time is thus a function of the release rate from the tissue and the elimination rate from the systemic circulation (either by excretion or by inactivation of the enzyme).

While many studies of drug-induced toxicity on various organs have utilized a single time point to differentiate the degree of damage, this analytical approach can cause potential problems. If the investigator chooses a single time point and it is the incorrect time for measuring the amount of enzyme in the serum, plasma, or whole blood, one may not be able to differentiate between the various treatments. It is most likely, in such a case, that the sampling time is too late and that all enzyme levels have returned to baseline values. An alternative method to better quantify the extent of tissue damage following the IM of a parenteral formulation would be to calculate the area under the serum enzyme activity curve. This area under the curve can be calculated using the trapezoidal rule or more complicated mathematical algorithms as described in any standard pharmacokinetic textbook (Gibaldi and Perrier 1982).

To characterize the entire enzyme activity versus time curve in an in vivo study, it is necessary to design the experimental procedure to ensure that one can sample the peak enzyme concentration and the entire profile until enzyme activity approaches baseline levels. The half-life of enzymes in serum from a variety of species can be quite divergent. The approximate half-life of a particular enzyme in each species can be estimated from the serum enzyme activity versus time curve. The relatively short half-life of CK in the rodent (approximately 2 to 4 h) versus the rabbit (ranging from 8 to 24 h) can explain why rodent studies can be conducted within 24 h versus a longer time frame for rabbits (48 to 72 h). The investigator must also decide if baseline enzyme levels are to be subtracted from each of the measured levels.

It is possible that the time of peak enzyme activity in blood is treatment and species dependent. We have noted in previous studies that the time of peak enzyme levels in the rabbit is dependent on the severity of the treatment, with more myotoxic treatments peaking at an earlier time compared with less myotoxic treatments (Brazeau and Fung 1990a). In the rodent model, in contrast, the time of peak enzyme activities seems to be formulation-independent, as discussed earlier. Consequently, it is possible that the differences in the myotoxicity can also be quantified using the serum CK levels at 2 h in the rodent model.

There is one caution that the experimenter should be aware of when conducting both in vitro or in vivo studies. The quantification of tissue damage in these studies often involves the measurement of enzyme activities in blood or the incubation medium. The simultaneous release of endogenous inhibitors into serum or the incubation medium from damaged tissues could cause the levels of enzymes to be lower than that actually released from the site of injury. Secondly, the total amount of enzyme available for release from the muscle may be affected by the treatment. An additional component of these studies should include, if possible, quantifying the remaining concentration of enzyme in the tissue at the injection site or in the isolated muscle. With this measurement, one could quantify the total mass balance of the enzyme being investigated. This has been reported as a useful method by Svendsen et al. (1985) in the rabbit model, and we have utilized it in the isolated rodent muscle model (Brazeau et al. 1995).

CONCLUSIONS

The models discussed in this chapter primarily provide a method to evaluate the extent to which short-acting parenteral formulations can be tested for their potential to cause acute muscle damage. The in vitro methods can be used to provide a rapid method to screen out potentially toxic drugs, components, or products during preformulation. The in vivo models provide a means to assess the extent to which long-acting injectables or repeated injections can damage muscle tissue. These systems primarily rely on measuring the release of cytosolic enzymes, a measure of an alteration in the muscle sarcolemma. In general, these methods have been shown to be predictive of clinical experiences with these formulations. Yet there are key assumptions and considerations a formulator must remember during the experimental design phase in order that his or her experimental findings to be valid and provide insight into the development of parenteral formulations with reduced muscle damage.

ACKNOWLEDGMENTS

We would like to thank Ms. Patricia Khan for her technical assistance and Dr. Pramod Gupta for his patience and understanding in this project.

REFERENCES

Al-Suwayeh, S. A., I. R. Tebbett, D. Wielbo, and G. A. Brazeau. 1996. In vitro-in vivo myotoxicity of intramuscular liposomal formulations. *Pharm. Res.* 13: 1384–1388.

Amelink, G. J., and P. R. Bär. 1986. Exercise-induced muscle protein leakage in the rat: Effects of hormonal manipulation. *J. Neurol. Sci.* 76:61–68.

Amelink, G. J., R. W. Koot, W. B. Erich, J. Van-Gijn, and P. R. Bär. 1990. Sex-linked variation in creatine kinase release, and its dependence on oestradiol, can be demonstrated in an in-vitro rat skeletal muscle preparation. *Acta Physiol. Scand.* 138:115–124.

Aktas, M. A., D. Augusta, D. Concordet, P. Vincalir, H. Letebvre., P. L. Toutain, and J. B. Braun. 1994. Creatine kinase in dog plasma, preanalytical factors of variation, reference values and diagnostic significance. *Res. Vet. Sci.* 56:30–36.

Bär, P. R. 1990. The influence of sex hormones on the plasma activity of muscle enzymes. *Int. J. Sports. Med.* 11:409–410.

Brazeau, G. A. 1998. Drug-induced muscle damage. In *Oxidative stress in skeletal muscle*, edited by A. Z. Reznick, L. Packer, C. K. Sen, J. O. Holloszy, and M. J. Jackson. Berlin, Germany: Birkhäuser Verlag, pp. 295–315.

Brazeau, G. A., and H. L. Fung. 1989a. An in vitro model to evaluate muscle damage following intramuscular injections. *Pharm. Res.* 6:167–170.

Brazeau, G. A., and H. L. Fung. 1989b. In vitro assay interferences of creatine kinase activity. *Biochem. J.* 257:619–621.

Brazeau, G. A., and H. L. Fung. 1989c. Use of an in-vitro model for the assessment of muscle damage from intramuscular injections: In vitro-in vivo correlation and predictability with mixed solvent systems. *Pharm. Res.* 6:766–771.

Brazeau, G. A., and H. L. Fung. 1990a. Effect of organic cosolvent-induced skeletal muscle damage on the bioavailability of intramuscular [^{14}C] diazepam. *J. Pharm. Sci.* 79:773–777.

Brazeau, G. A., and H. L. Fung. 1990b. Mechanisms of creatine kinase release from isolated rat skeletal muscles damaged by propylene glycol and ethanol. *J. Pharm. Sci.* 79:393–397.

Brazeau, G. A., and C. A. White. 1991. Use of an in vivo rodent model to evaluate muscle damage following intramuscular injection. *Pharm. Res.* 8:S168.

Brazeau, G. A., S. Al-Suwayeh, J. Peris, B. Hunter, and D. W. Walker. 1995. Creatine kinase release from isolated EDL muscles in chronic ethanol-treated rats. *Alcohol.* 12:145–149.

Brazeau, G. A., B. Cooper, K. A. Svetic, C. L. Smith, and P. Gupta. 1998. Current perspectives on pain upon injection of drugs. *J. Pharm. Sci.* 87:667–677.

Dempsey, R., J. Morgan, and L. Cohen. 1975. Reduction of enzyme efflux from skeletal muscle by diesthylstilbestrol. *Clin. Pharmacol. Therap.* 18:104–111.

Evans, L. A. F., P. E. Genereux, E. M. Gibbs, and S. C. Sutton. 1996. Predicting injection site muscle damage III. Evaluation of intramuscular formulations in the L6 cell line. *Pharm. Res.* 12:1585–1587.

Freshney, R. I. 1987. *Culture of animal cells: A manual of basic technique.* New York: Wiley-Liss, pp. 245–256.

Gibaldi, M., and D. Perrier. 1982. *Pharmacokinetics.* New York: Marcel Dekker, pp. 445–449.

Gloor, H. O., C. Vorburger, and J. Schädelin. 1977. Intramuskulär injektionen und serumkreatinphosphokinase-aktivität. *Schweiz. med. Wschr.* 107:948–952.

Hanid, A., G. Slavin, W. Mair, C. Sowter, P. Ward., J. Webb, and J. Levi. 1981. Fibre type changes in striated muscle of alcoholics. *J. Clin. Pathol.* 34:991–995.

Hescheler, J., R. Meyer, S. Plant, D. Krautwurst, W. Rosenthal, and G. Schultz. 1991. Morphological, biochemical and electrophysiological characterization of a clonal cell (H9C2) line from rat heart. *Circ. Res.* 69:1476–1486.

Keffer, J. H. 1996. Myocardial markers of injury: Evolution and insights. *Amer. J. Clin. Pathol.* 105:305–320.

Laska, D. A., P. D. Williams, J. T. Reboulet, and R. M. Morris. 1991. The L6 muscle cell line as a tool to evaluate parenteral products for irritation. *J. Parent. Sci. Technol.* 45:77–82.

Mejia-Alvarez, R., G. F. Tomaselli, and E. Marban. 1994. Simultaneous expression of cardiac and skeletal muscle isoforms of the L-type Ca^{2+} channel in a rat heart muscle cell line. *J. Physiol. London* 478:315–329.

Olling, M., K. VanTwillert, P. Wester, A. B .T. Boinck, and G. Rauws. 1995. Rabbit model for estimating relative bioavailability, residues and tissue tolerance of intramuscular products: Comparison of two ampicillin products. *J. Vet. Pharmacol. Ther.* 18:34–37.

Preedy, V. R., and T. J. Peters. 1988. Acute effects of ethanol on protein synthesis in different muscles and muscle protein fractions of the rat. *Clin. Sci.* 74:461–466.

Reed, K. W., and S. H. Yalkowsky. 1985. Lysis of red blood cells in the presence of various cosolvents. *J. Parent. Sci. Technol.* 39:64–69.

Richler, C., and D. Yaffe. 1970. The in vitro cultivation and differentiation capacities of myogenic cell lines. *Dev. Biol.* 23:1–22.

Sipido, K. R., and E. Marban. 1991. L-type calcium channels, potassium channels and novel nonspecific cation channels in a clonal muscle cell line derived from embryonic rat ventricle. *Circ. Res.* 69:1487–1499.

Steiness, E., F. Rasmussen, O. Svendsen, and P. Nielsen. 1978. A comparative study of serum creatine phosphokinase activity in rabbits, pigs and humans after intramuscular injection of locally damaging drugs. *Acta Pharmacol. et. Toxicol.* 42:357–364.

Svendsen, O. 1983. Intramuscular injections and local muscle damage: An experimental study of the effect of injection speed. *Acta Pharmacol et. Toxicol.* 52: 305–309.

Svendsen, O., F. Hojelse, and R. E. Bagdon. 1985. Tests for local toxicity of intramuscular drug preparations: Comparisons of in vivo and in vitro methods. *Acta Pharmacol. et. Toxicol.* 56:183–190.

Surber, C., and U. Dubach. 1989. Tests for local toxicity of intramuscular drug preparation. Comparison of in vivo and in vitro findings. *Arzneim.-Forsch./ Durg Res.* 39:1586–1589.

Surber, C., and H. Sucker. 1987. Tissue tolerance of intramuscular injectables and plasma activities in rats. *Pharm. Res.* 4:490–494.

Trounce, I., E. Byrne, and X. Dennett. 1990. Biochemical and morphological studies of skeletal muscle in experimental chronic alcoholic myopathy. *Acta Neurol. Scand.* 82:386–391.

Williams, P. D., B. G. Masters, L. D. Evans, D. A. Laska, and G. H. Hottendorf. 1987. An in vitro model for assessing muscle irritation due to parenteral antibiotics. *Fund. Appl. Toxicol.* 9:10–17.

Wu, A. H. 1998. Analytical and clinical evaluation of new diagnostic tests for myocardial damage. *Clin. Chim. Acta* 272:11–21.

9

Histological and Morphological Methods

Bruce M. Carlson
Robert Palmer

Department of Anatomy and Cell Biology
University of Michigan
Ann Arbor, Michigan

Many injected materials and solutions cause damage to skeletal muscle. At one extreme are certain snake and spider venoms, some of which cause massive muscle damage (Arce et al. 1991; Gutierrez et al. 1984; Harris et al. 1975; Maltin et al. 1983). A number of other materials, however, cause direct muscle damage as a side effect of their main action. The most widely studied of these are local anesthetics (Benoit and Belt 1970; Basson and Carlson 1980; Foster and Carlson 1980), but injection of a wide variety of other substances also causes muscle damage. Examples are diazepam and digoxin (Steiness et al. 1978), cis(Z)-clopenthixol (Svendsen 1983), certain antiphlogistic agents (Řeřabková 1983), and certain antibiotics (Gray 1967). In addition, certain binary solvent systems alone cause muscle fiber damage after injection (Brazeau and Fung 1989).

Regardless of the myotoxic agent, the lesions produced at the sites of injection typically fall into one of two pathological types—nonischemic and ischemic (Foster and Carlson 1980). For both of these types of lesions, morphological methods can be effectively employed in both detecting the areas of muscle damage and in following the progress of resolution of that damage. Because nonischemic and ischemic lesions of muscle have different characteristics and different courses of recovery, it is important to distinguish between them.

Nonischemic lesions retain the presence of an essentially intact microcirculation regardless of the topographical extent of the muscle damage. The most important characteristic of a nonischemic lesion is that the various stages of muscle degeneration and regeneration occur synchronously throughout the lesion. This is important not only for the analysis of the pathology but also in a practical sense because nonischemic lesions of muscle regenerate much more rapidly, and often more effectively, than do ischemic lesions.

Ischemic lesions of muscle are characterized by one or more areas in which the blood supply to the muscle has been interrupted. In many cases, actual damage to the muscle fibers can be directly attributable to the injectable agent, with the simultaneous direct disruption of the vasculature by the agent. On the other hand, the injectable agent could also act primarily on the local vasculature without directly damaging the muscle fibers. Under these circumstances, muscle fiber damage could still occur, but it would be secondary to prolonged ischemia instead of direct due to myotoxicity of the injectable agent.

The recovery of muscle from an ischemic lesion follows a topographically nonuniform path that depends principally on the time course and pattern of revascularization. Typically, there is a pronounced gradient of muscle fiber degeneration and regeneration that is closely related to the pattern of revascularization of the damaged area. Because of the delay in revascularization, the time course for total regenerative recovery can be considerably prolonged compared to the recovery of nonischemic lesions.

Stages in the overall course of muscle fiber degeneration and regeneration in a nonischemic lesion are summarized in Table 9.1. Muscle fibers in ischemic lesions undergo the same stages of degeneration and regeneration as those outlined in Table 9.1, but the progression of cell-mediated degeneration and subsequent regeneration only occurs when capillaries have grown into the area in question. Understanding the basic pathophysiology of these lesions is important in designing morphological approaches for the study of muscle lesions caused by injectable agents.

Table 9.1. Characteristic Phases in the Degeneration and Regeneration of Nonischemic Skeletal Muscle in the Rat

Days After Injection	Predominant Processes
0–1	Initial damage by injected agent.
	Intrinsic degeneration of muscle fibers.
1–3	Acute inflammation and macrophage-mediated phagocytosis of damaged muscle fibers.
2–3	Activation of satellite cells and establishing a population of myoblasts.
3–5	Early myotube stage of regeneration.
5–8	Late myotube stage of regeneration.
8–30+	Maturation of regenerating muscle fibers.

BASIC PRINCIPLES UNDERLYING MORPHOLOGICAL ANALYSIS

A fundamental reason for conducting morphological analysis of muscle that has been exposed to injectable agents is to determine whether or not these agents cause tissue damage, but much more specific information can also be obtained through such analysis. With appropriate sampling, the following information can be obtained through a routine morphological screening:

- *Whether or not muscle damage has occurred:* Assuming that the sample was collected from the region exposed to the injectable agent and that the sample was collected sometime during the interval between early muscle damage and late repair, documenting damage is readily accomplished through the standard histological techniques that are outlined below.

- *The time course of damage and its repair:* Determination of the time course of muscle damage may require an extensive series of sampling. Initial muscle fiber damage, for example, can be detected as early as 10 min after exposure to an exogenous agent by the examination of electron micrographs or semithin sections stained with toluidine blue. The time course of the various stages of degeneration and regeneration (see Table 9.1) can be normally determined through an examination of routine histological preparations.

- *The type of lesion:* Determination of whether a muscle lesion is ischemic or nonischemic can be made easily through routine histology if topographical sampling is accurate. Interpretation is facilitated if the sections are taken at several levels through the lesion. If only one section is examined, a tangential section through an ischemic lesion can be incorrectly diagnosed as a nonischemic lesion.

- *The types of cells and tissues affected:* Injectable agents can potentially damage any cell or tissue component of a muscle, including the microvasculature and nerves. Substantial damage to any tissue component can be determined by examination of histological sections, but specific histochemical or immunocytochemical markers may better define damage to certain cell or tissue types (e.g., vascular endothelium).

- *The extent of the lesion:* If great precision is required, determination of the extent (e.g., volume) of a lesion involves careful sampling and morphometric analysis of microscopic sections. For quantitative screening, biochemical methods, such as determination of serum levels of creatine kinase (CK), or whole muscle analysis of contractile properties may be more time-effective.

- *The extent of recovery:* For muscle, the best way to determine the extent of recovery is to use physiological methods, in particular the measurement of contractile properties (specifically, maximum tetanic force) of the muscle either in vivo or in vitro. One can obtain information about the extent of morphological recovery of damaged or regenerated muscle fibers through the measurement of cross-sectional areas of the muscle fibers.

The key to any accurate morphological analysis is sampling, both in time and in space. In small laboratory rodents, one can easily sample entire muscles, but in larger animals or in humans, even determining the region to be sampled can be challenging. In other words, a normal appearing set of histological sections could simply mean that the tissue sample was not taken through the site of an existing lesion. One method for localizing the tissue exposed to an injectable agent, especially for short-term sampling, is to mix into the injection medium a nontoxic dye, such as methylene blue. Unless the tissue is to be biopsied, it is relatively easy to determine the region of exposure. If biopsy samples are required, their sampling limitations must be recognized.

Techniques of Morphological Analysis

When contemplating the use of morphological methods for analyzing the effects of injectable agents on skeletal muscle, it is important to understand the strengths and limitations of these methods, as well as other factors, such as expense and sample preparation time. It is also important to view these techniques in relation to the level of analysis required. The requirements of a screening study for drug toxicity are quite different from those for clinical diagnostic sampling from a single patient or an in-depth research study.

Many of the techniques referred to below are listed in great detail in laboratory manuals (e.g., Dubowitz 1985; Loughlin 1993; Luna 1968; Mikel 1994; Sarnat 1983), and the intent of this chapter is not to provide that level of technical detail. Rather, categories of morphological methods will be discussed, with emphasis on why they might be appropriate or inappropriate for a particular purpose.

Electron Microscopic Methods

In the context of this chapter, electron microscopy will refer to both ultrastructural analysis and the light microscopic analysis of the semithin sections that are produced during the process of preparing the tissues for thin sectioning and actual electron microscopic examination. The obvious strength of electron microscopic analysis is the ability to detect structures, both normal and abnormal, below the level of resolution of the light microscope.

Electron microscopy can be important in the analysis of any stage of muscle damage and repair, but it is especially valuable in detecting the earliest manifestations of muscle fiber damage. At the survey level, damaged muscle fibers show dramatic differences from normal ones at the light microscopic level on semithin sections, often within minutes of exposure to an injected agent (Figure 9.1) or after an ischemic episode. Follow-up electron microscopy then allows the detection of damage to specific subcellular structures (Figure 9.2). Similarly, electron microscopic analysis can be valuable at any phase in the overall process of degeneration/repair, if fine structural detail is required (Figure 9.3).

Procedural Issues

One of the most important elements of an electron microscopic investigation is to ensure that the tissue is in good condition; otherwise, postmortem changes could be interpreted as reflecting tissue damage. The muscle tissue should be exposed to fixative within minutes of removal from the body to reduce the chances of postmortem artifacts. For laboratory animals, perfusion is often recommended as the best mode of introducing a fixative to

Figure 9.1. Toluidine blue-stained thick section of monkey thumb muscle 4 h after an injection of 0.75 percent bupivacaine into the area. This technique provides a dramatic differentiation between lightly stained damaged (arrows) and darkly stained nondamaged muscle fibers.

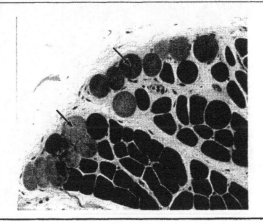

Figure 9.2. Electron micrograph of a monkey muscle fiber 4.5 h after exposure to 0.75 percent bupivacaine. Disruption of the cell membrane (arrows) is readily apparent by this technique. The basal lamina (arrowheads) is preserved.

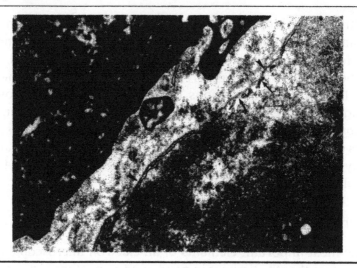

Figure 9.3. Electron micrograph of a cross-sectioned muscle fiber from the lateral rectus muscle of a rat 6 h after a retrobulbar injection of 35 μL of 2.0 percent mepivacaine. The micrograph shows a surviving satellite cell (S) associated with a muscle fiber that has extensive destruction of its mitochondria (asterisks) and other cytoplasmic contents. Intact basal lamina—arrowheads.

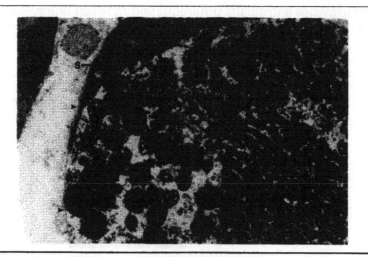

the tissues, but if an ischemic lesion is present, the fixative may not adequately penetrate the avascular region. An effective method of fixing rodent muscle is to expose the muscle in situ and bathe it in fixative for several minutes before it is removed from the animal. Then the muscle can be removed without danger of major contraction artifacts, and small pieces of tissue can then be removed and directly immersed into fixative. It is important that the pieces be not too large (1 mm or less in diameter and up to 3 mm long) or the fixative will not adequately penetrate the tissue sample. Standard fixation is in glutaraldehyde followed by osmium tetroxide postfixation. (For one protocol, see Dubowitz [1985], p. 17.)

Orientation of the tissue is another issue. For some purposes, examination of cross-sections provides more appropriate information; for others, longitudinal sections are preferable. For overall surveys of possible muscle damage, cross-sections usually provide the most information for initial screening, but if the integrity of the contractile apparatus is in question, longitudinal sections may be more appropriate. In typical cases of screening for possible muscle damage, examination of the tissue at low magnification (<2,500×) is most profitable. A number of immunocytochemical and histochemical techniques can be applied to muscle at the ultrastructural level, but these would normally be done only for specialized research purposes rather than for a general survey of muscle damage. Therefore, they will not be dealt with here.

Histological Methods

For broad screening for potential tissue damage caused by injectable agents, standard histological methods provide the most efficient approach. This is possible because one can scan a relatively large area of tissue, and the methods are sensitive enough to detect most types of tissue damage. General histological methods are least useful in detecting immediate subcellular damage or in detecting responses by different muscle fiber types very early or very late in regeneration. On the other hand, histology is the method of choice for examining the phases of overt muscle fiber breakdown, the associated inflammatory response, and the early stages of muscle fiber regeneration. For these stages, both the morphological clarity and the color information inherent in a standard hematoxylin and eosin stain (e.g., its ability to highlight cytoplasmic basophilia in early stages of the repair process) make such a preparation an ideal screening tool (Figure 9.4). Other special histological stains can highlight specific features that might be of importance in the tissue analysis. For example, most of the standard connective tissue stains (e.g., the trichrome stains that involve an aniline blue component) will cause deposits of collagen to stand out clearly, and a number of lipid stains will similarly highlight intracellular deposits of lipid or fat cells. Details of specific staining techniques are clearly laid out in

Figure 9.4. Hematoxylin and eosin-stained paraffin section through the tibialis anterior muscle of a rat two days after an injection of 2 percent xylocaine. This technique differentiated very well the damaged muscle fibers at the peak of the stage of phagocytosis (dark areas) and the surviving muscle fibers (light colored) around the periphery of the lesion.

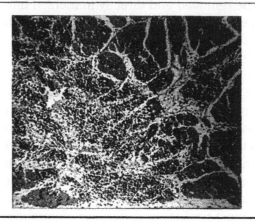

technique books, such as the *Armed Forces Institute of Pathology Manual* (Luna 1968).

Procedural Issues

One of the first decisions is how to treat the tissue once it is removed from the body. The two common options are quick freezing or fixation followed by embedding in paraffin. Both methods of tissue preparation can produce excellent sectioned material, but the overall appearance of the stained sections often looks surprisingly different when frozen and fixed tissues are compared side by side. The differences are especially prominent when muscle in stages of degeneration or early regeneration are compared. For routine screening purposes, it is better to use one method of tissue preparation so that interpretations and comparisons will be more consistent.

When removing the tissue from the body, it is important that it be fixed or frozen at approximately resting length, or the inherent contraction of the muscle fibers will cause longitudinal kinking of the muscle fibers. When working with rodents, one usually removes the entire affected muscle for histological analysis. Some investigators keep the muscle attached to the bone during fixation, but a much more convenient and entirely satisfactory method for use with fixation and subsequent paraffin embedding is to cut a thin strip from a 3 × 5 in. card and make slits at both ends. The tendons of the removed muscle can be wedged into the slits and the length of the muscle adjusted appropriately. When muscles are to be frozen, some investigators tie them to tongue blades to maintain them at the proper length. For biopsies of larger muscles, a variety of clamps have been used to maintain the muscle sample at the proper length.

Although ideally any tissue should be fixed or frozen as soon after removal from the body as possible, good quality hematoxylin and eosin preparations can be prepared from muscle fixed or frozen as late as 2 h after removal or death, if the tissue is kept cool (less than 15°C). Delayed fixation or freezing is not appropriate, however, for muscle on which histochemical examination is intended.

Rapid freezing is a standard technique in the processing of clinical muscle biopsies, because of the batteries of enzyme histochemical tests routinely employed. However, simple histological screening for indications of morphological damage and repair of rodent muscle after exposure to injectable agents is often better accomplished by fixation in Bouin's solution or buffered formalin and staining cross or longitudinal sections of muscle with hematoxylin and eosin. On the other hand, if the overall analysis of the muscle samples involves both routine histology and histochemistry, then it is most convenient to run all these techniques on sections from frozen muscle.

Histochemical Methods

Large numbers of histochemical methods have been adapted for use on skeletal muscle tissue. These have been extensively treated in muscle pathology books and manuals, and individual laboratory methods will not be dealt with in technical detail in this chapter (see Dubowitz 1985; Loughlin 1993; Mikel 1994; Sarnat 1983).

There are two principal uses for histochemical methods in muscle biology. One is to detect specific muscle fiber types. The other is to detect changes in metabolic properties of muscle fibers, especially in disease states.

Almost all muscles consist of mixed populations of fast and slow muscle fibers. Over the years, many histochemically based classifications of muscle fibers have been used, principally based on the histochemical reactions of muscle fibers for myosin adenosine triphosphatase (ATPase) activity at different pHs. (See Dubowitz [1985], pp. 56–64 for historical review.) On the basis of the staining reactions of cross-sectioned muscle fibers at pHs of 9.4 and 4.3 (Figure 9.5), skeletal muscle fibers have been subdivided into four principal types (Brooke and Kaiser 1970), specifically Types 1, 2A, 2B, and 2C, with Type 1 being slow muscle fibers and Types 2A through 2C being variants of fast muscle fibers.

Currently, histochemical classifications of muscle fiber types are being replaced by classifications based on immunocytochemical reactions (see below); but for certain types of screening (e.g., differentiating simply between fast and slow muscle fibers), they can still be useful. A principal application

Figure 9.5. Myofibrillar ATPase reaction on serial frozen sections of normal rat extensor digitorum longus muscle, showing the pH-dependent reversal of staining. A. pH 9.4, with fast (Type 2) muscle fibers staining dark, and slow (Type 1) muscle fibers staining light. B. pH 4.3, showing the reversal of staining, with slow muscle fibers dark and fast fibers light.

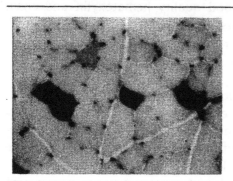 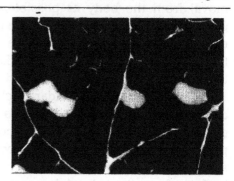

for such muscle fiber-typing methods in studies of reactions of muscles to injectable agents is in determining if, in the immediate postinjection period, there is evidence of differential susceptibility of fast or slow muscle fibers to the agent in question. Another potential application of such methods is in the analysis of muscle that has regenerated after being severely damaged by an injectable agent. A deviation from the normal proportion of fast and slow muscle fibers could indicate damage to nerve fibers as well as to muscle fibers, since in regeneration the type of motor nerve innervating the muscle fiber determines its type (Gutmann and Carlson 1975).

The other potential application of histochemical methods in investigating the effects of injectable agents on muscle is in investigations of the effects of the agent on a specific enzyme or metabolic pathway (e.g., Dolwick et al. 1977). Such investigations fall more into specific research applications rather than screening techniques, and they will not be covered in this chapter. Specific protocols for the more commonly used techniques are given in Mikel (1994).

Procedural Issues

The principal concerns with enzyme histochemical methods are preservation of structure and preservation of enzyme activity. Flash freezing is the standard method for treating the muscle. Immediate freezing after removal of the muscle is best, especially for certain enzymes; however, if the muscle is wrapped in gauze soaked in saline and kept cool, a delay of 1 or possibly up to 2 h before freezing is possible, especially for histochemical muscle fiber typing. Pieces of muscle should normally not be larger than 12 to 15 mm in length and 5 to 7 mm in diameter, because ice crystals may form in the center of larger pieces of muscle during the freezing process. Flash freezing is commonly accomplished by quickly immersing the tissue into a mixture of dry ice and isopentane or into a vial of isopentane immersed in liquid nitrogen. Isopentane is used because it conducts heat away from the muscle quickly enough to prevent the formation of ice crystals in the muscle fibers.

There are many ways of orienting and embedding the muscle during the freezing process so that it will be adequately supported during sectioning. Any of the standard technique books and manuals describe appropriate methods. Because the formation of ice crystals can make muscle sections unusable, it is important to avoid freezing and refreezing at all stages of the sectioning process. Once sections are made, they can be stored at –80°C in plastic boxes, which are then wrapped in a plastic wrap and surrounded with a wrap of aluminum foil. Sections treated in this way can be saved for many months without losing enzyme activity. Then sections collected at different times can be removed as a group for individual staining procedures. It is often easier to compare histochemical reactions on sections that have been stained during the same session.

Immunocytochemical Methods

For investigating possible muscle damage by injectable agents, immunocytochemical methods can be used for the precise localization of specific molecules or epitopes, or as a means of typing muscle fibers (Figure 9.6). The rationale for the immunocytochemical typing of muscle fibers is the same as that described in the previous section on histochemical methods. Because of their greater specificity, immunocytochemical methods can be used not only for the typing of mature muscle fibers, but also for identifying isozyme shifts of specific muscle proteins, such as developmental forms of myosin heavy chains (Schiaffino and Reggiani 1996). This can be useful in determining stages in the repair of damaged muscle fibers.

Immunocytochemical methods are also important in the localization of specific molecules of the extracellular matrix, such as laminin (see Figure 9.6), which can serve as a good marker of damage to basal laminae. Another specific localization that can be of considerable value in screening for muscle damage is factor VIII (von Willebrand factor), which is an excellent marker for vascular endothelium and can be used for the quantification of capillaries in cross-sections of muscle.

Procedural Issues

Many appropriate antibodies are available commercially; some are monoclonal and others are polyclonal. The best conditions for reacting the antibody with the tissue often depend on the specific antibody. Some require

Figure 9.6. Immunocytochemical preparation of normal rat tibialis anterior muscle reacted with antibodies against laminin and slow myosin heavy chain. The laminin stains the basal lamina around all muscle fibers. The slow muscle fibers are lightly stained, whereas fast muscle fibers are completely unstained.

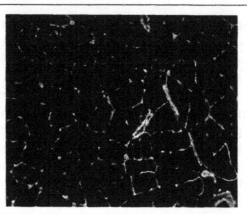

the use of frozen sections, others can be reacted successfully with appropriately fixed paraffin sections. Normally, the manufacturer will supply the investigator with the best conditions for using a particular antibody. The principles of immunocytochemistry and specific techniques are listed in a large variety of books (e.g., Cuello 1983), but a couple of strategic issues should be discussed here. The first concerns the nature of the chromophore on the secondary antibody that is used to demonstrate the reaction site of the primary antibody with the tissue in question. The second involves the use of control sections.

The standard indirect immunocytochemical reaction involves reacting a primary antibody (either monoclonal or polyclonal) against a specific molecule or epitope that is presumably present in the tissue and then reacting a secondary antibody against the primary antibody. Most commonly, the secondary antibody is conjugated with a fluorescent dye (typically fluorescein isothiocyanate [FITC] or rhodamine), which allows the antibody and its corresponding antigenic site to be readily localized with a fluorescence microscope. This technique is relatively rapid, and it can give very nice fluorescent images of multiple antibody localizations if different fluorochromes are used, but a major disadvantage is fading of the fluorescent marker. If one needs to conduct morphometric analysis or some other time-consuming procedure in the analysis of the sections, then it is often preferable to use a more permanent antibody-marking method, such as the immunoperoxidase method (Vandesande 1983).

Adequate controls are crucial for an immunocytochemical investigation. Both positive and negative controls are important. The positive control is usually a tissue that is known to be immunoreactive with the antibody that is being used. Such a control is very important if there is the chance that the antigen in question would be eliminated by some direct or indirect action of the injectable agent. The tissue used for a negative control is usually a serial section to the one used as the real test, and it is commonly placed on the same slide. For the negative control, the primary antibody is omitted, but the secondary antibody is applied to the section. Staining of the negative control section can indicate problems with specificity or cross-reactions with the secondary antibody.

Neuromuscular Staining Methods

Injectable agents can potentially affect the innervation of muscle. There many ways to assess neuromuscular disruption, from electromyography to morphology. Morphological methods of investigation of disturbances of the neuromuscular junction or of nerve fibers themselves are typically either very tedious, very capricious, or both, unless the nerve damage is very gross. Because of either the time and sampling constraints of techniques such as electron microscopy, or the fickle nature of many of the classical silver-based histological nerve stains, morphological methods would normally not be among the first techniques chosen for routine screening for neuromuscular damage.

Procedural Issues

Some staining reactions, such as those for acetylcholinesterase bound to the basal lamina of the neuromuscular junction, are relatively easy to perform and some can even be done on a whole muscle level. However, acetylcholinesterase is a very persistent enzyme that can often give a positive staining reaction even months after the muscle fiber beneath it is destroyed. Some techniques for demonstrating aggregates of acetylcholine receptors (e.g., alpha-bungarotoxin binding) on muscle fibers are moderately easy, but interpretation can be very difficult. This is because even in the absence of innervation, acetylcholine receptors can form and aggregate on a regenerating muscle fiber on the basis of molecular information contained in the basal lamina of the muscle fiber (Hansen-Smith 1986). All the above caveats aside, if, on the basis of preliminary screening, there is reason to suspect damage to the neuromuscular junctions or to axons of the intramuscular nerves themselves, the nature of the pathology can be further investigated by the judicious use of light and electron microscopic methods. Quantitation, however, remains difficult. Such investigations quickly become highly focused research operations for which very specialized techniques must be employed to demonstrate the suspected disturbed processes.

Summary of Strengths and Limitations of Morphological Techniques in Assessing Muscle Damage After Injections

The value and utility of morphological methods, in general, in assessing muscle damage after exposure to injected agents must first be viewed in relation to the strengths and weaknesses of other methods, such as physiological or biochemical measures. Morphological methods are typically more time-consuming than other methods that lend themselves to rapid assessments of the status of muscle. If done properly, the in vivo or in vitro determination of a battery of contractile properties of muscle is an excellent quantitative means of determining the functional capacity of a muscle, but one can only indirectly infer the nature of the damage by such methods. Biochemical methods, like determination of serum CK levels, are rapid and convenient sampling tools, but they are even less precise than physiological methods in allowing determination of the nature of the lesion in muscle. Although highly quantitative, their accuracy in assessing the level of muscle damage in a specific site, rather than throughout the entire body, is sometimes suspect. The principal strength of morphological methods is their ability to determine the nature of structural lesions accurately. Accurate quantitation is both time-consuming and difficult with most morphological methods.

Assuming that the use of morphological techniques is indicated, they should be viewed in two ways—those best suited for first-level screening and those that should be employed for obtaining specific detailed information. The best single technique for first-level screening for muscle damage is the examination of tissue sections stained with hematoxylin and eosin. From the examination of such material one can obtain a wealth of information about the nature of processes occurring at the cell and tissue level in all components of muscle, including the vasculature, innervation, and connective tissue.

Such information can be obtained from examination of suitably stained paraffin or frozen sections. The morphology is usually better in paraffin-embedded tissue, but if histochemical or immunocytochemical information is also desired, it may be more convenient and informative to process serial frozen sections for both hematoxylin and eosin staining and for the desired histochemical reactions. Especially if muscle fiber typing is required or desirable, the use of frozen tissue for the morphological analysis is the most appropriate. Another advantage of frozen sections is speed. With frozen sections, the time from removal to morphological examination can be as little as a few hours to a day, whereas fixation and paraffin embedding methods typically take several days to complete.

Electron microscopy is certainly the method for the finest resolution of morphology, but the major operational drawbacks of this method are the very limited sampling area and the time required from tissue removal to completion of specimen preparation, which is rarely less than a week to 10 days. High cost and the need for technical support are also major drawbacks of electron microscopic examination of tissue. Nevertheless, there are circumstances when only electron microscopic analysis will generate the required information.

Overall, morphological analysis of muscle is most important when one needs to know the cellular nature of a lesion, the response of a muscle to an injected agent or the process of recovery of the damaged muscle. By far, the most effective approach is a combined analysis involving morphological, physiological, and biochemical techniques, where each is used in a manner that exploits its strength.

REFERENCES

Arce, V., F. Brenes, and J. M. Gutierrez. 1991. Degenerative and regenerative changes in murine skeletal muscle after injection of venom from the snake *Bothrops asper*: A histochemical and immunocytochemical study. *Int. J. Exp. Pathol.* 72:211–226.

Basson, M. D., and B. M. Carlson. 1980. Myotoxicity of single and repeated injections of mepivacaine (Carbocaine) in the rat. *Anesth. Analg.* 59:275–282.

Benoit, P. W., and W. D. Belt. 1970. Destruction and regeneration of skeletal muscle after treatment with a local anesthetic, bupivacaine (Marcaine). *J. Anat.* 107:547–556.

Brazeau, G. A., and H.-L. Fung. 1989. Use of an in vitro model for the assessment of muscle damage from intramuscular injections: In vitro–in vivo correlation and predictability with mixed solvent systems. *Pharmaceut. Res.* 6:766–771.

Brooke, M. H., and K. K. Kaiser. 1970. Muscle fibre types: How many and what kind? *Arch. Neurol.* 23:369–379.

Cuello, A. C., ed. 1983. *Immunohistochemistry.* Chichester, UK: John Wiley & Sons.

Dolwick, M. F., F. M. Bush, H. R. Seibel, and G. W. Burke. 1977. Degenerative changes in masseter muscle following injection of lidocaine: A histochemical study. *J. Dent. Res.* 56:1395–1402.

Dubowitz, V. 1985. *Muscle biopsy,* 2nd. ed. London: Bailliere Tindall.

Foster, A. H., and B. M. Carlson. 1980. Myotoxicity of local anesthetics and regeneration of the damaged muscle fibers. *Anesth. Analg.* 58:727–736.

Gray, J. E. 1967. Local histologic changes following intramuscular injections. *Arch. Path.* 84:522–527.

Gutierrez, J. M., G. V. Ownby, and G. V. Odell. 1984. Pathogenesis of myonecrosis induced by crude venom and a myotoxin of *Bothrops asper*. *Exp. Mol. Pathol.* 40:367–379.

Gutmann, E., and B. M. Carlson. 1975. Contractile and histochemical properties of regenerating cross-transplanted fast and slow muscles in the rat. *Pfluegers Arch.* 353:227–239.

Hansen-Smith, F. M. 1986. Formation of acetylcholine receptor clusters in mammalian sternohyoid muscle regenerating in the absence of nerves. *Devel. Biol.* 118:129–140.

Harris, J. B., M. A. Johnson, and E. Karlsson. 1975. Pathological responses of rat skeletal muscle to a single subcutaneous injection of a toxin isolated from the venom of the Australian tiger snake, *Notechis scutatus scutatus. Clin. Exp. Pharmacol. Physiol.* 2:383–404.

Loughlin, M. 1993. *Muscle biopsy. A laboratory investigation. Oxford:* Butterworth-Heinemann.

Luna, L. G. 1968. *Manual of histologic staining methods of the Armed Forces Institute of Pathology,* 3rd. ed. New York: McGraw-Hill.

Maltin, C. A., J. B. Harris, and M. J. Cullen. 1983. Regeneration of mammalian skeletal muscle following the injection of the snake venom toxin, taipoxin. *Cell Tissue Res.* 232:565–577.

Mikel, U. V., ed. 1994. *Armed Forces Institute of Pathology, Advanced laboratory methods in histology and pathology.* Washington, D.C.: American Registry of Pathology.

Řeřabková, L. 1983. Podkoženi kosterního svalu intramuskularním podním protižanetlivych latek pyrazolidinového typu. *Sborník Lekarsky* 85 (6):161–166.

Sarnat, H. B. 1983. Muscle pathology and histochemistry. Chicago: American Society of Clinical Pathologists Press.

Schiaffino, S., and C. Reggiani. 1996. Molecular diversity of myofibrillar proteins: Gene regulation and functional significance. *Physiol. Revs.* 76:371–423.

Steiness, E., F. Rasmussen, O. Svendsen, and P. Nielson. 1978. A comparative study of serum creatine phosphokinase (CPK) activity in rabbits, pigs and humans after intramuscular injection of local damaging drugs. *Acta Pharmacol. et Toxicol.* 42:357–364.

Svendsen, O. 1983. Intramuscular injections and local muscle damage: An experimental study of the effect of injection speed. *Acta Pharmacol. et Toxicol.* 52:305–309.

Vandesande, F. 1983. Peroxidase-antiperoxidase techniques. In *Immunohistochemistry,* edited by A. C. Cuello. Chichester, UK: John Wiley & Sons, pp. 101–119.

10

Conscious Rat Model to Assess Pain Upon Intravenous Injection

John M. Marcek

Animal Health Toxicology
Pharmacia and Upjohn, Inc.
Kalamazoo, Michigan

Many factors must be considered during the course of developing new and innovative pharmaceutical materials. Chief considerations during formulation development include the need to preserve the pharmacologic properties of agents being developed, assessing and improving manufacturing processes, minimization of impurity and by-product formation during manufacturing, minimization of inherent problems associated with solubility and instability of compounds, and the ability of the patient to tolerate the formulation. Additionally, developers must consider the cost-effectiveness of the manufacturing and formulation processes and address marketing concerns for the long-term goals of a particular entity as required by the sponsoring company. Thus, while formulation science may be driven by the physicochemical properties of new entities, many factors outside this realm need to be considered before formulations are finalized. Final product formulations are rarely the best in all of the categories mentioned, but are chosen because they represent the best compromise given such an array of considerations.

It is in this environment that pharmaceutical companies are required to operate. Changes made in formulations throughout the development process have the potential to change formulation characteristics with regard to any of a wide variety of considerations including the effectiveness and/or safety of a compound. Additional safety and efficacy testing is required if the sponsoring company makes formulation changes during development because of the potential effects on efficacy and safety. Additional testing requires additional development expense, both in terms of resources required and delays in product introduction. In today's highly competitive marketplace, delays can have profound effects on both the profitability of the product and, hence, the company. In effect, development delays may cause a company to cease development of a potentially useful compound based on business, not scientific or medical, criteria. Therefore, it is in the best interest of pharmaceutical developers to identify and solve potential formulation problems as early in the development process as possible.

An additional effect of costly delays initiated by a formulation change is the potential to stifle research into new and promising technologies. Additional studies that may be required to demonstrate the safety of new excipients may be bypassed if acceptable, but potentially suboptimal, formulations already exist. In the interest of getting a product to market in acceptable development time, it is tempting to try to fit new compounds into existing and already approved formulations that are more easily accepted by regulatory agencies.

Intravenous (IV) drugs play a very important role in the pharmaceutical armortmentaria. Advantages of IV administration of drugs include rapid absorption and distribution, preclusion of first-pass metabolism, and the fastest onset of systemic pharmacologic effects, as is needed in critical care situations. Antibiotic drugs may be given intravenously to achieve higher blood concentrations than are possible by other routes. Pain in humans has been noted following IV injection of diazepam (Hussey et al. 1990; Siebke et al. 1976), potassium chloride (Pucino et al. 1988), erythromycin lactobionate (Putzi et al. 1983), propofol (Klement and Arndt 1991a), and other anesthetics and sedatives (Kawar and Dundee 1982). While pain upon injection may not be of paramount concern during pharmaceutical development, particularly in the case of life-saving drugs or drugs intended for unmet medical needs, early investigation into the pain-producing potential of formulations may reduce the need for later reformulation and costly delays in development. Competitive advantage may also play a role if a similar product is developed without this unwanted side effect. To this end, we have developed a model that objectively measures the pain or discomfort experienced by laboratory rats following IV administration of new pharmaceutical entities. The objective is to identify superior formulations, in terms of pain-producing potential, early in the preclinical testing phase of IV drug development.

The measurement of pain in animal models has been difficult for researchers to quantitate. Underlying the presumption of animal pain is the assumption that pain responses in animals and humans are identical. That is, if a procedure is painful to humans, it should also be distressing to animals. However, because of the subjectivity of the response and the inability for any direct means of communication with animals, quantification and qualification of pain experiences in animals are inherently difficult to measure. Indeed, pain in man is difficult to measure even with the ability to communicate more directly. Scoring systems, such as the Visual Analog Scale (VAS), have been developed in an effort to quantify pain experiences in humans. However, correlation between VAS scores made simultaneously by trained medical staff and patients was poor (Grossman et al. 1991), and considerable variation was also reported between children's self-report of pain and parent and nurse ratings (Manne et al. 1992). This type of scoring system has been proposed for use in animals. However, due to a lack of specific external indicators of pain and the subjective nature of this system, practical difficulties are associated with its implementation. As already noted, variation in pain assessment among observers can be a common problem.

Because animals are not able to communicate directly, one must rely on behavioral and physiological indices of pain. More objective tests have been developed that rely on behavioral reactions to stimuli that are presumed to be painful to animals. Other tests rely on the experimenter's subjective assessment of an often variable series of responses. Some of the reactions to noxious stimuli that have been used to assess pain reactions include reflexive escape responses (tail-flick test, hot-plate test, pinch test), conscious escape (flinch-jump test), prolonged protective activity (fleeing or fighting), and retreat and withdrawal (Vierck and Cooper 1984). These tests are generally used to measure the efficacy of analgesic compounds and are not specific for pain observed with the IV administration of test substances.

Recent toxicology studies in our laboratory showed that rats reacted to IV infusion of new compounds and/or vehicles by vocalizing and struggling in the restraint tube (Marcek et al. 1992). The rapid onset of signs following the initiation of injection and the disappearance of signs concomitant with the completion of injection led to the interpretation that these signs were an indication of pain caused by the test formulation (active substance and/or vehicle). The objective of the studies discussed here was to develop a screening process to rapidly and objectively evaluate the pain produced during IV administration of new compounds and formulations. Additionally, compounds outside the normal physiologic osmolality and pH range were studied to investigate the contribution of these factors in the elicitation of a pain response. Several compounds known to be painful following IV infusion in humans were also studied to determine the effectiveness of this model in identifying known human irritants as painful when administered intravenously to rats. Finally, the effect of the rate of dose administration was studied to determine its effect on the pain response. A search of the current literature revealed no in vitro model that could be used to study this complex phenomenon.

EXPERIMENTAL PROCEDURES

Rats were cared for and used in accordance with the *Guide for the Care and Use of Laboratory Animals* (DHEW 1985 and subsequent amendments).

Protocols were reviewed and approved by the Corporate Animal Welfare Committee.

Test substances were administered to a rat placed in a large Broome restraint tube (7.5 cm outside diameter) that had been modified to respond to the activity of the rat. The modifications included cutting a slot halfway up the junction between the tube and the end partition, and the addition of an electronic circuit (a strain gauge bridge) on the surface of the tube to monitor the tube's flexion. Flexion of the tube changes the resistance through the strain gauge, resulting in a measurable change in voltage across the strain gauge bridge. Strain gauge output was recorded directly on a personal computer via a data acquisition board and appropriate software. A detailed description of the methodology used can be found elsewhere (Marcek et al. 1992).

In order to distinguish pain induced by dosing solutions from those due to needle stick, a polyethylene cannula (PE-10, Clay Adams, Parsippany, N.J.) was inserted into the lateral tail vein as previously described (Rhodes and Patterson 1979). Rats were allowed to recover after cannula placement prior to injection. Rats were placed in the restraint tube and allowed to become acclimated to the environment. Immediately following the acclimation period, 1 mL of test solution was administered over 1 min. Response to injection was measured by calculating the variance (variation around the mean strain gauge output for each response interval) of the output (10 samples/sec) during the 1 min time period immediately preceding the injection and during the 1 min infusion time period. Because of the possible effects of learning on response, animals were dosed once and were not reused.

Experiment 1

Five groups of 10 male Sprague Dawley rats [Crl:CD(BR), Charles River Laboratories, Portage, Mich; approximately 400 g each] were given a single IV injection of saline control or one of several solutions known to produce clinical signs of pain in rats and/or humans (anecdotal evidence). Substances tested included a sodium acetate vehicle (1 mL contained 2.42 mg sodium acetate, 0.00184 mL glacial acetic acid, 6.955 mg sodium chloride, q.s. ad USP (U.S. Pharmacopeia) Water for Injection, pH adjusted to 4.51 with 10 percent sodium hydroxide), an hydrochloric acid (HCl) vehicle (a 10 percent solution of HCl in USP Water for Injection, sufficient to make a 0.05 N solution, pH 1.3), a citric acid vehicle (1 mL contained 4.5 mg sodium chloride, 0.936 mg sodium citrate, 3.84 mg citric acid in USP Water for Injection, sufficient to make 0.02 M solution, pH 2.8), and 0.1 M potassium chloride (KCl) (1 mL contained 7.45 mg KCl in USP Water for Irrigation, pH 4.7). All reagents used were analytical or reagent grade.

Experiment 2

In order to investigate the sensitivity of the system, 5 groups of 5 male Sprague Dawley rats each received a single IV injection of saline control or 0.0125, 0.025, 0.05, or 0.1 M KCl. Rats were prepared and substances administered as described above.

Experiment 3

The objective of this study was to evaluate the response of rats given an analgesic substance (morphine) prior to exposure to IV administration of a substance known to produce clinical signs of pain (KCl). Two groups of 4 male Sprague Dawley rats were given intraperitoneal injections of morphine sulfate (2 or 4 mg/kg) 15 min before administration of 0.05 M KCl. Two additional groups received no morphine pretreatment prior to administration of saline control or 0.05 M KCl. Rats were prepared and substances administered as described above.

Experiment 4

The objective of this study was to examine the rats' response to IV infusion of solutions of various osmolalities. Five groups of 5 male Sprague Dawley rats each received a single IV injection of a saline solution prepared at concentrations of 0.3 (physiologic saline), 1.0, 2.0, 3.0, or 4.0 osmol/kg at a constant pH (7.4). Rats were prepared and test substances were administered as described above.

Experiment 5

The objective of this study was to examine the rats' response to IV infusions of solutions of various pHs. Five groups of 5 male Sprague Dawley rats each received a single IV injection of a saline solution prepared at pH 3, 5, 7, 9, or 11. Solutions were made with normal saline and pH was adjusted to the desired level by the addition of sodium hydroxide (NaOH) or HCl. Rats were prepared and substances administered as described above.

Experiment 6

The objective of this study was to examine the response to IV infusions of various compounds known to cause pain in humans. Five groups of 5 male Sprague Dawley rats each received a single IV injection of saline control, propofol (Diprivan®, 1 percent, 10 mg/mL, Zeneca Pharmaceuticals, Wilmington, Del.), diazepam (Valium®, 5 mg/mL, Hoffman-LaRoche, Inc.,

Nutley, N.J.), erythromycin lactobionate (8.3 mg/mL, Lederle Parenterals, Inc., Carolina, Puerto Rico), or 0.05 M KCl (positive control). Injection volume was 1 mL with the exception of propofol where 0.5 mL was administered due to toxicologic considerations (LD50, 42 mg/kg [Iswaran et al. 1993]). Rats were prepared and substances administered as described above.

Experiment 7

In order to determine if infusion rate has a potential to influence results, 2 groups of 5 rats were given 2 IV injections of 0.3 osmol/kg saline or 4 osmol/kg saline. The first injection was given over a 60 sec period and was followed by a brief (approximately 5 min) recovery period. The second injection was given over a 30 sec period. The injection volume for both injections was 1 mL.

Statistical Analyses

Preliminary examination of the data from the first experiment indicated departures from normality and heterogeneous variances among treatment groups. Therefore, log transformations were made on data from all experiments, and treatment group differences were analyzed using analysis of variance. For statistically significant variables, treatment groups were compared to the appropriate control group using the least significant difference method. Results from experiment seven were analyzed using a two-way analysis of variance.

RESULTS

Initial examination of the data revealed several potential variables to be considered as the primary indicator of a positive response. Factors considered included the area under the curve (AUC), frequency of peaks, and variance of the data set. AUC was determined not to be an accurate measure of the responsiveness of an individual, since the body position of the animal within the restraint tube, and the ability of the animal to shift and change its position at any point during the pretreatment or infusion period, could induce a change in the baseline output. Changes in baseline values would result in altered AUC measurement, leading to incorrect interpretation of the data. Frequency of peaks as a response variable was rejected due to inadequate definition of peaks. Animals that reacted positively to infusion of the test material struggled in the tube as a result of the discomfort and pain of the injection. Increased movement caused fluctuation in output and a concomitant increase in variance of the data set. Therefore, variance (variation of the data set around the mean strain gauge output for each response interval) was a more accurate indicator of the rat's reaction to administration of the test substance than the other variables. Typical negative (0.3 osmol/kg saline) and positive (4 osmol/kg saline) individual responses are presented in Figure 10.1.

Mean output variance for each dose group in the first experiment is presented in Figure 10.2. No difference was observed between treated and control groups during the pretreatment period ($p = 0.6216$). No increase in variance was observed in the saline-treated group when pretreatment variance was compared to infusion period variance ($p = 0.07$—analysis of the change in response using a single sample paired ttest). This suggests that

Figure 10.1. Response of rats 21 and 42 to infusion of 1 mL of 0.3 osmol/ kg and 4 osmol/kg saline, respectively. The top line represents the event marker and indicates the beginning of the pretreatment period and the beginning and end of the infusion period.

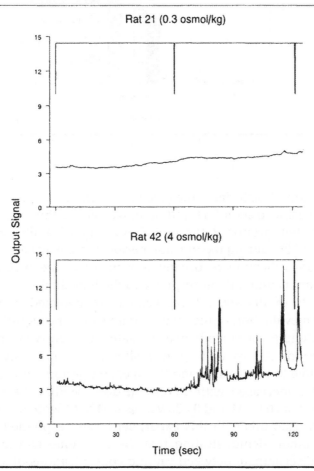

Figure 10.2. Mean variance of strain gauge output for the first experiment. Time period refers to pretreatment (Pretrt) and infusion periods (Infusion). Bars with different letters differ ($p < 0.01$). From Marcek et al. (1992), reprinted with permission from Plenum Publishing Corp.

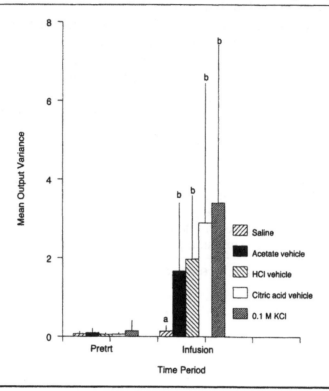

the act of infusion of material at the given rate was not perceived as an unusual effect causing discomfort and/or movement within the tube. Variance of treatment groups 2 through 5 was significantly greater than controls ($p = 0.0006$) during the infusion period. Increased variance was interpreted as an indication of greater movement in the tube due to increased discomfort and pain in response to the injection.

The results of the second experiment are depicted graphically in Figure 10.3. An evaluation of the results again shows no significant difference in strain gauge variance between treatment groups during the pretreatment period. All treated groups show a significantly increased response relative to controls during the injection period, and the intensity of the response increased with increasing dose. Within the KCl–treated groups, 0.10 versus 0.05 M and 0.025 versus 0.0125 M were not statistically different from each other. In this experiment, rats responded in a dose-dependent manner, demonstrating that the technique had an adequate sensitivity to discriminate between varying concentrations of an irritating

Figure 10.3. Mean variance of strain gauge output for the second experiment. Bars with different letters differ ($p < 0.05$). From Marcek et al. (1992), reprinted with permission from Plenum Publishing Corp.

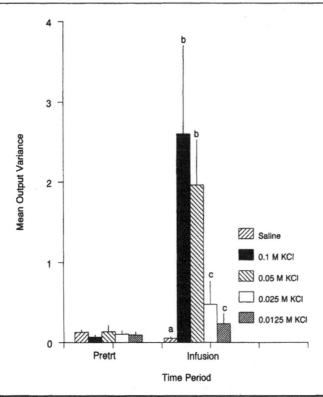

material. Based on these results, the positive control dose was changed to 0.05 M KCl.

The results of experiment three are depicted graphically in Figure 10.4. No significant differences in strain gauge variance between treatment groups was observed during the pretreatment period. A significant treatment response was noted for rats given 0.05 M KCl when compared to controls. Rats in both morphine-treated groups showed no significant difference from controls during the treatment period, and the response of both groups was significantly lower than that of KCl–treated rats. These results demonstrate that the administration of morphine ablates or reduces the sensation responsible for increased activity following IV administration of KCl.

The results of experiment four are shown in Figure 10.5. As in other studies, no significant differences were observed in strain gauge variance between treatment groups during the pretreatment period. A numerical increase in mean variance was noted at all dose concentrations relative

Figure 10.4. Mean variance of strain gauge output for experiment three. Bars with different letters differ ($p < 0.05$). From Marcek et al. (1992), reprinted with permission from Plenum Publishing Corp.

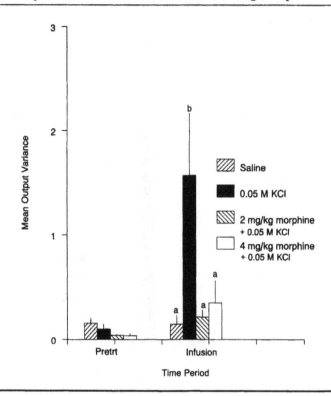

to 0.3 osmol/kg saline; however, responses were not dose dependent. Significant responses relative to 0.3 osmol/kg saline were observed at 2, 3, and 4 osmol/kg. The results of this experiment indicate that a threshold response exists and that the threshold was identified.

The results of experiment five are shown in Figure 10.6. No significant differences were observed in strain gauge variance between treatment groups during the pretreatment period. The results show no increase in strain gauge variance during the infusion period at any pH level tested.

The results of experiment six are shown in Figure 10.7. No significant differences were observed in strain gauge variance between treatment groups during the pretreatment period. Positive and negative control materials (0.05 M KCl and saline, respectively) performed as expected in the infusion period. Changes in strain gauge output were evident in 3 of 5 animals treated with propofol while anesthetic effects (lethargy, somnolence) were more apparent in the 2 animals that did not respond (see Figure 10.8). No evidence of an increase in strain gauge output variability was

Figure 10.5. Mean variance of strain gauge output for experiment four. Bars with different letters differ ($p < 0.05$).

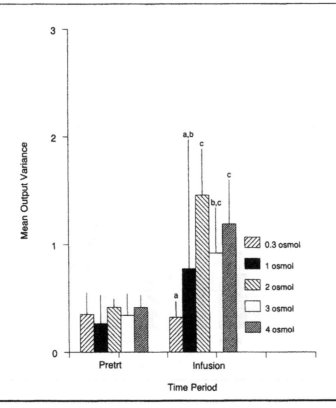

noted during the infusion period for rats treated with diazepam. Transient changes in output were noted in most diazepam-treated animals; however, responses lasted only a brief period. Anesthetic effects were noted beginning approximately 30 sec into the infusion period and were profound by the completion of infusion (1 min) (see Figure 10.9). A positive pain response was noted in all rats treated with erythromycin, resulting in a significant increase in strain gauge variance.

The results of experiment seven are shown in Figure 10.10. No differences were observed in strain gauge variance between treatment groups during the pretreatment period, and no difference was observed in response to 0.3 osmol/kg saline administered over the 2 time periods. Strain gauge variance was increased when 4 osmol/kg saline was administered over a 30 sec interval relative to a 60 sec interval; however, the change was not statistically significant (time effect $p = 0.7813$).

Figure 10.6. Mean variance of strain gauge output for experiment five.

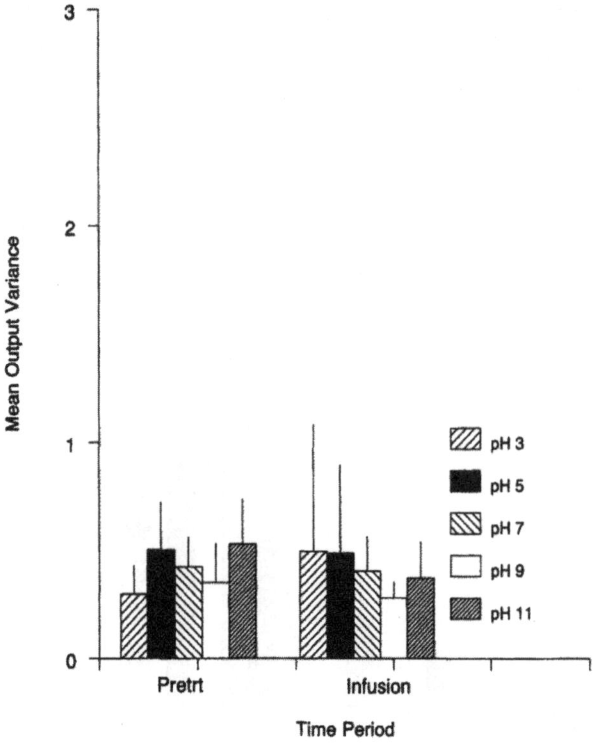

DISCUSSION

The results of experiments one through three have been reported previously (Marcek et al. 1992) and are included here as the basis for validating the conscious rat IV pain model. The results demonstrate (1) the ability of the model and the statistical analysis used to measure objectively the pain response to intravenously administered substances, (2) the ability of the model to discriminate between varying concentrations of a material known to cause pain when administered intravenously, and (3) the absence of a pain response following administration of a known centrally acting analgesic. In order to provide further evidence of the usefulness of this model, the additional studies described were conducted.

Experiments four and five were conducted to examine some of the physicochemical properties of compounds and formulations. Unphysiologic osmolality and pH have been demonstrated to cause pain following injection in isolated vein segments in humans (Klement and Arndt 1991b). The results of current studies with the conscious rat IV pain model did not

Figure 10.7. Mean variance of strain gauge output for experiment 6. Bars with different letters differ ($p < 0.05$).

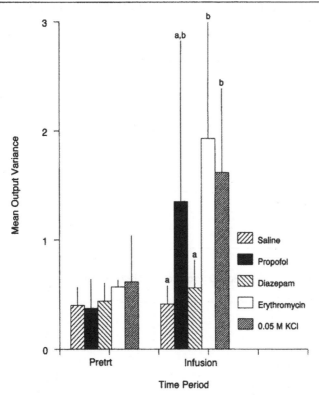

duplicate the isolated human vein segment results; however, positive results were obtained following IV administration of solutions with osmolality above 2 osmol/kg, similar to results obtained following injection of hyperosmolar solutions in humans (Klement and Arndt 1991b). A lack of further increase in response variance to solutions above 2 osmol/kg indicates that the pain threshold was achieved; however, dilution of test solutions in tail vein blood probably occurred rapidly enough and to the extent that further increases in response were not seen. Similarly, the use of intact and not isolated vein segments, can explain why no response to solutions of various pHs was observed. The high buffering capacity of blood rapidly neutralized the effect of saline, which has minimal buffering capacity at any pH.

The conscious rat IV pain model was not modified in any way in order to attempt to isolate the vein segment to be used. Modifications made in studies using isolated vein segments in humans (Klement and Arndt 1991b) included insertion of two Teflon® cannulae into a vein segment

Figure 10.8. Response of rats 6 and 10 to infusion of 0.5 mL of propofol (10 mg/mL). The top line represents the event marker and indicates the beginning of the pretreatment period and the beginning and end of the infusion period.

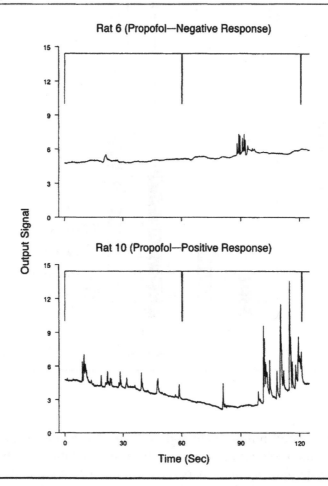

between two valves on the dorsal side of the hand. The vein segment between the cannulae was isolated from the systemic circulation by external occluders, and the hand was raised above the level of the heart to further minimize blood flow. Physiologic saline was infused into the isolated vein segment to simulate flow in a normally patent vein. Modification of the conscious rat IV pain model to attempt to mimic those conditions would likely require further restraint of the rat in order to prevent the animal's movement from disturbing occluding devices or other equipment necessary to maintain an isolated segment. Further restraint of the subject is

Figure 10.9. Response of rat 15 to infusion of 1 mL of diazepam (5 mg/mL). The top line represents the event marker and indicates the beginning of the pretreatment period and the beginning and end of the infusion period.

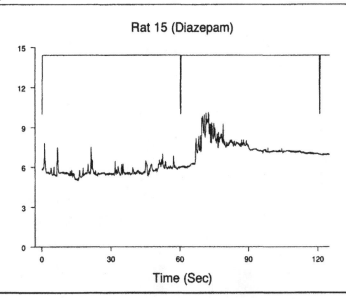

unacceptable, since the movement induced by IV injection is the primary response variable. Similarly, the size of the cannulae used is sufficient to occlude the majority of blood flow through the lateral tail vein; therefore, test materials should be in close contact with the vein wall for sufficient time to allow nociceptive responses. The results of experiments four and five suggest that, although the lateral tail vein may be significantly occluded, collateral veins can provide sufficient volume for dilution of test materials, and the potent buffering capacity of blood may exceed the ability of the test solutions used to elicit a response.

While use of an isolated vein segment appears to have some advantage over the conscious rat IV pain model, disadvantages of this technique also exist. Beyond the likely further restraint required to maintain an isolated vein segment as mentioned above, the use of this preparation does not allow for an assessment of reactions to formulations as they would be encountered in preclinical or clinical settings. Therefore, while the use of an isolated vein segment may be advantageous in investigating components of the pain response, the conscious rat model may be better suited to assess reactions in a complete, physiologically whole setting where dilution and buffering of test substance by blood occurs. Additionally, the use of a relatively small vein in the conscious rat model provides a worst-case

Figure 10.10. Mean variance of strain gauge output for experiment seven.

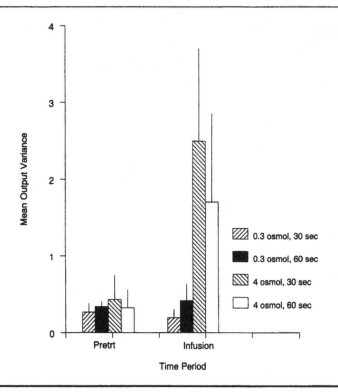

scenario, ensuring maximal contact between the test material and the vein wall. Many currently used IV formulations specify use in larger or central veins in order to minimize pain and/or thrombotic effects.

Experiment six was conducted to examine the performance of the conscious rat IV pain model following IV injection of various compounds known to cause pain in humans. Administration of propofol or diazepam did not increase mean strain gauge variance above that of the negative control. These negative results are most likely due to the rapid onset of anesthetic effects of the test materials in rats. Lack of motor activity and flat strain gauge ouput tracings were observed following dose administration in most propofol-treated and all diazepam-treated rats. Closer examination of individual animal results revealed positive responses (changes in strain gauge output) in 3 of 5 rats treated with propofol, as well as transient responses in several diazepam-treated rats (see Figures 10.8 and 10.9). It is tempting to consider these positive and/or transient responses as the result of pain experienced by the animal prior to anesthetic effect, and thus draw some correlation between human and animal experience. However, excitatory effects have been reported during induction of anesthesia in up to

20 percent of patients receiving propofol (Mackenzie and Grant 1985), and paradoxical stimulation has been reported during IV administration of diazepam (Ashton 1994). Therefore, it is not possible to distinguish between pain experienced by the animal, or excitatory effects brought on by systemic administration of these two test materials.

Results of IV administration of erythromycin lactobionate appear more clear, with all animals showing evidence of changes in strain gauge output during the infusion period. However, it is not possible to rule out systemic effects of the test material, since abdominal cramps and nausea have been reported during dose administration in humans (Putzi et al. 1983, Siefert et al. 1989). If similar side effects are experienced by rats, changes in strain gauge output would be expected. It should be noted that infusion time was substantially longer in humans (10–30 min) than in the current study and that gastrointestinal side effects were not noted until some time after the completion of infusion (Siefert et al. 1989). These observations support the idea that the increase in variance observed in rats was in response to painful stimuli of the stimuli.

Experiment seven was conducted to determine if the rate of infusion of a solution known to be irritating in the conscious rat IV pain model has the potential to affect responses. Positive responses were observed in 5 of 5 rats following infusion of 4 osmol/kg saline for 30 sec and in 3 of 5 rats following infusion of 4 osmol/kg saline for 60 sec. Strain gauge variance was substantially greater after the 30 sec infusion relative to the 60 sec infusion; however, the increase was not statistically significant. No difference in response at the 2 infusion times was observed for rats treated with 0.3 osmol/kg saline, indicating that potential stetching of the lateral tail vein with possible activation of mechanoreceptors in the vein wall did not contribute to the change in response.

APPLICATIONS

Development of a rapid, inexpensive, and effective screen for the assessment of the pain produced by new compounds and formulations would enhance pharmaceutical development by providing information affecting the acceptability, and potentially the development course, of a new product. While a great many factors need to be considered in choosing a potential drug candidate and during the candidate's formulation development, it would be a great advantage to gather information on the pain-producing potential of new materials early in the development process. Results of current studies with the conscious rat IV pain model discussed here indicate where this model may be used to best advantage should formulation alternatives exist.

The results of the current studies revealed further characteristics of the conscious rat IV pain model that should be understood if the model is to be successfully employed. Studies with solutions of unphysiologic osmolality and pH show that systemic administration of materials can be affected by dilution and the buffering capacity of blood. Additionally, infusion of materials known to be painful in humans illustrates that the time period involved for infusion allows for demonstration of systemic or side effects of test materials.

These factors appear to limit the applicability of this model to basic pain research and attempts to elucidate the mechanisms of action involved in pain perception. However, these factors do not preclude the use of the model in an applied setting, where the objective may be to provide information on the total effect of new compounds and formulations or to provide comparisons between materials. For these reasons, it may be best to consider using the conscious rat IV pain model in a preclinical setting, where tolerance of animals to formulations and successful multiple administrations of test formulations are required.

The objective measurement of pain in animals is problematic for researchers not only from the scientific perspective but also from moral and ethical perspectives as. One benefit of the conscious rat IV pain model is its ability to limit pain experienced by animals during preclinical drug development trials. Early consideration and selection of the best test formulation may limit the pain experienced by a significant number of animals used to assess the safety and efficacy of a new material prior to its introduction to humans. Public opinion and government regulations are becoming more concerned with the number of animals used for the development of pharmaceutical materials, as well as the types of experiences animals undergo. The use of this model with a relatively small number of animals would provide evidence of the intent of the industry to minimize the pain and distress experienced by animals during drug development. Thus, public relations for the industry as a whole would benefit from improved perception of researchers as individuals who are committed to the best use of the resources available.

SUMMARY AND CONCLUSIONS

The results of these experiments indicate that the pain response observed in the conscious rat pain model objectively measures reactions to IV injection of test substances. However, since systemic exposure to test materials does occur, buffering and dilution effects of blood, systemic effects of test compounds, and the rate of IV infusion all need to be considered in interpreting results. Use of this model may best serve in selecting formulations to pursue in preclinical settings, where tolerance of animals to formulations and successful multiple administrations of test formulations are required. These studies also show limitations in the ability of the rat IV pain model to predict responses in humans accurately.

ACKNOWLEDGMENTS

The author gratefully acknowledges William Seaman for his guidance and support, R. John Weaver for statistical analyses, and David Gleason and Larry Jones for their excellent technical assistance. This research was funded through Pharmacia and Upjohn, Inc.

REFERENCES

Ashton, H. 1994. Guidelines for the rational use of benzodiazepines. *Drugs* 48:25–40.

DHEW. 1985. *Guide for the care and use of laboratory animals*. Publication (NIH) 85-23 and subsequent amendments. Departmnet of Health, Education, and Welfare. Washington, DC.

Grossman, S. A., V. R. Sheidler, K. Swedeen, J. Mucenski, and S. Piantadosi. 1991. Correlation of patient and caregiver ratings of cancer pain. *J. Pain and Symptom Manage.* 6:53–57.

Hussey, E. K., G. E. Dukes, J. A. Messenheimer, K. L. R. Brouwer, K. H. Donn, T. F. Krol, and L. J. Hak. 1990. Correlation of delayed peak concentration with infusion-site irritation following diazepam administration. *DICP Ann. Pharmacother.* 24:678–681.

Iswaran, T. J., N. Izumi, P. G. Morrissey, and M. Wormald. 1993. Studies on single dose and multiple dose administration of propofol to animals. *Jpn. Pharmacol. Ther.* 21:11–26.

Kawar, P., and J. W. Dundee. 1982. Frequency of pain on injection and venous sequelae following the I.V. administration of certain anaesthetics and sedatives. *Br. J. Anaesth.* 54:935–938.

Klement, W., and J. O. Arndt. 1991a. Pain on injection of propofol: Effects of concentration and diluent. *Br. J. Anaesth.* 67:281–284.

Klement, W., and J. O. Arndt. 1991b. Pain on I.V. injection of some anaesthetic agents is evoked by the unphysiological osmolality or pH of their formulations. *Br. J. Anaesth.* 66:189–195.

Mackenzie, N., and I. S. Grant. 1985. Comparison of propofol with methohexitone in the provision of anesthesia for surgery under regional blockade. *Br. J. Anaesth.* 57:1167–1172.

Manne, S. L., P. B. Jacobsen, and W. H. Redd. 1992. Assessment of acute pediatric pain: Do child self-report, parent ratings and nurse ratings measure the same phenomenon? *Pain* 48:45–52.

Marcek, J. M., W. J. Seaman, and R. J. Weaver. 1992. A novel approach for the determination of the pain-producing potential of intravenously injected substances in the conscious rat. *Pharm. Res.* 9:182–186.

Pucino, F., B. D. Danielson, J. D. Carlson, G. L. Strommen, P. R. Walker, C. L. Beck, D. J. Thiege, and D. S. Gill. 1988. Patient tolerance to intravenous potassium chloride with and without lidocaine. *Drug Intell. Clin. Pharm.* 22:676–679.

Putzi, R., J. Blaser, R. Lüthy, R. Wehrli, and W. Siegenthaler. 1983. Side-effects due to the intravenous infusion of erythromycin lactobionate. *Infection* 11:161–163.

Rhodes, M. L., and C. E. Patterson. 1979. Chronic intravenous infusion in the rat: A nonsurgical approach. *Lab. Anim. Sci.* 29:82–84.

Siebke, H., B. B. Ellertsen, and B. Lind. 1976. Reactions to intravenous injections of diazepam. *Br. J. Anaesth.* 48:1187–1189.

Siefert, C. F., R. J. Swaney, and R. A. Bellanger-McCleery. 1989. Intravenous erythromycin lactobionate-induced severe nausea and vomiting. *DICP Ann. Pharmacother.* 23:40–44.

Vierck, C. J. Jr., and B. Y. Cooper. 1984. Guidelines for assessing pain reactions and pain modulation in laboratory animal subjects. In *Advances in pain research and therapy,* vol. 6, edited by L. Kruger and J. C. Liebeskind. New York: Raven Press, pp. 305–322.

Section C

APPROACHES IN THE DEVELOPMENT OF LESS-PAINFUL AND LESS-IRRITATING INJECTABLES

11

Cosolvent Use in Injectable Formulations

Susan L. Way

Boehringer Ingelheim Pharmaceuticals, Inc.
Ridgefield, Connecticut

Gayle Brazeau

University of Florida
Gainesville, Florida

Formulators today must routinely deal with progressively more water-insoluble compounds. This makes developing solution dosage forms particularly challenging. Identification and utilization of clinically acceptable excipients—as well as scalable methods to formulate solubilized compounds—has been, and continues to be, a subject of great importance to formulation scientists.

One of the most common approaches used in parenteral formulation of water-insoluble compounds is the use of organic cosolvent systems. These systems utilize certain organic solvents combined with physiologically compatible aqueous solutions. These systems are primarily used to provide higher solubility for poorly water-soluble compounds, which allows for these compounds to be administered in solution form. The ability to administer compounds in solution form by the parenteral route eliminates particle size considerations and dissolution barriers, generally providing for complete bioavailability of poorly absorbed and/or highly metabolized compounds by avoiding hepatic first-pass effects. Cosolvents may also be used to improve the chemical stability of compounds prone to hydrolytic or photolytic degradation, or occasionally to decrease the aqueous solubility of a given compound when administered intramuscularly. There are numerous products on the market for parenteral use that utilize cosolvent systems. Table 11.1 lists a number of these products with their cosolvent compositions (Trissel 1996).

Table 11.1. Cosolvent Composition of Selected Marketed and Investigational Parenteral Products (Trissel 1996)

General Name	Trade Name	Manufacturer	Route	Cosolvent Composition
Digoxin	Lanoxin®	Burroughs Wellcome	IM, IV	40% PG, 10% EtOH, pH 6.8
Trimethoprim-sulfamethoxazole	Septra®	Glaxo Wellcome	IV	40% PG, 10% EtOH, 0.3% diethanolamine, 1% BA
Phenytoin	Dilantin®	Parke-Davis	IV	40% PG, 10% EtOH, pH 12
Diazepam	Valium®	Roche	IM, IV	40% PG, 10% EtOH, 1.5% BA
Lorazepam	Ativan®	Wyeth-Ayerst	IV	41% PG, 9% PEG 400, 2% BA
Pentobarbital	Nembutal®	Abbott	IV	40% PG, 10% EtOH, pH 9.5
Chlordiazepoxide HCl	Librium®	Roche	IM	20% PG, 1.5% BA
Etoposide	VePesid®	Bristol-Myers Squibb	IV	65% PG, 30.5% EtOH, 8% Tween 80®, 3% BA
Miconazole	Monistat®	Janssen	IV	11.5% Cremophor® EL
Secobarbital sodium	Tubex® cartridge	Wyeth-Ayerst	IM, IV	50% PEG, pH 9.5-10.5
Nitroglycerin	Nitro-Bid®	Hoechst Marion Roussel, Abbott	IV	70% EtOH, 4.5% PG
Multivitamins	M.V.I.®-12	Astra	IV	30% PG, 1.6% Tween 80®, 0.028% Tween 20®
Investigational Compounds				
9-Amino-camptothecin			IV	2% DMA, 50% PEG 400
Bryostatin			IV	60% PEG 400, 30% dehydrated alcohol, 10% Tween 80®
Diaziqoune			IV	10% DMA, pH 6.5

Abbreviations: IV: Intravenous; IM: Intramuscular; PG: propylene glycol; PEG: polyethylene glycol; EtOH: ethanol; BA: benzyl alcohol; DMA: dimethylacetamide

In terms of solubility enhancement, the use of cosolvents is one of the most powerful methods available to formulators. The solubilizing potential of cosolvents compares very favorably to other generally accepted techniques used for solubilization of water-insoluble compounds, including micellar solubilization, complexation, prodrugs, and salt formation. In many instances, cosolvents may be the technique of choice for parenteral applications given that (1) micellarization using surface active agents could likely be problematic from an irritation/toxicity perspective, (2) suitable complexing agents may not be appropriate for the compound of interest, (3) formation of either prodrugs or salt forms may not be possible for a given compound, and (4) appropriate cosolvent vehicle selection may reduce tissue irritation.

Numerous factors must be considered before a cosolvent system is selected. Ideally, the water-miscible organic solvent must be nontoxic; should cause minimal or no hemolysis, irritation, or muscle damage on injection; and should be nonsensitizing. The solvent should also be devoid of any inherent pharmacological activity that may interfere with that of the drug itself. Obviously, the cosolvent formulation should provide the desired pharmaceutical/biopharmaceutical profiles and should allow for a reasonable shelf life following manufacture. These solvents are rarely used undiluted due in part to their inherent properties, for example, viscosity and tonicity. Therefore, the physicochemical properties of the cosolvent system must also be considered (viscosity, pH, lipophilicity), as well as the safety of the various solvents used. A summary of some of the physicochemical properties of common solvents used in parenteral formulations is given in Table 11.2.

Ideally, it is best to select and use solvents that would maximize the solubility of the compound. Maximizing the solubility of a compound in a particular cosolvent system would result in lower total levels of the nonaqueous solvent(s) being administered to the patient, thereby lowering the chance for potential side effects. This will also reduce the chance of precipitation of the solution on administration, which is a major concern when administering doses via the IV route. There are numerous reports in the literature regarding cosolvency theory, and potentially useful methods based on various physicochemical properties for predicting solubilities in various solvents and solvent mixtures, as well as the effects of cosolvent systems on the physicochemical properties of compounds solubilized in them (Hildebrand 1916, 1917, 1919; Hildebrand and Scott 1950; Higuchi et al. 1953; Edmonson and Goyan 1958; Moore 1958; Paruta et al. 1962, 1964; Gorman and Hall 1964; Fedors 1974; Martin et al. 1980, 1982; Yalkowsky et al. 1976; Martin and Miralles 1982; Yalkowsky and Roseman 1981; Rubino and Yalkowsky 1985, 1987; Yalkowsky and Rubino 1985; Rubino et al. 1984; Rubino 1987, 1990; Rubino and Berryhill 1986; Rajagopalan et al. 1988; Grisson et al. 1993; Bendas et al. 1995; Darwish and Bloomfield 1995; Vitkova et

Table 11.2. Physicochemical Parameters for Commonly Used Organic Solvents (at 25°C)

Solvent	Molecular Weight (g)	Dielectric Constant, ε	Solubility Parameter, δ (cal/cm^3)	Density (g/mL)	Boiling Point (°C)	Interfacial Tension (dyne/cm)
DMF	73	36.7[a]	12.1[a]	0.94[b]	153[b]	6.9[a]
DMA	87	37.8[a]	10.8[a]	0.94[b]	165[b]	4.6[a]
PEG 400	380–420	13.6[a]	11.3[a]	1.13[c]	—	11.7[a]
EtOH	46	24.3[a]	12.7[a]	0.79[b]	78.5[b]	0.5[a]
PG	76	32.0[a](20°)	12.6[a]	1.04[b]	189[b]	12.4[a]
Benzyl alcohol	108	13.1[d]	—	1.04[b]	204.7[b]	—
Glycerin	92	42.5[a]	17.7[a]	1.26[b]	290[b] (dec)	32.7[a]
Water	18	78.5[a]	23.4[a]	1.00[b]	100[b]	45.6[a]
DMSO	78	46.7[a]	—	1.10[a]	189[a]	—

Dec: decomposition
a: Rubino and Yalkowsky (1987)
b: Budavari (1989)
c: Wade and Weller (1994)
d: Weast and Tuve (1967)

al. 1995). Therefore, this chapter focuses more on the conventional solvents and use levels encountered in parenteral dosage forms, safety/toxicity of these cosolvents, and ways in which to minimize cosolvent-related side effects.

COMMONLY USED SOLVENTS

There are numerous solubilizing agents available to formulators, particularly for use in preclinical work. However, the solubilizers available to formulators for use in humans are considerably more limited, usually on the basis of available safety/toxicity data. The most common organic solvents encountered in cosolvent systems for human clinical/commercial use include PEG 400, PG, glycerol, and ethanol. In general, these solvents are considered to possess a low order of toxicity. This is essential, and obvious, since parenteral administration can result in fairly large amounts of these solvents being placed in the body over a short period of time.

Although the solvents used in cosolvent formulations are generally considered to be of low orders of toxicity, there have been numerous reports of adverse effects related to the vehicles themselves (Carpenter 1947;

Wang and Kowal 1980; Singh et al. 1982; Smith and Dodd 1982; American Academy of Pediatrics Committee on Drugs 1985; Demey et al. 1988; Golightly et al. 1988; Lolin et al. 1988; Andersen et al. 1989; Napke and Stevens 1990; Doenicke et al. 1992; Rhodes et al. 1993; Windebank et al. 1994; Farooqui et al. 1995). These adverse effects may result from administration of high doses of a single cosolvent formulation or concurrent administration of different formulations that contain similar cosolvent systems. It is important to note that any side effects associated with these usually well-tolerated solvent systems may be much more serious when administered to pediatric patients (Sweet 1958; Martin and Finberg 1970; Brown et al. 1982; Gershanik et al. 1982, Lorch et al. 1985; MacDonald et al. 1987; Huggon et al. 1990). Summaries of single dose LD_{50} values and reported human exposures for organic solvents commonly used in parenteral formulations are presented in Tables 11.3 and 11.4. It has been suggested that these solvents should be used at levels of no more than 25 percent of the LD_{50} value in order to avoid any unwanted pharmacological or toxicological effects, although they may be used at considerably higher concentrations depending on the purpose of the study (Bartsch et al. 1976). Others recommend that certain organic solvents should not be used in pharmacological or toxicological studies at concentrations above 10 percent (Singh et al. 1982). The following discussion addresses the reported safety/toxicity data reported in the literature for many of the solvents used in parenteral formulations.

Polyethylene Glycols

PEGs are polymers of ethylene oxide with the general formula

$$HO\text{-}CH_2\text{-}(CH_2\text{-}O\text{-}CH_2)_n\text{-}CH_2OH$$

where n represents the number of oxyethylene groups. The PEGs are designated by a numerical value, which is indicative of the average molecular weight for a given grade. Molecular weights below 600 are liquids, and molecular weights above 1,000 are solids at room temperature. These polymers are readily soluble in water, which make them quite useful for parenteral dosage forms. Only PEG 400 and PEG 300 are utilized in parenteral products, typically at concentrations up to 30 percent (v/v) (Wade and Weller 1994). These polymers are generally regarded as nontoxic and nonirritating. There are numerous reviews regarding the pharmaceutical and toxicological properties of these polyols (Smyth et al. 1950; Rowe and Wolf 1982).

PEGs have been shown to possess marked central nervous system (CNS) effects following IV administration (Lockard and Levy 1978; Lockard et al. 1979). Klugmann and coworkers (1984) found that pretreatment of mice with 15 percent PEG 400 at 20 mL/kg given three hours prior to the

Table 11.3. Single Dose LD$_{50}$ Values in Rodents for Various Organic Solvents Commonly Encountered in Parenteral Formulations

	Parenteral LD$_{50}$ Values (g/kg) for Various Species						
	Mouse			Rat			References
Solvent	ip	sc	iv	ip	sc	iv	
PEG 300				17		7.1	Rowe and Wolf (1982); Carpenter and Shaffer (1952)
PEG 400	13.2–14.5		8.6	12.3–14.7		4.7–7.3	Budden et al. (1978); Rowe and Wolf (1982); Bartsch et al. (1976)
PG	9.6–11.4	18.5	6.6–8.0	6.7–13.5		6.4–6.8	Davis and Jenner (1959); Bartsch et al. (1976); Latven and Molitor (1939)
EtOH	1.2–3.2	8.3–10.5	2.0–2.5	4.1–5.0		1.4–1.8	Latven and Molitor (1939); Bartsch et al. (1976); Trèmolières and Lowy (1964)
Glycerin	8.7–9.0	0.09–10.0	4.3–6.2	8.7	0.10	5.6	Budden et al. (1978); Latven et al. (1939); Anderson et al. (1950); Bartsch et al (1976); Tao et al. (1983)
DMA	2.3–3.5		2.5–3.0	2.8–4.4	5.3	2.6–4.8	Davis and Jenner (1959); Sherman et al. (1978), Bartsch et al. (1976); Auclair and Hameau (1964); Wiles and Narcisse (1971); Thiersch (1962)
DMF	1.2–5.9		2.8–3.5	4.4–6.1	6.1	2.8–5.7	Davis and Jenner (1959); Bartsch et al. (1976); Auclair and Hameau (1964); Wiles and Narcisse (1964); Theirsch (1962)
Cremophor® EL			2.6-4.2				BASF (1988)
DMSO	2.5–13.9		3.4–7.6	8.2–10.1		5.4–8.1	Bartsch et al (1976); Wiles and Narcisse (1971); Willson et al. (1965)
BA	1.0		< 0.52			0.05– 0.08	McCloskey et al. (1986);
0.9%			> 52			> 41.6	Kimura et al (1971)

Table 11.4. Human Exposures to Selected Organic Solvents Commonly Encountered in Parenteral Formulations

Solvent	Dose	Route	Administered As	Clinical Observations	References
DMSO	1 gm/kg	IV	10 to 40% solutions	Hemoglobinuria observed following administration of 20–40% solutions, which cleared within 2–3 h post-infusion: No indication of short-term nephrotoxicity following evaluation of beta-2-microglobulin.	Bennett and Muther (1981)
DMA	100–610 mg/kg/day for 2–5 days	IV	10% solution administered over 5 to 10 min	Dose-related side effects included nausea and vomiting within 14 h of administration, anorexia; liver toxicity as indicated by increased SGOT levels (5–7 days after start of therapy), returning to normal within 2–5 days after achieving peak levels; altered CNS function—depression, lethargy, confusion, hallucinations—returning to normal within several days after therapy; hypotension and high fever observed at high doses.	Weiss et al. (1962)
Cremo-phor® EL	2–20 mL	IV	Incremental doses administered every 4 min, each over a 30 sec period	Small transient fall in blood pressure and rise in pulse rate following each dose. No marked changes in respiratory rate and no consistent alterations in central venous pressure observed. Statistically significant effects only observed after the 20 mL dose.	Savege et al. (1973)
PG	5–21 g/day	IV	Administered as an infusion over a 4 h period	No alterations in plasma osmolality, free hemoglobin, or haptoglobin.	Speth et al. (1987)
BA	130–405 mg/kg/day	IV	0.9% BA (bacteriostatic concentration)	*Neonates:* Progressive metabolic acidosis, bradycardia, gasping respirations, seizures, and subsequent death in low birth weight neonates. *Adults:* No clinically significant changes observed in healthy males (hematology, vital signs, electrocardiograms, EEG, laboratory parameters), shown to be as well tolerated as same formulation preserved with parabens.	Brown et al. (1982); Santiero (1989); Evens (1975); Gershanik (1982); Novak et al. (1972)

administration of adriamycin (a potent antineoplastic agent) resulted in alleviation of some of the toxicity associated with the compound. They also showed that PEG 400 decreased both the acute high-dose and chronic low-dose adriamycin-associated lethality, as well as afforded protection against cardiomyopathy—one of the dose-limiting side effects observed in patients. Additionally, PEG 400 did not interfere with the antitumor activity of the compound. Laine et al. (1995) reported nephrotoxicity due to PEG 400 secondary to chronic high-dose intravenous administration of lorazepam.

PEG 300, PEG 400, and PEG 4000 administered intraperitoneally have been shown to have adverse effects on rat gastrointestinal physiology (Cho et al. 1992). The PEGs caused a decrease in gastric mucosal blood flow (GMBF) as well as gastric secretory function. They also exacerbated ethanol-induced gastric damage in a dose-dependent manner. The gastric damage appeared to be inversely related to molecular weight (PEG 300 > PEG 400 > PEG 4000). Other investigators have shown that the PEGs affect cardiovascular and autonomic systems. PEG 300, PEG 400, and PEG 600 administered intravenously and intra-arterially to dogs produced a dose-dependent enhancement of the blood pressure response to epinephrine and acetylcholine (Heilman et al. 1972). PEG 300 has also been implicated as the causative agent responsible for fatalities and near fatalities due to severe metabolic acidosis in patients (Sweet 1958).

Smith and Cadwallader (1967) evaluated the behavior of erythrocytes in PEG–water solutions. They observed that solutions of PEG 300 in water were hemolytic. They also observed that solutions of water–PEG 400 or water–PEG 600 could afford some protection from hemolysis. They concluded that polyethylene glycols could protect both rabbit and human erythrocytes in the order (MW): 200 < 300 < 400 < 600. The ability of the PEGs to contribute to the tonicity of the resulting solutions was also observed to be inversely related to molecular weight—low molecular weight PEGs contributed to tonicity, and the higher molecular weight species did not. They suggested that this lack of contribution to tonicity was related to decreased membrane permeability of the higher molecular weight species.

Nishio and coworkers (1982) investigated the effects of PEG 300 and PEG 400 on erythrocytes. They showed that incubation of erythrocyte suspensions in the presence of PEG–saline solutions resulted in the release of potassium ions and hemoglobin. They found that hemolysis and potassium ion loss decreased with increasing concentrations of PEGs, and that no loss was observed in iso-osmotic and hyperosmotic concentrations following a 2 min incubation time. However, longer incubation times (through 2 h) resulted in potassium loss and hemolysis in iso-osmotic and hyperosmotic solutions (PEG 300 > PEG 400).

Fort and coworkers (1984) evaluated the hemolytic potentials of mixtures of ethanol and water or saline with PEG 400 by both in vitro and in vivo methods. They showed that a PEG 400:ethanol:water mixture of 3:2:5 resulted in no hematuria in vivo in rats, while partial hemolysis was observed in vitro using dog blood. All other mixtures resulted in hematuria and hemolysis. Reed and Yalkowsky (1985) reported that the in vitro hemolytic LD_{50} value (total volume percent cosolvent required to produce 50 percent hemolysis of healthy erythrocytes) for PEG 400 was 30.0 (total volume percent). This indicated that red blood cells were relatively tolerant of PEG 400.

Propylene Glycol

PG, a dihydroxy alcohol, is one of the more common solvents encountered in pharmaceutical cosolvent formulations, for both parenteral and nonparenteral dosage forms. PG is generally regarded as nontoxic. It is more hygroscopic than glycerin and has excellent solubilizing power for a wide variety of compounds. In addition, it has excellent bacteriocidal and preservative properties (Heine et al. 1950).

PG is metabolized to carbon dioxide and water via lactic and pyruvic acid intermediates; therefore, it is not prone to the severe toxicities associated with the use of other glycols, such as ethylene glycol (Huff 1961; Lehman and Newman 1937a, b). It is approximately one-third as intoxicating as ethanol (Seidenfeld and Hanzlik 1932). It is a generally recognized as safe (GRAS) listed material (*Federal Register* 1982). The World Health Organization (WHO) has established an acceptable daily intake (ADI) at 25 mg/kg body weight (FAO/WHO 1974).

When used in large concentrations, PG has been associated with marked hyperosmolality (Bekeris et al. 1979; Glasgow et al. 1983; Flinger et al. 1985); metabolic acidosis due to the formation of lactic acid (Kelner and Bailey 1985; Pesola et al. 1990); CNS depression (Arulanatham and Genel 1978; Lolin et al. 1988); intoxication (Cate and Hendrick 1980; Demey et al. 1984); augmentation of muscle twitch induced by benzodiazepines (Driessen et al. 1985); contact dermatitis in sensitive individuals (Fisher 1995); cerebral ischemia (Drummond et al. 1995); renal compromise (Levy et al. 1995); and cardiovascular side effects, including hypotension, bradycardia, atrial and ventricular conduction abnormalities (Gross et al. 1979), as well as allergic reactions leading to hypersensitivity myocarditis. These complications can be particularly serious in infants. Other investigators have suggested that the main toxic effect of PG is depression of the CNS (Martin and Finberg 1970; Zarolinski et al. 1971). Additionally, there have been numerous reported side effects following nitroglycerin (Hill et al. 1981; Col et al. 1985; Demey et al. 1988) and etomidate therapies (Morgan et al. 1977; Doenicke et al. 1982; Fellows et al. 1983; Bedichek and Kirschbaum 1991; Doenicke et al 1994; Moon 1994; Levy et al. 1995; Van de Wiele et al. 1995).

There are numerous reports regarding the use of PG based on safety/ toxicity data (Seidenfeld and Hanzlik 1932; Braun and Cartland 1936;

Weatherby and Haag 1938; Morris et al. 1942; Dominguez-Gil and Cadorniga 1971a, b; Zarolinski et al. 1971; Ruddick 1972). Seidenfeld and Hanzlik (1932) reported single fatal doses of PG administered intramuscularly and intravenously to rats and rabbits. No symptoms were reported in rats and rabbits until IM doses exceeded 6.3 to 7.4 g/kg. Increased respiratory rate, loss of equilibrium, depression, and subsequent coma and death were observed. IM fatal doses were 14 g/kg and 7 g/kg in rats and rabbits, respectively. IV fatal doses were 16 g/kg and 5 g/kg in rats and rabbits, respectively. Braun and Cartland (1936) indicated that the minimum fatal IV dose to rats was 18.9 g/kg. They also noted that administration of undiluted PG destroyed the veins, making subsequent administration very difficult, and that PG was better tolerated than glycerol by IM and subcutaneous (SC) routes. There are numerous reports of convulsions following intraperitoneal (IP) administration in mice (Lampe and Easterday 1953; Braun and Cartland 1936).

The hemolytic potential of PG has been well documented by numerous investigators (Weatherby and Haag 1938; Randolph and Mallery 1944; Potter 1958; Brittain and D'Arcy 1962). Weatherby and Haag (1938) evaluated hemolysis of various PG–saline mixtures using an in vitro method. They observed hemolysis in cases where the PG concentration was greater than or equal to 0.14 M. They believed that PG permeated the erythrocytes so rapidly that it did not exert an appreciable osmotic effect on the cell. Brittain and D'Arcy (1962) later evaluated hematologic effects following IV administration of PG to rabbits. The rabbits were given a single dose of 4 mL/kg of either 12.5, 25, or 50 percent PG in normal saline via the marginal vein. They observed no effect on red blood cell count, total white cell count, or hemoglobin concentration. However, they observed a marked decrease in clotting times with an associated increase in platelet count. They also reported no effect of the PG concentrations on fragility of the red blood cell membranes. Fort and coworkers (1984) evaluated hemolysis due to PG–containing formulations by both in vitro (using dog blood) and in vivo (rats) methods. The compositions evaluated ranged from 10 to 60 percent PG, 0 to 40 percent ethanol diluted with either water or 0.9 percent NaCl. All of these formulations caused hemolysis in vitro. However, only the 1:3:6 PG:ethanol:saline mixture resulted in no hematuria when administered to rats, while all other compositions caused hematuria. Reed and Yalkowsky (1985) determined the in vitro red blood cell hemolytic LD_{50} for PG to be 5.7, which indicated that it was fairly hemolytic relative to the other solvents tested. Only glycerin and DMSO were found to be more hemolytic than PG by this method.

There has been some work conducted in humans evaluating hemolysis following administration of PG–containing solutions. In the work by Speth and coworkers (1987) evaluating the pharmacokinetics of PG in humans, they reported no alterations in plasma osmolality, free hemoglobin or haptoglobin following IV infusion (4 hour) of total PG levels ranging from 5.1 to 21.0 g/day, with C_{max} values up to 425 µg/mL. They found that PG exhibited nonlinear pharmacokinetics and that clearance was dose and concentration dependent (saturable) in the dose range of 3 to 15 g/m^2, with a mean elimination half-life of 2.3 hours. There were no signs of metabolic acidosis or changes in osmolality in these patients, even though the plasma levels were in the range where these effects had been previously reported. The absence of effects could have been due to the slow rate of administration, or to the presence of additional excipients in the formulation (soybean lecithin, 0.5 mg/mL; PEG 300, 75 mg/mL; and PG, 25 mg/mL).

Ethanol

Ethanol (EtOH) is typically used as a solvent in pharmaceutical applications; however, it also possesses some antimicrobial properties. Parenteral products typically use 95 percent or 96 percent rather than absolute alcohol at use levels up to 50 percent. However, these levels typically are associated with pain on injection. EtOH is a component of commercial parenteral formulations for such compounds as diazepam, phenytoin, and digoxin. However, parenteral administration of EtOH–containing formulations has been associated with various complications. Such cases have been reported with IV administration of nitroglycerin (Shook et al. 1984). Intoxication was observed in several elderly patients receiving high doses of IV nitroglycerin. These patients received up to 20.7 mL EtOH/h during their course of therapy, which exceeded the average adult rate of EtOH metabolism of 10 mL/h (Hill et al. 1981). These effects would likely be more pronounced in patients with compromised hepatic function and myocardial ischemia or low cardiac output. Others reported that rapid infusion of EtOH may be cardiotoxic, in that it possesses both atrial and ventricular arrhythmogenic properties, as well as negative inotropic effects (Ahmed et al. 1973; Delgado et al. 1975; Child et al. 1979).

The toxicity of EtOH has been well documented (Lehman 1937b; MacGregor et al. 1964; Maling 1970; Wiberg et al. 1970). It is fairly toxic when administered intraperitoneally. Heistand (1952) reported that mortality increased with increasing concentrations of ethanol injected intraperitoneally when the amount of alcohol was held constant. Wiberg et al. (1970) showed that high concentrations of EtOH (20 percent w/v) produced a fatal chemical peritonitis. Maling (1970) determined the IV LD_{50} to be 2.0 g/kg and 4.2 g/kg in mice and rats, respectively. The LD_{50} following subcutaneous administration to mice was determined to be 8.3 g/kg. Lethal doses in dogs following subcutaneous and IV administration were found to be 6.0 to 8.0 g/kg and 5.4 g/kg, respectively. A comprehensive list of effects of EtOH as a function of blood level in humans is also listed.

EtOH is a well-known CNS depressant. The result of ingestion is intoxication, with associated loss of muscle coordination, slurred speech, or more severe effects including lethargy, stupor, coma, respiratory depression, and possibly death. These same effects have been observed following IV administration. There are also reports of fatalities in neonates and children following IV administration of ethanol (Gettler and St. George 1935; Jung et al. 1980).

Fort et al. (1984) evaluated hemolysis due to various EtOH–containing concentrations ranging from 30 to 40 percent diluted in either water or 0.9 percent NaCl. They found that all mixtures caused hemolysis in vitro; however, the 3:7 EtOH:0.9 percent NaCl caused no hematuria in vivo. Reed and Yalkowsky (1985) determined the in vitro hemolytic LD_{50} to be 21.2 (total volume percent) for EtOH, indicating that it was fairly well tolerated by erythrocytes.

Glycerin

Glycerin (glycerol) is one of the oldest and most widely used excipients in pharmaceutical products. It is a clear, colorless liquid that is miscible with water and alcohol. Glycerol is hygroscopic, stable to mild acidic and basic environments, and can be sterilized at temperatures up to 150°C. It is well known as both a taste masking and cryoprotective agent, and as an antimicrobial agent. It has good solubilizing power and is a commonly used solvent in parenteral formulations. It is considered to be one of the safest excipients used since it is metabolized to glucose or to substances that are involved with triglyceride synthesis or glycolysis (Frank et al. 1981). It is a GRAS–listed excipient and is typically used at levels of up to 50 percent in parenteral formulations (Wade and Weller 1994).

Glycerol is a naturally existing sugar alcohol that is endogenous to humans. It is broken down to triglycerides, glucose by the gluconeogenesis pathways or to pyruvate by the glycolytic pathway. It has also been used in parenteral formulations as an energy source (Fairfull-Smith et al. 1982; Jones 1982; Tao et al. 1983). Glycerol has been used clinically to treat Reye's syndrome (Mickell et al. 1977), traumatic intracranial hypertension (Wald and McLaurin 1982), brain edema in stroke patients (Tourellotte et al. 1972; Macdonald and Uden 1982), reduce intraocular pressure in cataract surgery (Guindon et al. 1981), and improve hearing loss associated with Meniere's disease (Angleborg et al. 1982; Lunsford 1982).

Somewhat surprisingly, there are numerous reports of adverse effects following administration of this endogenous substance, including hemolysis, hemoglobinuria, renal damage, hyperglycemia, hyperosmolality, and convulsions. A fairly extensive review of adverse reactions resulting from IV administration of glycerol is given by Frank et al. (1981). There are reports that glycerol is approximately 20 times more toxic when administered intraperitoneally or subcutaneously, as compared to the IV route (Tao et al. 1983). However, some of this sensitivity to IP administration may be related to strain differences (Uche et al. 1987).

Patients with acute cerebral infarction received 10 percent glycerol solutions administered daily for 7 to 10 days over a 6 h period (Welch et al. 1974). In these reports, there were no reported side effects even with prolonged administration, with the exception of "transient hemoglobinuria" in cases where the glycerol content of the solutions was 30 percent or greater. However, side effects, including hematuria, hemoglobinuria, and hemolysis have been reported by other physicians (Cameron and Finchk 1956; Potter 1958; MacCannel 1969; Hagnevik et al. 1974). Hagnevik and coworkers (1974) reported that administration of 20 percent glycerol in normal saline to three patients during intracranial surgery resulted in either (1) no effect; (2) massive hemolysis and hemoglobinuria that dissipated quickly; or (3) severe hemolysis and hemoglobinuria, as well as serious renal damage. However, the rates of administration that resulted in these side effects were more rapid—60 g/15 min, 70 g/30 min, and 80 g/60 min—than those used previously (wherein the dose was infused over 6 h). The resulting hemolytic side effects were most likely due to the rapid rate of administration.

Early studies by Smith (1950) reported that glycerol did not have a direct toxic effect on erythrocytes, which seems reasonable since it is used as a cryoprotectant to prevent hemolysis during freeze-thaw studies. These studies showed that no hemolysis resulted from diluting blood with 30 percent glycerol in Ringer's solution (1:1 ratio), followed by freezing at -70°C. No hemolysis was reported for up to 8 weeks. The same results were obtained when the glycerol solution was prepared in normal saline. It should be noted that the absence of hemolysis could have been in part due to the presence of the various salt solutions.

However, glycerol is known to permeate red blood cells rapidly, causing fluid influx and subsequent hemolysis (Tourtellotte et al. 1972). Early work by Husa and Adams (1944) showed that glycerol was hemolytic even at iso-osmotic concentrations, and that the addition of NaCl reduced its hemolytic potential. Similar findings were observed by other investigators (Hammarlund and Pedersen-Bjergaard 1961; Zanowiak and Husa 1959). Cadwallader and coworkers (1963, 1964) calculated the isotonic coefficients for glycerin solutions and showed that the addition of increasing amounts of NaCl afforded some protection from hemolysis, again indicating that the degree of hemolysis resulting from IV administration was dependent on the tonicity of the glycerol-saline solutions. Reed and Yalkowsky (1985) reported that glycerol was the most hemolytic of the 15 organic solvents evaluated, with a hemolytic LD_{50} value of 3.7 (total volume percent).

Cremophors

The cremophors are water soluble polyoxyethylene derivatives of castor oil that are nonionic surface-active agents. Several grades are used in pharmaceutical formulations, particularly Cremophor® EL (Polyoxyl 35 castor oil) and Cremophor® RH40 (Polyoxyl 40 hydrogenated castor oil).

However, Cremophor® EL is the grade used for parenteral applications in humans. These substances are mixtures of hydrophilic and hydrophobic components, composed primarily of ricinoleic acid esters and fatty acid esters of glycerol/polyglycol and polyglycols. The main component of Cremophor® EL is glycerol–polyethylene glycol ricinoleate. Cremophor® EL is a pale yellow, oily liquid that forms clear solutions when mixed with water. It is also readily soluble in water-alcohol mixtures. It can be heat sterilized at a temperature of 120°C for 30 min, but it may be prone to hydrolysis if heated in the presence of strong acid or basic substances (BASF 1988).

The most common adverse effect reported following administration of cremophor-containing formulations are severe reactions related to histamine release. The cremophors have been implicated in anaphylactoid reactions, typically following rapid IV injections (Dye and Watkins 1980; Hopkins 1988; Reynolds and Aronson 1992; Dorr 1994). Hopkins (1988) and Reynolds and Aronson (1992) reported anaphylactoid responses following IV administration of vitamin K in a cremophor solution. However, Havel et al. (1987) reported that this formulation was well tolerated in patients. Patients treated with miconazole preparations containing cremophors have also presented unusual serum lipoprotein patterns, hypercholesterolemia, and hypertriglyceridemia (Golightly et al. 1988). There are numerous reports in the literature relating to anaphylactic reactions following administration of althesin and propanidid (Watkins 1979; Watkins et al. 1976, 1978; Forrest et al. 1977; Dye and Watkins 1980). Windebank and coworkers (1994) reported that cremophor was a potential neurotoxic agent since a total dose 0.1 percent (v/v) produced axonal swelling and degeneration of dorsal root ganglion neurons, and 0.001% (v/v) produced demyelination in vitro.

Earlier studies in dogs showed that Cremophor® EL caused histamine-like responses accompanied by marked hypotension in dogs. Studies were subsequently conducted to evaluate whether these cardiorespiratory effects occurred in normal human volunteers following IV administration of Cremophor® EL (Savege et al. 1973). Subjects were given incremental dose volumes ranging from 2 to 20 mL (administered every 4 min, each over a 30 sec period). Following administration of each dose of Cremophor® EL, there was a small, transient reduction in blood pressure and a rise in pulse rate. However, none of these changes were statistically significant, with the exception of the high dose (20 mL). These studies showed no marked change in respiratory rate or pattern and no consistent alterations in central venous pressure.

Benzyl Alcohol

Benzyl alcohol (BA) is a bacteriostatic agent used against gram-positive bacteria, yeasts, molds and fungi, and it is commonly used as a preservative in parenteral products. It also has anesthetic properties at levels of approximately 1 percent. The bacteriostatic activity is reduced in the presence of nonionic surface-active agents. It also has good solubilizing power, and is typically used in concentrations up to 2 percent as a preservative and up to 5 percent as a solvent. BA is commonly found as a preservative in intravascular flush solutions at a level of 0.9 percent. The WHO has established an ADI of 5 mg/kg (FAO/WHO 1980).

BA is metabolized in the body to benzaldehyde via alcohol dehydrogenase and subsequently to benzoic acid via aldehyde dehydrogenase. However, the reported toxicities, particularly acute toxicity, appeared to be associated with the parent compound and not the metabolite. Studies using the enzyme inhibitors pyrazole (alcohol dehydrogenase inhibitor) and disulfiram (aldehyde dehydrogenase inhibitor) showed that marked lethality was observed with increased plasma levels of BA, and not with benzaldehyde levels (McCloskey et al. 1986). These elimination pathways are saturable, indicating that additional amounts of BA would likely result in significantly higher plasma levels once the metabolic capacity has been exceeded.

Toxicity studies in adult and neonatal mice were conducted following IP administration of single doses of BA ranging from 500 to 1500 mg/kg administered in maximum dose volumes of 0.28 mL and 0.07 mL for adult and neonates, respectively (McCloskey et al. 1986). The data showed that the acute LD_{50} for BA was 1,000 mg/kg for both adult and neonatal groups after 4 h. However, deaths were observed in the adult group at day seven, resulting in a revised LD_{50} value of 650 mg/kg.

Macht (1920) reported on the toxicity of intravenously administered alcohols to cats. He reported that BA was approximately 8 times more toxic than ethanol, with lethal doses of 5.0 mL/kg and 0.6 mL/kg, respectively. Kimura et al. (1971) investigated the parenteral toxicity data for BA, finding that a 0.9 percent solution was quite safe following administration of 1 mL/kg to dogs and monkeys. They found no changes in complete blood counts or blood chemistry values. They also reported that rapid IV injections of 0.9 percent BA could be safely given to mice to a maximum volume of 50 mL/kg. Kimura et al. (1971) reported that BA was significantly more toxic than ethanol when administered at the same doses to mice, rats, and dogs.

Most of the early studies evaluating the toxicity of BA indicated that it was a relatively harmless substance with regard to humans. However, numerous incidences of BA toxicity following parenteral administration of solutions containing levels of only 0.9 percent have subsequently been reported in the literature. Reported toxicities of BA include hypersensitivity reactions, hemolysis, sedation, dyspnea, loss of motor function, and possible death. Toxicity has been reported following exposure to catheter flush solutions containing very low levels of BA (0.9 percent). However, the most severe toxic effects, including death, have occurred in neonates (Gershanik et al. 1982; Jarvis et al. 1983; Benda et al. 1986; Wilson et al. 1986; Hiller et al. 1986; González de la Riva Lamana 1987; and Santeiro 1989). Its use has been implicated as the causative agent in "gasping syndrome" in neonates (Gershanik et al. 1982). This syndrome is characterized by a progression of symptoms from gradual neurological deterioration, severe metabolic acidosis, gasping respiration, hematologic abnormalities, skin breakdown, hepatic and renal failure, hypotension, to cardiovascular collapse.

Several investigators have reported that BA caused hemolysis of erythrocytes (Kimura et al. 1971; Ohmiya and Nakai 1978; McOrmond et al. 1980). Ohmiya and Nakai (1978) later reported that the hemolytic potential of BA was time, dose, and temperature dependent. They also showed that the concentration of erythrocytes had a profound effect on the amount of hemolysis observed. They determined that the hemolytic in vitro LD_{50} using their method was 100 mM following incubation for 60 min at 37°C. Kimura and coworkers (1971) evaluated blood chemistry profiles following administration of 0.9 percent solutions of BA to rats, mice, and dogs, and determined that these concentrations were completely nonhemolytic in dogs and monkeys at a dose level of 1 ml/kg. They determined that the lethal IV dose of 0.9 percent BA in dogs was 0.83 to 1.06 g/kg. Additionally, they showed that slow IV administration of up to 40 mL/kg 0.9 percent BA to rats resulted in no fatalities.

Amide Solvents

N,N-Dimethylacetamide

N,N-dimethylacetamide (DMA) is a clear liquid that is used as a solvent for poorly water-soluble compounds in the pharmaceutical industry. It is miscible with water and alcohols and very soluble in organic solvents and mineral oil. It is mildly hygroscopic, stable to heat and hydrolysis, and has a low vapor pressure. DMA is sequentially metabolized to monomethylacetamide, and subsequently to acetamide (Kim 1988).

Caujolle et al. (1970) reported "maximum doses never fatal" (MDNF) and "minimum doses always fatal" (MDAF), for DMA as 2.5 g/kg and 6.0 g/kg for mice, and 2.5 g/kg and 3.7 g/kg for rats, respectively. They also reported 24 h LD_{50} values for DMA as 4.19 g/kg and 3.84 g/kg for mice and rats, respectively. Testicular injury was reported following a single IP dose of up to 3 g/kg DMA. However, subchronic administration of 36 IP injections at low doses did not show any toxicity or histopathology.

Wiles and Narcisse (1971) evaluated the parenteral toxicity of DMA by IV and IP administration to mice and rabbits. They observed the same signs of toxicity by both routes of administration, which included decreased activity, weakness, anesthesia, analgesia, labored breathing, cyanosis, collapse, and convulsions accompanied by hemorrhage prior to death. They found that toxicity was dose related, with faster onset of toxic signs following administration of higher doses. IV administration of 708 to 1,480 mg/kg DMA to rats resulted in a rapid period of hypotension, followed by a long-lasting hypertensive period. IV administration of DMA to dogs and cats at a dose of 95 mg/kg caused no changes in blood pressure. At 236 mg/kg, mild hypotension was observed over a 5 min period. A dose of 472 mg/kg was lethal to cats (Auclair and Hameau 1964).

DMA has been used as a solvent for numerous pharmaceutical preparations, including oxytetracycline, chloramphenicol, and reserpine (Spiegel and Noseworthy 1963). DMA has also been used as a solvent for certain anticancer compounds, including amsacrine. In vehicle studies conducted in mice, the single IV dose LD_{50} was found to be 2,341 mg/kg.

DMA was believed to possess some inherent antitumor activity and was subsequently taken into Phase I clinical trials in 17 patients as a potential antitumor agent (Weiss et al. 1962). DMA was administered at doses ranging from 100 mg/kg/day to 610 mg/kg/day from a 10 percent solution over 5 to 10 min for 3 to 5 days. Toxicity—specifically gastrointestinal, hepatic, and CNS—was observed at the high doses. However, all signs of toxicity appeared to be reversible, returning to normal following completion of the therapy. Gastrointestinal signs of toxicity included nausea, vomiting, and anorexia. Hepatic toxicity was manifested by elevated serum glutamic-oxaloacetic acid transaminase (SGOT) levels up to several days after the completion of therapy, which returned to normal 2 to 5 days after reaching peak levels. No evidence of hepatic toxicity was observed on biopsy 3 weeks after therapy was completed. CNS effects (including depression, lethargy, occasional confusion and disorientation) were observed after the second or third day of therapy. The degree of lethargy and confusion ranged from mild to severe. Some patients developed hallucinations, perceptual distortions, and, at times, became delusional at high doses of DMA (above 400 mg/kg). CNS symptoms preceded more severe side effects, including hypotension and high fever, in 3 patients. However, typical use levels for parenteral applications are approximately 30 mg/kg, and would not be expected to cause these side effects (Spiegel and Noseworthy 1963).

Reed and Yalkowsky (1985) determined that DMA was very non-hemolytic with an in vitro hemolytic LD_{50} value of 37.0 (total volume percent). Only dimethylisosorbide was found to be less hemolytic (39.5).

N,N-Dimethylformamide

N,N-dimethylformamide (DMF) is a widely used organic solvent with excellent solubilizing capacity. It has been referred to as the "universal organic solvent" due to its small size, electron-donating properties, and high dielectric constant (Budavari 1989). It is a colorless liquid that is miscible with water and other organic solvents.

Following parenteral administration, DMF is metabolized in vivo to either monomethylformamide or N-(hydroxymethyl)-N-methylformamide. It is primarily excreted in the urine as either of the metabolites, with relatively small amounts excreted as intact parent compound (Kennedy and Short 1986).

Generally, the formamides possess a relatively low order of toxicity following single-dose administration. Kutzsche (1965) determined the acute toxicity (LD_{50} values) of DMF following IV administration in dogs, guinea pigs, and rabbits to be 0.47 g/kg, 1.0 g/kg, and 1.8 g/kg, respectively. However, liver damage has been reported in rats following single IP doses of 0.6, 0.9, or 1.2 g/kg DMF. Davis and Jenner (1959) reported the LD_{50} values following IP administration to mice to be 1.1 g/kg. Reported IP LD_{50} values in rats are 1.3 g/kg (Massmann 1956) and 2.5 g/kg (Thiersch 1962).

Montaguti et al. (1994) evaluated the relative hemolytic potentials of several organic solvents, including DMF, dimethylsulfoxide (DMSO), EtOH, PEG 400, and BA, in several different mouse strains. They found that DMF was well tolerated in terms of hemolytic and precipitation potentials (in vitro tests). Hemolytic potential was evaluated following incubation of the solvent with blood at 37°C for 45 min. In general, DMF was the best tolerated of the solvents evaluated in both of these studies. DMF has been reported to be hemolytic when incubated with human erythrocytes for 45 min at 37°C (Cadwallader and Phillips 1969). These amides have been shown to readily penetrate the red blood cell membrane and afford little to no protection from hemolysis.

Dimethylsulfoxide

DMSO is a colorless, aprotic solvent that has a relatively high dielectric constant. It is miscible with water and many common organic solvents, including glycerol, acetone, and EtOH, in all proportions. DMSO is also very hygroscopic, capable of absorbing over 70 percent of its own weight at 20°C/65 percent relative humidity (RH) (Willson et al. 1965). Additionally, it has excellent solubilizing properties. Pharmacological evaluations showed that drugs administered systemically in DMSO did not significantly alter their lethality or cellular penetration (Dixon et al. 1965).

Toxicity studies have shown that DMSO possesses a relatively low order of toxicity. Willson et al. (1965) evaluated both acute and multiple dose toxicity from IV and IP injections in mice, rats, and dogs. Anemia and peritoneal inflammation were observed following 24 daily injections of DMSO to rats. No fatalities were observed in dogs receiving 1.2 g/kg or less daily by IV injection for 24 days. They observed perivascular inflammation and intravascular thrombosis, which was attributed to repeated administration of undiluted DMSO. However, dilution of DMSO prior to administration eliminated these unwanted effects. Additionally, hemolytic anemia, which was found to be reversible, was observed in rats and dogs following repeated IV injections of DMSO.

Studies conducted in humans at doses of 1 gm/kg administered intravenously from 10 to 40 percent solutions resulted in transient hemoglobinuria, which resolved within 2 to 3 hours (Bennet and Muther 1981). These studies also showed no short-term nephrotoxicity.

DMSO has been shown to exert cryoprotective effects in the preservation of red blood cells, platelets, bone marrow, and tissue culture cells (Lovelock and Bishop 1959; Pyle and Boyer 1962; Porterfield and Ashwood-Smith 1962). Additionally, DMSO in concentrations up to approximately 20 percent has been shown to reduce the hemolytic activity of various antimicrobial preservatives, including phenols, BA, thimerosal, and benzalkonium chloride (Ansel and Leake 1966; Ansel and Cabre 1970).

However, there are numerous in vitro and in vivo reports of the hemolytic nature of DMSO. Cadwallader and Drinkard (1967) evaluated the behavior of human erythrocytes in the presence of water–DMSO cosolvent systems ranging from 5 to 40 percent DMSO. They found that hemolysis occurred in all DMSO–containing solutions, and those with compositions greater than 35 percent DMSO resulted in discoloration and precipitation. Norred et al. (1970) speculated that DMSO was capable of removing fatty acids from the erythrocyte membrane in a concentration-dependent manner. The leaching of fatty acids led to the formation of lesions, which subsequently disrupted the integrity of the membrane. Reed and Yalkowsky (1985) determined the in vitro hemolytic LD_{50} value for DMSO to be 5.1 (total volume percent). Only glycerin was found to be more hemolytic than DMSO of the 15 solvents tested in the study. Montaguti and coworkers (1994) reported marked hemolytic activity of DMSO, tested in dose ranges from 1.0 to 5.66 mL/kg in 3 inbred mouse strains. These reports were consistent with previous reports indicating high hemolytic potential in mice, rats, cats, and dogs (Rosenkrantz et al. 1963; DiStefano and Klahn 1965; Willson et al. 1965). These effects have been reported to be markedly reduced when the DMSO solutions were diluted with saline.

HEMOLYTIC POTENTIAL OF SOLVENTS/COSOLVENTS

It is preferable to utilize injectables that are totally biocompatible with body fluids. However, the incorporation of cosolvents into parenteral formulations has long been recognized as having the potential to destroy red blood cells, as does the addition of water alone. These solvents have the ability to hemolyze cells via either membrane disruption/interaction or by osmotic action. Early investigators have shown that the composition of parenteral dosage forms directly influenced the hemolysis of erythrocytes (Husa and Rossi 1942; Easterly and Husa 1954; Grosicki and Husa 1954; Hartman and Husa 1957; Cadwallader and Husa 1958; Thomasson and Husa 1958; Ansel and Husa 1959; Marcus and Husa 1959; Winters and Husa 1960; Schnell and Husa 1962; Cadwallader 1963; Ansel 1964, 1965; Ku and Cadwallader 1975). These authors have also shown that the effect on the erythrocytes depends not only on the concentration of the organic in the cosolvent but also its ability to penetrate or disrupt the cell membrane. Therefore, there have been numerous investigations as to which vehicles are more tolerated for parenteral applications. Tables 11.5a and 11.5b summarize the in vitro hemolytic LD_{50} values for several common organic solvents encountered in parenteral formulations and the effects of increasing concentrations of NaCl on the observed hemolytic potentials (Reed and Yalkowsky 1985, 1986).

Table 11.5a. LD_{50} Values Expressed as Total Volume Percents of Various Cosolvents for Lysis of Erythrocytes (Reed and Yalkowsky 1985)

Cosolvent	LD_{50}
Glycerin	3.7
DMSO	5.1
PG	5.7
10% EtOH, 40% PG	10.3
EtOH	21.2
PEG 400	30.0
DMA	37.0
DMI	39.5

Table 11.5b. Effect of Increasing Sodium Chloride Concentrations on LD_{50} Values Expressed as Total Volume Percents of Various Cosolvents for Lysis of Erythrocytes (Reed and Yalkowsky 1986)

Cosolvent	Aqueous NaCl Concentration			
	0.9%	1.8%	2.7%	3.6%
Glycerin	3.3	8.3	12.7	11.9
PG	6.2	14.7	20.0	19.3
PEG 200	10.2	22.4	26.6	27.9
DMA	36.6	40.4	39.3	36.9
PEG 400	29.6	33.5	27.6	23.9
DMI	17.9	16.6	15.9	9.6
EtOH	20.5	20.0	20.5	19.7

There is a great deal of information available in the literature regarding the hemolytic potential of various solvents/cosolvents. However, much of this information is contradictory as to whether a particular cosolvent system is hemolytic or nonhemolytic. The discrepancies regarding hemolytic potential of a particular solvent system apparently result from the differences in the test methods used to evaluate the degree of hemolysis, particularly relating to volume ratios of blood to cosolvent, incubation/contact times, and whether the systems are static or dynamic (Banziger 1967; Wickliffe et al. 1968; Fort et al. 1984; Obeng and Cadwallader 1989; Krzyzaniak et al. 1997a, b, c). The temperature at which samples are maintained has also been shown to have a direct effect on the observed degree of hemolysis, with lower temperatures resulting in lesser extents of hemolysis (Cadwallader et al. 1964; Kimura et al. 1971). Additionally, it is also important to note that there may also be some species and/or strain differences relating to how susceptible blood cells might be to hemolysis (Montaguti et al. 1994).

Reed and Yalkowsky (1985, 1986) performed numerous studies addressing the effect of various cosolvents on hemolysis using an improved hemolytic method that would be suitable for use in the presence of cosolvent systems. They used terminology that expressed the ratio of blood to cosolvent volume as a concentration (i.e., total volume percent of cosolvent). A blood to cosolvent ratio of 9:1 would be expressed as a 10 percent cosolvent. They determined the LD_{50} values for various cosolvent systems. They found that EtOH, PEG 400, DMA, and dimethyl isosorbide (DMI) were considerably less hemolytic than DMSO and PG (Table 11.5a). The 10 percent EtOH–40 percent PG vehicle commonly used in marketed products (and well accepted as a parenteral vehicle) had an LD_{50} value approximately twofold greater than the very hemolytic solvents DMSO and PG.

Reed and Yalkowsky (1985, 1986) investigated the hemolysis resulting from increasing amounts of various cosolvents in water, as well as the importance of the ratios of blood to test solution. They showed that hemolysis was clearly a function of the concentration of the organic component present in the cosolvent mixture. DMSO and PG cosolvent mixtures were found to be quite hemolytic, even at relatively low cosolvent fractions. Surprisingly, some solvents were well tolerated even when tested undiluted (DMA, DMI, PEG 400) at blood:test solution ratios of 9:1. Reed and Yalkowsky (1987) continued to investigate cosolvent-induced hemolysis in an attempt to determine the relationship between structure and hemolytic potential for the above cosolvents. They concluded that the simple alcohols became more hemolytic with increasing chain length, consistent with other reports for simple alcohols (Ku and Cadwallader 1984) and both anionic and cationic detergents (Ross and Silverstein 1954). They also observed that decreasing steric bulk attached to the hydroxyl groups, and decreasing the number of hydroxyl groups resulted in a decreased hemolytic potential.

Although they were unable to determine a relationship between LD_{50} values and physicochemical properties for all of the solvents tested, they did observe a good correlation between LD_{50} values and log partition co-efficient (PC) values when only the simple alcohols were included in the regression analysis. Similar attempts to correlate physical parameters with hemolytic potential have been made for drug molecules using dielectric constants, pH values, hydrogen bonding numbers, van der Waals volume, pK_a, octanol-water partition coefficients, and lipid spin labeling. However, no clear association has been made between any single parameter and resulting damage to the erythrocytes.

Ward and Yalkowsky (1992) later proposed that the hemolytic potential of a cosolvent was most accurately described by a single parameter, the effective concentration (EC), which could be used to generate dose-response hemolysis curves. They used the data obtained by Obeng and Cadwallader (1989) for PG cosolvent systems as the basis for their work. They defined the EC as the concentration in the final mixture of aqueous PG cosolvent solution and blood:

$$EC = \frac{PG \text{ concentration} \times \left(\dfrac{solution \ volume}{injection \ time} \right)}{blood \ flow \ rate}$$

They proposed that use of this term essentially condensed several parameters (including vessel diameter, blood flow rate, injection volume, concentration and rate of administration) into a single parameter. They demonstrated with the PG system that there was a relationship between hemolytic potential and effective concentration, and that these kinetic factors must be considered in order to evaluate hemolysis in an in vitro system accurately.

Krzyzaniak et al. (1997a, b) showed that the degree of solvent-induced hemolysis was not only dependent on the ratio of formulation to blood but also to the amount of time in which the formulation was in contact with blood. Their in vitro method of determining hemolysis incorporated factors relating to the dynamics of an IV injection. The fundamental basis for this was that once a cosolvent formulation is injected into a vein, it is immediately mixed (and subsequently diluted) with blood, resulting in a decreased concentration of cosolvent formulation to which the erythrocytes will be exposed. Initially, the effect of contact time and volume of water and various concentrations of salt solutions were evaluated (Krzyzaniak et al. 1997a). Research showed that longer contact times resulted in greater degrees of hemolysis, with more hemolysis observed for systems where the ratio of test solvent to blood was increased. Subsequent evaluations were focused on various cosolvent systems, using EtOH, glycerol, PG, and PEGs (Krzyzaniak et al. 1997b). They determined a hemolytic potential rank order for these tested solvents to be: glycerin > PG > PEG 300 > EtOH, although there was no difference between PEG 300 and EtOH at short contact times. For all cosolvent systems tested the observed extent of hemolysis increased as a function of cosolvent composition as well as contact time.

Krzyzaniak and coworkers (1997c) pointed out the range of conditions utilized in the most common in vitro methods, and the differences as to whether hemolysis occurred in the presence of a given cosolvent. The conditions used in the various models were so different, it is not surprising that there were inconsistencies with regard to hemolysis caused by cosolvents. The amount of hemolysis resulting from an IV injection of any given cosolvent depends on the initial concentration of the cosolvent, the concentration of the formulation after initial mixing with blood, and the amount of time to be completely diluted by the total blood volume.

In Vitro/In Vivo Hemolysis Comparisons

Fort and coworkers (1984) investigated the hemolysis of aqueous PEG 400, PG, and EtOH combinations in vivo and in vitro. Hemolysis was evaluated following a 2-week period of IV administration of a PG:EtOH:water solution (5:1:4) to rats and dogs. After 2 weeks, observations included decreases in hematocrit, hemoglobin, and number of erythrocytes, as well as marked hematuria. Further evaluation of urine samples showed that they were positive for occult blood, bilirubin, ketones, and protein. Several cosolvents (PG, PEG 400, and EtOH) of varying compositions were also evaluated in vivo in rats and in vitro in dog blood. It was found that any combination of EtOH and water with PG (10–30 percent) resulted in hematuria and complete in vitro hemolysis in all tested ratios. The same results were obtained when 0.9 percent NaCl was substituted for water with the exception of 10:30:60 (PG:EtOH:saline), which did not cause hematuria in vivo, but caused complete hemolysis in vitro. They also found that 40 percent EtOH in the presence or absence of normal saline caused hemolysis. Lower concentrations of EtOH (30 percent or less) in solutions containing normal saline did not cause hematuria even though some hemolysis in vitro was observed. The solution containing PEG:EtOH:water (3:2:5) was found to be nonhemolytic. Fort et al. (1984) concluded that intravenously administered PEG solutions were less hemolytic than similar solutions containing PG.

Krzyzaniak and coworkers (1997c) compared hemolysis using nine different in vitro methods, including a dynamic method which represented a more realistic picture of what happens to the formulation in vivo following an injection. They found that the hemolysis data generated by their dynamic model was much more representative of what was observed in vivo as compared to data generated by the other in vitro methods (Table 11.6). Excellent agreement was observed when comparing hemolysis data obtained from their dynamic in vitro method to that observed in vivo. Several

Table 11.6. Detection of Hemolysis by In Vivo and In Vitro Methods (Krzyzaniak 1997a)

Number	Formulation Composition	Hemolysis Observed in vivo	In Vitro Method (% Hemolysis Detected)			
			Husa and Adams (1944)	Fort et al. (1984)	Reed and Yalkowsky (1985)	Krzyzaniak et al. (1997c)
1	Normal saline (NS)	no[a,b,c]	0.0	0.0	0.0	0.0
2	10% EtOH in NS	no[c]	1.7	1.7	0.0	0.7
3	30% EtOH in NS	no[a]	92.4	89.2	0.0	0.5
4	40% PG in NS	yes[c]	50.7	23.3	61.0	5.6
5	60% PG in water	yes[a]	87.3	100.0	100.0	9.5
6	10% PG + 30% EtOH in NS	no[a]	82.3	85.3	0.0	1.2
7	10% EtOH + 20% PG in water	no[b]	89.5	81.3	8.8	2.0
8	10% EtOH + 40% PG in water	yes[a,b]	63.0	78.9	69.2	10.3
9	20% EtOH + 30% PEG 400 in water	no[a]	44.1	37.4	0.0	0.3

a: Fort et al. (1984)

b: Gerald (1988)

c: Turitto (1996)

of the vehicles tested by the static in vitro methods gave false-positive results when compared to results obtained from in vivo hemolysis studies (due to the high ratio of formulation to blood and the long incubation times). Although these static in vitro methods were not accurate in assessing the degree of hemolysis in vivo, they can be useful in assessing potential cellular damage resulting from IM injections, where there is a prolonged contact time between the vehicles and the tissues.

Methods to Reduce Hemolysis

Use of Additives. Numerous investigators have reported that the addition of various salts, including NaCl and sodium sulfate (Na_2SO_4), affords partial to full protection from hemolysis. It is well known that solutions of various therapeutic compounds (such as ammonium chloride, urea, boric acid, EtOH, and glycerin) fail to prevent hemolysis even when used at isotonic levels, indicating marked differences between iso-osmotic and isotonic values for compounds that can affect the red blood cell membrane (Husa and Rossi 1942; Husa and Adams 1944; Easterly and Husa 1954; Grosicki and Husa 1954; Hartman and Husa 1957; Cadwallader and Husa 1958; Thomasson and Husa 1958; Ansel and Husa 1959; Marcus and Husa 1959; Zanowiak and Husa 1959; Winters and Husa 1960; Hammarlund and Pedersen-Bjergaard 1961; Schnell and Husa 1962; Cadwallader 1963; Ansel 1964; Cadwallader et al. 1964). This is due to the fact that some of these additives may permeate the red blood cell membrane, causing an influx of water, resulting in hemolysis. Therefore, whether an additive has protective effects on erythrocytes will depend on its ability to penetrate the cell membrane. Such cosolvent compositions that are iso-osmotic with blood (0.9 percent or 0.15 M NaCl isotonic comparators) include 2.6 percent glycerin in water, 2.0 percent PG in water, 8.7 percent PEG 300, and 11.6 percent PEG 400.

Over the years, Husa and coworkers found that hemolysis occurred in solutions containing less than 0.45 percent NaCl, and that it was prevented with the use of concentrations from 0.45 to 0.9 percent. Hemolysis also resulted from solutions containing 1 to 2 percent dextrose, partial hemolysis at 3 percent dextrose, and solutions containing 4 to 5 percent dextrose resulted in no hemolysis. They showed that the 9 substances tested fell into 3 categories: prevents hemolysis (NaCl, dextrose), induces hemolysis (ammonium chloride, boric acid, carbitol) and those of moderate hemolytic potential (EtOH, PG, glycerin, diethylene glycol). Ammonium chloride, boric acid, and carbitol appear to cause hemolysis by a mechanism other than osmotic effects, probably by changing the permeability of the erythrocyte membrane.

Hammarlund and Pedersen-Bjergaard (1958, 1961) evaluated the effect of iso-osmotic solutions on erythrocyte hemolysis. They evaluated various salts for their potential for protecting erythrocytes from hemolysis.

They showed that monovalent amine salts typically resulted in hemolysis, whereas divalent and trivalent amine salts usually protected from hemolysis. They also showed that the addition of either NaCl or Na_2SO_4 was able to prevent hemolysis of erythrocytes exposed to various iso-osmotic solutions of ephedrine. They found that an iso-osmotic solution of EtOH (1.39 percent) required 0.5 percent NaCl to prevent hemolysis. Cadwallader and Drinkard (1967) also showed that the addition of isotonic amounts of various compounds (NaCl, calcium chloride, dextrose, lactose, potassium bromide, sodium citrate, sodium bromide, sodium iodide, and sodium salicylate) prevented hemolysis in aqueous solutions containing 5 to 40 percent DMSO. These studies again illustrate the difference between iso-osmotic concentrations and isotonic concentrations.

Cadwallader (1963) calculated "hemolytic" isotonic coefficients for several polyhydric alcohol-water solutions (PG, glycerol). These data showed that water-glycerin and water–PG mixtures should not be assumed to be hypertonic with respect to blood. In fact, all mixtures studied were found to be hypotonic with respect to rabbit and human erythrocyte membranes. Therefore, isotonicity calculations were not valid for these applications. They also showed that PG was more hemolytic than glycerin, consistent with Jacobs and coworkers' (1935) observation that each additional hydroxyl group added to the propane molecule decreased the rate of penetration into erythrocytes.

Reed and Yalkowsky (1986) showed the effect of increasing amounts of NaCl on the hemolytic LD_{50} values of the common organic solvents found in parenteral formulations (Table 11.5b). They showed differences in the degrees of protection afforded by NaCl between the various solvents. For example, the presence of NaCl had essentially no effect on the LD_{50} value for EtOH, whereas it decreased the LD_{50} value for glycerol by almost fourfold.

Fu et al. (1987) investigated several parenteral vehicles for hemolytic potential both in vitro and in vivo following IV administration to rats. The animals were dosed daily with a single bolus dose of 2.5 mL/kg through the tail vein for 2 weeks. They reported a high degree of hemolysis for a 15 percent PG solution, which was significantly reduced by the addition of either 1.8 percent NaCl or 20 percent sorbitol (concentrations higher than those yielding isotonic solutions). They also showed that PEG 400 had the ability to reduce the hemolytic potential of a 15 percent PG solution from approximately 80 percent hemolysis (with no added PEG 400) to approximately 20 percent hemolysis with addition of 20–45 percent PEG 400. This is useful to formulators in that it makes the vehicle more biocompatible, as well as provides increased solubilization power for the cosolvent system.

Use of Slow Infusion Rates. One of the easiest ways to minimize hemolytic consequences of administration of parenteral products containing cosolvents is to administer these doses as slow infusions, as opposed to bolus injections. This results in lower effective concentrations of cosolvent in the plasma. Slow administration of the dose also reduces the chance of precipitation of the drug in the vascular compartment by allowing for gradual dilution with the plasma components.

Welch et al. (1974) reported that glycerol has been used successfully in the treatment of more than 500 patients with acute cerebral infarctions when administered daily for 7 to 10 days infusing 500 mL of 10 percent glycerol in normal saline over 6 h with none of these adverse effects. This study did report that hemolysis was seen when the solution was administered as a rapid infusion. However, Hagnevik et al. (1974) reported hemolytic changes ranging from hemolysis and mild to marked hemoglobinuria following administration of 20 percent glycerol at rates of 60 g/15 min, 70 g/30 min and 80 g/60 min to 3 patients undergoing intracranial surgery. As one can see, there were enormous differences in the rates of administration of the glycerol solutions between these reports. The side effects were associated with much faster infusions than those used by others to treat stroke patients (Meyer et al. 1971). Therefore, one can observe that the rate of administration has a tremendous effect on the glycerol-related hemolysis observed following IV administration. These data from Welch and coworkers suggest that it would be entirely possible to greatly reduce or eliminate the hemolysis when administering such solutions slowly.

Obeng and Cadwallader (1989) evaluated the effect of various parameters on the observed degree of hemolysis. These included flow rate of red blood cells at the site of injection, internal diameter, distance downstream from the site of injection, injection volume, rate of administration, and cosolvent composition. This method was a more realistic model for hemolysis, since it allowed for mixing of the cosolvent with blood at the site of injection and a relatively short contact time between the test solution and the blood. These studies clearly showed that the kinetic factors (rate of administration, blood flow rate) affected the degree of hemolysis associated with various cosolvents and recommended that solutions having known hemolytic potentials be administered slowly via large veins.

The *Physicians Desk Reference* (PDR 1994) recommends slow administration for many cosolvent-containing compounds that have been associated with various complications following IV administration. Such compounds include phenytoin, digoxin, diazepam, pentobarbital, lorazepam, and etoposide. Typically, the recommendations are to administer these doses slowly as infusions, with rates not to exceed 2 to 50 mg/min, depending on the compound. When administering doses to neonates or children, the rates of administration may need to be even slower, as is the case with phenytoin (not to exceed 1 to 3 mg/kg/min for neonates, compared to 50 mg/kg for adults). Slow administration allows for adequate mixing with blood and minimizes the risk of precipitation of the dose.

MUSCLE DAMAGE

Administration of formulations by the IM and SC routes is somewhat more flexible than formulations administered by the IV route because solutions or suspensions, either aqueous or oily, can be given. Use of these formulations tends to result in a more controlled release of drug. Cosolvents are frequently used to reduce the aqueous solubility of a given compound, such that it precipitates upon administration into tissues. The precipitation is followed by a resolubilization of the compound over time as the compound is slowly absorbed. The rate of solubilization is dependent on the properties of the tissues, such as pH and blood flow (Evans et al. 1973), and the vehicles used to administer the compound. Local muscle damage may result from direct damage to the sarcolemma membrane of the muscle fibers, or by some toxic effect of either the drug or the vehicle on myofibril intracellular organelles and membranes. Muscle damage may also contribute to the pain at the site of injection.

Hem and coworkers (1974–1975) evaluated the tissue irritation (muscle damage) and injectability of 23 potential nonaqueous parenteral vehicles. They found that several vehicles caused very little irritation (benzyl benzoate, 1,3-butylene glycol, ethyl oleate, glyceryl triacetate, sesame oil: benzyl benzoate [1:1], sesame oil) and were well absorbed; several caused moderate irritation (butyl lactate, castor oil, glyceryl monoricinoleate) and were not absorbed; and a number that caused necrosis (ethyl formate, isoamyl formate, octyl alcohol, polyoxyethylene oleyl ether, n-propyl alcohol, propylene carbonate, sorbitan trioleate). They included DMA in the study, finding that it was very well absorbed from the site of injection but caused moderate irritation that was found to dissipate within 7 days postinjection. Oshida and coworkers (1979) evaluated the physicochemical properties and local toxic effects of 335 parenteral formulations. They evaluated pH, osmotic ratio, hemolytic potential, cytotoxic effects on cultured cells, and muscle lesions following IM administration of 0.5 mL to the vastus lateralis or sarcospinalis muscle of rats. They showed there was a close correlation between the hemolytic potential of the formulation and the severity of muscle damage observed.

Svendson (1983) and Svendson and coworkers (1985) evaluated the muscle damage resulting from IM injections of several neuroleptic drugs in aqueous and oil vehicles, including Viscoleo®, sesame oil, methyl oleate, and squalane. They observed the injection site three days after IM administration of 2 mL of the various formulations. The most damage was observed with cis-(Z)-clopenthixol, regardless of formulation. Postmortem findings showed well-defined, relatively large areas of muscle necrosis in all of the animals administered aqueous formulations. These areas were considerably larger than those observed in the oil-treated animals. Generally, Viscoleo® (a triglyceride vegetable oil composed of short chain and saturated fatty acids, caprylic acid, capric acid, and lauric acid) resulted in much less damage than the aqueous solutions. Formulation of haloperidol, cis-(Z)-clopenthixol, or chlorpromazine in any of the oil vehicles essentially eliminated the observed muscle damage that resulted from administration of the aqueous solutions—necrotic areas were reduced from 5- to 34-fold when the oily vehicles were used instead of the aqueous formulations.

It has been observed that one of the consequences of IM injections is release of the enzyme creatine kinase (CK) into plasma, which is found in large amounts in skeletal muscle. This enzyme has been used as a marker of muscle damage (Attar and Matta 1971; Anderson and Damsgaard 1976; Greenblatt et al. 1976; Steiness et al. 1974, 1978; Svendson et al. 1979; Diness 1985). Steiness et al. (1974) reported that the size of the resulting necrotic area following IM administration of digoxin or the vehicle control to pigs was related to the injection volume (ranging from 1.5 to 4.0 mL). The necrotic areas resulting were, however, much smaller for the vehicle groups than those receiving the digoxin formulation, indicating that the drug itself contributed greatly to the necrosis.

Several investigators evaluated the effects of PG and glycerol formal vehicles on muscle necrosis (Rasmussen and Svendson 1976; Svendson et al. 1979). Svendsen et al. (1979) evaluated the effects of different dilutions of PG or glycerol formal in distilled water or 0.9 percent saline on the measured CK activity in muscle taken from the injection area and the contralateral uninjected site for up to 72 h postinjection. They showed that CK depletion from the muscle, which subsequently appeared in the plasma, was dependent on the PG or glycerol formal content of the vehicle—higher cosolvent compositions led to higher plasma CK levels, with PG causing greater CK release than glycerol formal. They also showed that local muscle damage (as indicated by weight of the isolated damaged muscle tissue) correlated with relative CK activity depletion in the muscle.

Brazeau and Fung (1989a, c) also evaluated PEG 400, PG, and EtOH cosolvent mixtures for their myotoxic potential using an in vitro model that they developed. This model measures cumulative release of CK as a marker of muscle damage, and the values can be compared to positive and negative control values. The specific details of this model are discussed in other chapters in this volume. They showed that at moderate cosolvent concentrations (20–40 percent, v/v), PG was considerably more myotoxic than PEG 400 or EtOH (PG > EtOH > PEG 400). This seemed to correlate with hemolytic potentials of the cosolvent mixtures as reported by Reed and Yalkowsky (1985). These results were compared to those obtained in vivo in rabbits, evaluating serum CK levels following IM administration of 40 percent PG, 40 percent PEG 400, or normal saline. They showed that in all cases serum CK levels increased following the injection. However, the levels were much higher for the cosolvent formulations (PG >> PEG 400 > saline). They observed that it took 3 days to return to normal serum CK levels.

In more recent studies, we have investigated the in vitro myotoxicity of DMA, Cremophor® EL, polysorbate 80, safflower oil, and Labrafil® using the isolated muscle model as above. The results from these studies are shown in Table 11.7 and are compared to our historical positive and negative control values (Dilantin® injection and normal saline, respectively). The toxicity of all these solvents, with the exception of safflower oil and 30% Cremophor® EL (very close to the negative saline control value), was intermediate between the positive and negative control values. This would be consistent with an oily vehicle being less toxic to tissues versus an aqueous vehicle. It is unclear as to why there was no concentration-myotoxicity response between the concentrations of Cremophor® EL. Of all these solvents, DMA and polysorbate 80 were found to be the most toxic. This could be attributed to their ability to solubilize the muscle membrane leading to release of CK.

In an attempt to elucidate the factors responsible for muscle damage, Brazeau and Fung (1989c) evaluated how physicochemical properties of the vehicle composition affected muscle damage following IM administration of various cosolvents, including PG–water, EtOH–water and PEG 400–water mixtures. The properties that were evaluated were dielectric constant, apparent pH, surface tension, and viscosity. They made several notable observations, including (1) as the hydrophilicity of the cosolvent mixtures increased, myotoxicity decreased; (2) there was no defined pH range where muscle damage could be minimized; and (3) that, unlike hemolysis, the addition of NaCl had no protective effect on muscle damage produced. They concluded that myotoxicity was not exclusively related to a single parameter or a combination of the four parameters evaluated.

Table 11.7. Myotoxicity of Selected Solvent Vehicles

Vehicle	Myotoxicity – Cumulative CK Release over 2 h Mean CK (× 100) and (SEM); $n = 4$–6
20% DMA	9.50 (2.60)
30% DMA	13.4 (2.10)
20% Cremophor® EL	6.87 (1.69)
30% Cremophor® EL	4.94 (0.83)
5% Tween 80®	20.1 (3.21)
Safflower oil	2.89 (1.47)
20% Labrafil®	7.90 (1.65)
30% Labrafil®	8.94 (1.69)
Positive control Dilantin® injection	70.1 (4.71)
Negative control normal saline injection	5.06 (0.50)

Chu and Brazeau (1994) also showed that PG and PEG 400 had different effects on skeletal muscle sarcoplasmic reticulum calcium uptake and release. They showed that 10.5 percent PEG 400 stimulated calcium uptake without significantly altering the adenosine triphosphatase (ATPase) activity of the calcium pump. However, at 10.5 percent PG, there was no significant effect on either calcium uptake or ATPase activity of the pump. These findings further supported the role of calcium in mediating cosolvent-induced muscle damage, as suggested earlier (Brazeau and Fung 1990b). They also provided a possible explanation for the differences in the two cosolvents in their potentials to cause muscle damage, based on increased myoplasmic calcium removal and reduced calcium release.

COSOLVENT-RELATED PAIN ON INJECTION

The use of parenteral routes of administration may result in pain and irritation at the site of injection. This may be related to the injection itself or the properties of the drug substance. However, the pain and irritation many times appears to be associated with the formulation vehicle, particularly those that contain high fractions of cosolvents or those that have high osmolalities. In general, comparisons between solutions containing lower or different cosolvent compositions or lower osmolalities have shown fewer incidences of pain on injection, as well as reduced local toxicity (Bjork et al. 1969; Almèn and Tragardh 1973; Almèn et al. 1977; Tillman et al. 1979).

There have been numerous methods and guidelines published relating to the assessment of pain (Beecher 1957; Woodforde and Merskey 1972; Ohnhaus and Adler 1975; Celozzi et al. 1980; Vierck and Cooper 1984; Comerski et al. 1986; Marcek et al. 1992; Gupta et al. 1994). These methods can be characterized as reflexive (tail-flick, paw-lick, hot plate, or pinch test), conscious escape (flinch-jump test), prolonged protective activity (fleeing/fighting), and retreat/withdrawal responses. These models vary in the degree of subjectivity of the pain assessment and are discussed elsewhere in this book.

Cosolvents Known to Cause Pain

Glycerin has been recognized as an irritating agent that caused pain and inflammation at the site of injection. Van Metre et al. (1996) reported pain and dermal reactions caused by the administration of glycerin in immunotherapy solutions. Such solutions come prepared in 50 percent glycerin to preserve potency for 2 to 3 years. The solutions are supposed to be diluted prior to administration to levels between 10 to 30 percent glycerin and administered in volumes ranging from 0.1 to 1.0 mL. Their results showed that

pain scores of subjects given glycerin increased significantly as both glycerin concentration and dose volume increased.

When used undiluted, PG can cause considerable pain and irritation
at the site of injection. These effects have been reported for parenteral administration of nitroglycerin (Demey et al. 1984; Shook et al. 1984; Col et al.
1985; Demey et al. 1984,1988); etomidate (Bedichek and Kirschbaum 1991;
Levy et al 1995), multivitamins (Glasgow et al. 1983), and phenytoin (Hitot-
sumatsu et al. 1995). Other investigators have shown that altered formulations of various cosolvent-containing preparations, containing either
reduced organic fractions or using a mixture of different organic solvents
to minimize the load of a particular solvent, were less painful than when administered in the traditional formulation (Burton et al. 1974). Many of these
studies have shown that pain on injection was associated with the formulation vehicle, particularly when containing relatively high amounts of PG.

Diazepam, which contains 40 percent PG, has been associated with
many incidences of pain on injection, which has been related to the composition of the formulation vehicle. Pain on injection has been reported in
up to 22 percent of patients, with subsequent development of venous
sequelae (phlebitis, thrombosis, or thrombophlebitis) appearing in up to
30 percent of patients (McClish 1966; Brown and Dundee 1968). It is suspected that precipitation of the poorly water-soluble drug on administration is at least partially responsible for these side effects. Langdon et al.
(1973), however, did not observe any correlation between pain on injection
and development of venous sequelae.

While evaluating pain and irritation following injection of various parenteral formulations using the rat paw-lick model, Gupta and coworkers
(1994) suggested that there was a pain "threshold limit" in terms of observed number of paw licks related to the concentration of a pain-inducing
component, at least in the case of PG–containing formulations. In these
studies, concentrations above this "threshold limit" did not result in increases in the pain responses, making predictions using this model somewhat problematic. These data showed that administration of formulations
containing 50 percent PG caused less pain than formulations containing
40 percent PG, in both the presence and absence of 5 percent EtOH. The
same observation was made for PG solutions containing 15 percent EtOH,
whereby more pain was observed at 35 percent PG, as compared to preparations containing 40 or 50 percent PG. Analysis of CK levels following
these injections showed that they increased (indicative of muscle damage)
as a function of the cosolvent composition. Therefore, one must be cautious
when interpreting data from these pain models, since pain may not correlate with damage resulting from the injection of the formulation.

Methods to Minimize Pain

There have been numerous investigations as to how to reduce the pain following parenteral administration of various formulations. In many cases, these methods are similar to those used to minimize hemolysis. The most common methods used to minimize pain on injection are (1) administration of the dose via a large vessel; (2) dilution of the formulation in some manner that does not result in precipitation, or similarly, administration of the dose as a slow infusion to reduce the effective concentration of cosolvent in the system at a given period of time; (3) formulation of the compound using solvents that are less irritating; or (4) prior or coadministration of an anesthetic or analgesic agent, such as lidocaine or morphine, to reduce the pain.

Administration Via Large Vessels

Kawar and Dundee (1982) investigated the effect of choice of injection site, including the variables of vein size and location. They observed that the greatest incidence of pain occurred when administering various formulations via small to medium sized veins, and that using the hand and wrist veins caused more pain than those in the antecubital space (Table 11.8). The use of large veins rather than small veins, and selecting the antecubital space rather than the back of the hand or wrist consistently showed better tolerability, regardless of whether the formulation contained 0.9 percent saline or various cosolvents.

Similarly, Langdon et al. (1973) reported that venous sequelae occurred less frequently when administering IV doses of diazepam through larger veins. They noticed that phlebitis almost always resulted when administering the doses through small veins. The incidence of pain resulting from administration of propofol, an anesthetic agent, has been reported to range from 25 to 100 percent if given via a vein on the dorsal side of the hand (Hynynen et al. 1985; Stark et al. 1986; Sebel 1989; Stokes et al. 1989; Johnson et al. 1990), and only 3 to 36 percent if injected into larger, proximal veins in the antecubital fossa (McCulloch and Lees 1985; Scott et al. 1988; Gehan et al. 1991).

Dilution of the Formulation

Dilution of cosolvent formulations has been shown to reduce the incidences of both pain and venous sequelae. However, precipitation of a poorly water-soluble drug is likely to result if diluted into an aqueous medium (water, saline, or even plasma). Precipitation may be immediate or may develop over time. Van Metre and coworkers (1996) showed that pain resulting from subcutaneous injections of glycerol solutions (0, 10, 20, and 30 percent glycerol with dose volumes ranging from 0.1 to 1.0 mL) to

Table 11.8. Frequency of Pain on Injection and Venous Sequelae Following Administration of Various Test Formulations (Total Number of Patients Evaluated in Parenthesis) (Kawar and Dundee 1982)

Drug/Formulation	Primary Solvent	% Frequency of Pain on Injection	% Frequency of Venous Sequelae	% Sequelae Related to Vein Size		% Sequelae Related to Vein Site	
				Large	Small + Medium	Antecubital Fossa	Back of Hand + Wrist
0.9% Saline	Water	0 (50)	2 (50)	0 (18)	3 (32)	0 (23)	4 (27)
2.5% Thiopentone	Water	9 (100)	4 (50)	5 (20)	3 (30)	17 (12)	0 (38)
1.0% Methohexitone	Water	12 (100)	10 (50)	12 (24)	8 (26)	12 (33)	6 (17)
1.0% ICI 35868 (Disoprofol)	Cremophor® EL	4 (50)	10 (50)	12 (24)	8 (26)	8 (48)	50 (2)
0.5% Diazepam							
Valium®	Propylene glycol	37 (100)	40 (50)	18 (28)	32 (22)	17 (30)	50 (20)
Diazemuls®	Soya bean oil	0 (50)	2 (50)	0 (31)	5 (19)	0 (32)	6 (18)
0.5% Midazolam	Water	1 (400)	8 (100)	11 (65)	3 (35)	11 (70)	0 (30)

15 subjects increased significantly as a function of both injection volume and glycerol concentration.

Alteration of the Vehicle Composition

In efforts to minimize both pain and venous sequelae, alternative formulation vehicles have been used for administering diazepam to patients. Burton and coworkers (1974) used a solution of 1 percent Cremophor® EL in saline to dilute diazepam to a final concentration of 1 mg/mL. Following administration of this formulation to over 400 patients, it was reported that incidences of pain on injection were essentially eliminated, even when injected into small veins, and incidences of venous sequelae in these patients were reduced to less than 1 percent. This eliminated precipitation of the solution, which was observed in the traditional formulation (Jusko et al. 1973). They also observed that if pain was observed following IV administration, flushing the vein with 5 mL saline or 10 mg of heparin sodium through the same needle diminished the incidence of venous sequelae.

Kortilla et al. (1976) evaluated the effects of PG following IM injection in humans, comparing pain, muscle damage and precipitation for the following diazepam formulations: Valium® (Roche), Diapam® (Orion) and an experimental formulation 301-K 2/74 (Orion). The 301-K 2/74 formulation contained a lower concentration of PG (20 percent) with 60 percent PEG 300. The Valium® and Diapam® formulations contained the same cosolvent composition (41 percent PG, 8.5 percent EtOH). These formulations provided no statistical differences in plasma levels following IM administration, although the levels for Valium® tended to be lower than for the other formulations. At doses of 0.15 mg/kg, they found that pain was significantly greater in the Valium® and Diapam® formulations than in the 301-K 2/74 or placebo (301-K 2/74 with no drug) in double blind crossover studies. This is consistent with earlier rat studies showing a lack of irritation after IM injections of the PG/PEG vehicle. They also showed that the PG/PEG formulation was less likely to precipitate as compared to the Diapam® formulation. Addition of 10 mg (2 mL) of Diapam® to 100 mL of 5 percent glucose caused precipitation, whereas up to 25 mg (5 mL) of the PG/PEG formulation could be added before precipitation was observed.

Kawar and Dundee (1982) evaluated the pain on injection of several preparations that were formulated in different solvent systems in a patient population. They evaluated factors such as composition, size of the vessel through which the dose was administered, and the frequency of venous sequelae. They found that the formulation causing the most irritation was the Valium® formulation containing 40 percent PG and 10 percent EtOH. The same compound formulated in an oil-based system caused no pain on administration. The other formulations composed of either water or Cremophor® EL caused less pain. Additionally, the PG formulation caused the highest percentage of venous sequelae as compared to the other vehicles. Diazepam formulated in the oil-based vehicle was essentially the same as the saline controls, suggesting that these sequelae were the result of the cosolvent.

Administration of Anesthetic/Analgesic Agents

The use of anesthetic/analgesic agents to minimize pain following injection of various parenteral formulations has been studied using agents ranging from aspirin to morphine (Comerski et al. 1986; King et al. 1992; Marcek et al. 1992; Doenicke et al. 1996). Comereski et al. (1986) observed that coadministration of lidocaine (0.5 to 1 percent) offered protection from pain but not from the associated muscle damage resulting from the injection. Marcek and coworkers (1992) reported the effect of morphine administered 15 min prior to being given an infusion of an irritating solution (0.05 M potassium chloride). They found that administration of morphine (ranging from 2 to 4 mg/kg) virtually eliminated the pain associated with the test solution alone. Celozzi and coworkers (1982) also showed that coadministration of a local anesthetic (lidocaine) reduced the pain associated with subplantar administration of antibiotic solutions. They showed that the administration of the anesthetic reduced the pain to approximately the same level as the control water injections. It is typically thought that pain on injection is related to muscle damage caused by the administration of the dose.

Propofol (Diprivan®) has a very high incidence of pain on IV injection. Several investigators showed that the use of various anesthetic/analgesic agents resulted in abatement of pain caused by the administration of propofol (Bahar et al. 1982; Brooker et al. 1985; Helbro-Hansen et al. 1988; Gehan et al. 1991; King et al. 1992). King and coworkers (1992) showed that coadministration of lidocaine (ranging from 5 to 20 mg doses) resulted in the reduction of both the incidence of pain and its severity. In this study of 368 patients, the incidence of pain following administration of lidocaine was 32 percent, relative to 73 percent following saline injection. The degree to which the pain was alleviated was found to be dose responsive. However, 6 percent of patients treated with 20 mg lidocaine still reported unpleasant pain.

CONCLUSIONS

The use of cosolvents as solubilization enhancers in parenteral formulations has been, and continues to be, a valuable tool for the formulation scientist. However, it becomes crucial for the formulator to understand prior to the selection or use of these cosolvent systems that they differ widely in their physicochemical properties, which in turn can result in varying degrees of adverse effects such as hemolysis, muscle damage, and pain at the injection site. The most commonly used cosolvents in parenteral formulations—including the polyethylene glycols, propylene glycol, ethanol, glycerin, cremophors, benzyl alcohol, dimethylacetamide, and dimethylsulfoxide—have been highlighted in this chapter. Furthermore, cosolvent-related factors, mechanisms, and approaches to offset the hemolysis, muscle damage, or pain following injection have been generally presented so that the formulator can rationally select and incorporate these agents into the design of injectables.

REFERENCES

Ahmed, S. S., G. E. Levinson, and T. J. Regan. 1973. Depression of myocontractility with low doses of ethanol in normal man. *Circulation* 48:378–385.

Almèn, T. and B. Tragardh. 1973. Effects of non-ionic contrast media on the blood flow through the femoral artery of the dog. *Acta Radiologica* 14 (supp):197–202.

Almèn, T., E. Boijsen, and S. E. Lindell. 1977. Metrizamide in angiography. *Acta Radiologica Diag.* 18:33–38.

American Academy of Pediatrics Committee on Drugs. 1985. Inactive ingredients in pharmaceutical products. *Pediatrics* 76 (4):635–643.

Andersen, K. E., and T. Damsgaard. 1976. The effect on serum enzymes of intramuscular injections of digoxin, pentazocine and isotonic sodium chloride. *Acta Med. Scand.* 99:317–319.

Andersen, T. H., K. B. Hindsholm, and J. Fallingborg. 1989. Severe complication to phytomenadione after intramuscular injection in woman in labor. *Acta Obstet. Gynecol. Scand.* 68:381–382.

Anderson, R. C., P. N. Harris, and K. K. Chen. 1950. Toxicological studies on synthetic glycerin. *J. Am. Pharm. Assoc. Sci. Ed.* 39:583–385.

Angleborg, C., I. Klockhoff, H-C. Larsen, and J. Stahle. 1982. Hyperosmotic solutions and hearing in Meniere's disease. *Am. J. Otol.* 3 (3):200–202.

Ansel, H. C. 1964. Intravenous solutions and the erythrocyte. *Am. J. Hosp. Pharm.* 21:25–30.

Ansel, H. C. 1965. Influence of polyethylene glycols on the hemolytic activity of phenolic preservatives. *J. Pharm. Sci.* 54:1159–1162.

Ansel, H. C., and G. E. Cabre. 1970. Influence of dimethyl sulfoxide on the hemolytic activity of antimicrobial preservatives I. *J. Pharm. Sci.* 59:478–481.

Ansel, H. C., and W. J. Husa. 1959. Isotonic solutions. VII. The permeability of red corpuscles to various salts of gluconic acid. *J. Am. Pharm. Assoc. Sci. Ed.* 48:516–521.

Ansel, H. C., and W. F. Leake. 1966. Hemolysis of erythrocytes by antibacterial preservatives III. Influence of DMSO on the hemolytic activity of phenol. *J. Pharm. Sci.* 55:685–688.

Arulanatham, K., and M. Genel. 1978. Central nervous system systemic toxicity associated with ingestion of propylene glycol. *J. Pediatr.* 93:515–516.

Attar, A. M., and C. Mata. 1971. Increased levels of creatinine phosphokinase after intramuscular injections. *Med. Annals D.C.* 40 (2):92–93.

Auclair, M., and N. Hameau. 1964. Toxicité et pharmacologie de deux solvants organiques: La diméthylacétamide et la diméthylformamide. *Soc. de Biologie.* 158:245-248.

Bahar, M., E. McAteer, J. W. Dundee, and L. P. Briggs. 1982. Aspirin in the prevention of painful intravenous injection of di-isopropofol (ICI 35 868) and diazepam (Valium®). *Anesth.* 37:847–848.

Banziger, R. 1967. Hemolysis testing in vivo of parenteral formulations. *Bull. Parent. Drug Assoc.* 21:148–151.

Bartsch, W., G. Sponer, K. Dietmann, and G. Fuchs. 1976. Acute toxicity of various solvents in the mouse and rat. *Arzneim.-Forsch.* 25 (8):1581–1583.

BASF Corporation. 1988. Cremophor EL. Technical leaflet.

Bedichek, E., and B. Kirschbaum. 1991. A case of propylene glycol toxic reaction associated with etomidate infusion. *Arch. Intern. Med.* 151:2297–2298.

Beecher, H. K. 1957. The measurement of pain: Prototype for the quantitative study of subjective responses. *Pharmacol. Rev.* 9:59–209.

Bekeris, L., C. Baker, J. Fenton, D. Kimball, and E. Bermes. 1979. Propylene glycol as a cause of elevated serum osmolality. *Am. J. Clin. Path.* 72 (4):633–636.

Benda, G. I., J. L. Hiller, and J. W. Reynolds. 1986. Benzyl alcohol toxicity: Impact on neurological handicaps among surviving very low birth weight infants. *Pediatrics* 77 (4):507–512.

Bendas, B., U. Schmalfuss, and R. Neubert. 1995. Influence of propylene glycol as cosolvent on mechanisms of drug transport from hydrogels. *Int. J. Pharm.* 116:19–30.

Bennett, W. M., and R. S. Muther. 1981. Lack of nephrotoxicity of intravenous dimethylsulfoxide. *Clin. Tox.* 18 (5):615–618.

Bjork, L., U. Erikson, and B. Ingelman. 1969. Clinical experiences with a new type of contrast medium in peripheral arteriography. *Am. J. Roentgenology* 106 (2): 418–424.

Braun, H. A., and G. F. Cartland. 1936. The toxicity of propylene glycol. *J. Am. Pharm. Assoc. Ed.* 25 (9):746–749.

Brazeau, G. A., and H. L. Fung. 1989a. An in vitro model to evaluate muscle damage following intramuscular injections. *Pharm. Res.* 6 (2):167–170.

Brazeau, G. A., and H. L. Fung. 1989b. Physicochemical properties of binary organic cosolvent-water mixtures and their relationships to muscle damage following intramuscular injection. *J. Parent. Sci. Tech.* 43 (4):144–149.

Brazeau, G. A., and H. L. Fung. 1989c. Use of an in vitro model for the assessment of muscle damage from intramuscular injections: In vitro-in vivo correlation and predictability with mixed solvent systems. *Pharm. Res.* 6 (9):766–771.

Brazeau, G. A., and H. L. Fung. 1990a. Effect of organic cosolvent-induced skeletal muscle damage on the bioavailability of intramuscular [14C]diazepam. *J. Pharm. Sci.* 79 (9):773–777.

Brazeau, G. A., and H. L. Fung. 1990b. Mechanisms of creatinine kinase release from isolated rat skeletal muscles damaged by propylene glycol and ethanol. *J. Pharm. Sci.* 79 (5):393–397.

Brittain, R. T., and P. F. D'Arcy. 1962. Hematologic effects following the intravenous injection of propylene glycol in the rabbit. *Tox. Appl. Pharm.* 4:738–744.

Brooker, J., C. J. Hull, and M. Stafford. 1985. Effect of lignocaine on pain caused by propofol injection. *Anesth.* 40:91–92.

Brown, S. S., and J. W. Dundee. 1968. Clinical studies of induction agents XXV: Diazepam. *Brit. J. Anaesth.* 40:108–112.

Brown, W. J., N. R. M. Buist, H. T. C. Gipson, R. K. Huston, and N. G. Kennaway. 1982. Fatal benzyl alcohol poisoning in a neonatal intensive care unit. *Lancet* i:1250.

Budavari, S., ed. 1989. *The Merck index,* 11th ed. Rahway, N.J., USA: Merck and Co, Inc.

Budden, R., U. G. Kuhl, and G. Buschmann. 1978. Ausgewahlte untersuchungen zur pharmakodynamischen eigenwirkung verschiedener losungsvermittler. *Arzneim.-Forsch.* 28:1579–1586.

Burton, G. W., R. J. Lenz, T. A. Thomas, and M. Midda. 1974. Cremophor EL as a diluent for diazepam. *Brit. Med. J.* 7:258.

Cadwallader, D. E. 1963. Behavior of erythrocytes in various solvent systems. I. Water-glycerin and water-propylene glycol. *J. Pharm. Sci.* 52 (12):1175–1180.

Cadwallader, D. E., and J. P. Drinkard. 1967. Behavior of erythrocytes in various solvent systems. IV. Water-dimethylsulfoxide. *J. Pharm. Sci.* 56:583–586.

Cadwallader, D. E. Jr., and H. J. Husa. 1958. Isotonic solutions. VI. The permeability of red corpuscles to various salts of organic acids. *J. Am. Pharm. Assoc. Sci. Ed.* 47:705–711.

Cadwallader, D. E., and J. R. Phillips. 1969. Behavior of erythrocytes in various solvent systems. V. Water-liquid amides. *J. Pharm. Sci.* 58(10):1220–1224.

Cadwallader, D. E., B. W. Wickliffe, and B. L. Smith. 1964. Behavior of erythrocytes in various solvent systems II. Effect of temperature and various substances on water-glycerin and water-propylene glycol solutions. *J. Pharm. Sci.* 53:927–931.

Cameron, G. R., and E. S. Finckh. 1956. The production of an acute haemolytic crisis by the subcutaneous injection of glycerol. *J. Path. Bact.* 71:165–172.

Carpenter, C. P. 1947. Cellosolve. *JAMA.* 135:880.

Carpenter, C. P., and C. B. Shaffer. 1952. A study of polyethylene glycols as vehicles for intramuscular and subcutaneous injection. *J. Am. Pharm. Assoc. Sci. Ed.* 41:27–29.

Cate, J. C. IV, and R. Hedrick. 1980. Propylene glycol intoxication and lactic acidosis. *NEJM.* 303:1237.

Caujolle, F., P. H. Chanh, N. Dat-Xuong, and M. C. Azum-Gelade. 1970. Toxicological studies upon acetamide and its N-methyl and N-ethyl derivatives. *Arzneim.-Forsch.* 20 (9):1242–1246.

Celozzi, E., V. J. Lotti, E. O. Stapley, and A. K. Miller. 1980. An animal model for assessing pain-on-injection of antibiotics. *J. Pharm. Meth.* 4:285–289.

Child, J. S., R. B. Kovick, J. A. Levisman, and M. L. Pearce. 1979. Cardiac effects of acute ethanol ingestion unmasked by autonomic blockade. *Circulation* 59 (1): 120–125.

Cho, C. H., W. M. Hui, N. X. Liao, X. G. Liu, S. K. Lam, and C. W. Ogle. 1992. Polyethylene glycol: Its adverse gastric effects in rats. *J. Pharm. Pharmacol.* 44:518–520.

Chu, A., and G. A. Brazeau. 1994. Solvent-dependent influences on skeletal muscle sarcoplasmic reticulum calcium uptake and release. *Tox. Appl. Pharmacol.* 125:142–148.

Col, J., C. Col-Debeys, E. Lavenne-Pardonge, L. Hericks, M. C. Broze, and M. Moriau. 1985. Propylene glycol-induced heparin resistance during nitroglycerin infusion. *Am. Heart J.* 110 (1):171–173.

Comerski, C. R., P. D. Williams, C. L. Bregman, and G. H. Hottendorf. 1986. Pain on injection and muscle irritation: A comparison of animal models for assessing parenteral antibiotics. *Fund. Appl. Toxicol.* 6:335–338.

Darwish, R. M., and S. F. Bloomfield. 1995. The effect of co-solvents on the antibacterial activity of paraben preservatives. *Int. J. Pharm.* 119:183–192.

Davis, K. J., and P. M. Jenner. 1959. Toxicity of three drug solvents. *Tox. Appl. Pharm.* 1:576–578.

Delgado, C. E., N. J. Fortuin, and R. S. Ross. 1975. Acute effects of low doses of alcohol on left ventricular function by echocardiography. *Circulation* 51:535–540.

Demey, H. E., R. A. Daelmans, M. E. DeBroe, and L. Bossaert. 1984. Propylene glycol intoxication due to intravenous nitroglycerin. *Lancet* i:1360.

Demey, H. E., R. A. Daelmans, G. A. Verpooten, M. E. De Broe, C. M. Van Campenhout, F. V. Lakiere, P. J. Schepens, and C. C. Bossaert. 1988. Propylene glycol induced side effects during intravenous nitroglycerin therapy. *Int. Care Med.* 14:221–226.

Diness, V. 1985. Local tissue damage after intramuscular injections in rabbits and pigs: Quantitation by determination of creatinine kinase activity at injection sites. *Acta Pharmacol. et Toxicol.* 56:410–415.

DiStefano, V., and J. J. Klahn. 1965. Observations on the pharmacology and hemolytic activity of dimethyl sulfoxide. *Tox. Appl. Pharm.* 7:660–666.

Dixon, R. L., R. H. Adamson, M. Ben, and D. P. Rall. 1965. Apparent lack of interaction between dimethyl sulfoxide (DMSO) and a variety of drugs. *Proc. Soc. Exp. Biol. Med.* 118:756–759.

Doenicke, A., B. Loffler, J. Kugler, H. Suttmann, and B. Grote. 1982. Plasma concentration and EEG after various regimens of etomidate. *Br. J. Anaesth.* 54:393–400.

Doenicke, A., A. E. Nebauer, R. Hoernecke, M. Mayer, and M. F. Roizen. 1992. Osmolalities of propylene glycol-containing formulations for parenteral use: Should propylene glycol be used as a solvent? *Anesth. Analg.* 75:431–435.

Doenicke, A., M. F. Roizen, A. E. Nebauer, A. Kugler, R. Hoernecke, and H. Berger-Hintzen. 1994. A comparison of two formulations for etomidate, 2-Hydroxypropyl-β-cyclodextrin (HPCD) and propylene glycol. *Anesth. Analg.* 79:933–939.

Doenicke, A. W., M. F. Roizen, J. Rau, W. Kellermann, and J. Babl. 1996. Reducing pain during propofol injection: The role of the solvent. *Anesth. Anal.* 82 (3): 472–474.

Dominguez-Gil, A., and R. Cadorniga. 1971a. Toxicidad muscular de los polioles, Part IV. *Il Farmaco-Ed. Pr.* 26 (9):535–543.

Dominguez-Gil, A., and R. Cadorniga. 1971b. Los polioles. Caracteristicas farmacotecnicas y toxicologicas. *Il Farmaco-Ed. Pr.* 26 (7):394–404.

Dorr, R. T. 1994. Pharmacology and toxicity of Cremophor EL diluent. *Ann. Pharmacother.* 28:S11–S14.

Driessen, J. J., T. B. Vree, J. van Edmond, L. H. D. J. Booji, and J. F. Crul. 1985. Interaction of some benzodiazepines and their solvents with vecuronium in the in vivo rat sciatic nerve-tibialis anterior muscle preparation. *Arch. Int. de Pharmacodynam. Therapie.* 273:277–288.

Drummond, J. C., D. J. Cole, P. M. Patel, and L. W. Reynolds. 1995. Focal cerebral ischemia during anesthesia with etomidate, isoflurane or thiopental: A comparison of the extent of cerebral injury. *Neurosurg.* 37:742–748.

Dye, D., and J. Watkins. 1980. Suspected anaphylactic reaction to Cremophor EL. *Br. Med. J.* 60:1353.

Easterly, W. D. Jr., and W. J. Husa. 1954. Isotonic solutions. IV. Urea and urea derivatives. *J. Am. Pharm. Assoc. Sci. Ed.* 43:750-754.

Edmonson, T. D., and J. E. Goyan. 1958. The effect of hydrogen ion and alcohol concentration on the solubility of phenobarbital. *J. Am. Pharm. Assoc. Sci. Ed.* 47:810–812.

Evans, E. F., J. D. Proctor, M. Fratkin, J. Valandia, and A. J. Wasserman. 1973. Differences in blood flow to human muscle groups as a possible determinant of drug absorption. *Clin. Pharm. Ther.* 14:134–135.

Evens, R. P. 1975. Toxicity of intravenous benzyl alcohol. *Drug Intel. Clin. Pharm.* 9:154–155.

Fairfull-Smith, R. J., D. Stoski, and J. B. Freeman. 1982. Use of glycerol in peripheral parenteral nutrition. *Surgery* 92 (4):728–732.

FAO/WHO. 1974. Toxicological evaluation of certain food additives with a review of the general principles and of the specifications. 17th Report of the FAO/WHO Expert Committee on Food Additives. *Tech. Rep. Ser. Wld. Hlth. Org.*, No. 539.

FAO/WHO. 1980. Evaluation of certain food additives: 23rd report of the joint FAO/WHO expert committee on food additives. *Tech. Rep. Ser. Wld. Hlth. Org.*, No. 648.

Farooqui, M. Y. H., B. Ybarra, J. Piper, and A. Tamez. 1995. Effect of dosing vehicle on the toxicity and metabolism of unsaturated aliphatic nitriles. *J. Appl. Tox.* 15 (5):411–420.

Federal Register. 1982. Food and Drug Administration (FDA. GRAS status of propylene glycol and propylene glycol monostearate. *Federal Register* 47:27810.

Fedors, R. F. 1974. A method for estimating both the solubility parameters and molar volumes of liquids. *Polym. Eng. Sci.* 14 (2):147–154.

Fellows, W., M. D. Bastow, A. J. Byrne, and S. P. Allison. 1983. Adrenocortical suppression in multiple injured patients: A complication of etodimate treatment. *Br. Med. J.* 287:1835–1837.

Fisher, A. A. 1995. Systemic contact dermatitis due to intravenous valium in a person sensitive to propylene glycol. *Cutis.* 55 (6):327–328.

Fligner, C. L., R. Jack, G. A. Twiggs, and V. A. Raisys. 1985. Hyperosmolality induced by propylene glycol. A complication of silver sulfadiazide therapy. *JAMA.* 253:1606–1609.

Forrest, A. R. W., K. Watrasiewicz, and C. J. Moore. 1977. Long term Althesin infusion and hyperlipidemia. *Br. Med. J.* 2:1357–1358.

Fort, F. L., I. A. Heyman, and J. W. Kesterson. 1984. Hemolysis study of aqueous polyethylene glycol 400, propylene glycol and ethanol combinations in vivo and in vitro. *J. Parent. Sci. Tech.* 38 (2):82–87.

Frank, M. S., M. C. Nahata, and M. D. Hilty. 1981. Glycerol: A review of its pharmacology, pharmacokinetics, adverse reactions and clinical use. *Pharmacother.* 1:147–160.

Fu, R. C-C., D. M. Lidgate, J. L. Whatley. and T. McCullough. 1987. The biocompatibility of parenteral vehicles—in vitro/in vivo screening comparison and the effect of excipients on hemolysis. *Bull. Parent. Drug Assoc.* 41 (5):164–167.

Gehan, G., P. Karoubi, F. Quinet, A. Leroy, C. Rathat, and J. L. Pourriat. 1991. Optimal dose of lignocaine for preventing pain on injection of propofol. *Br. J. Anesth.* 66:324–326.

Gerald, M. C., and F. V. O'Bannon. 1988. *Nursing pharmacology and therapeutics,* 2nd ed. Englewood Cliifs, N.J., USA: Appleton and Lange.

Gershanik, J., B. Boecler, H. Ensley, S. McCloskey, and W. George. 1982. The gasping syndrome and benzyl alcohol poisoning. *New Eng. J. Med.* 307 (22): 1384–1388.

Gettler, A. O., and V. St. George. 1935. Toxicology in children. *Am. J. Clin. Pathol.* 5 (6):466–488.

Glasgow, A. M., R. L. Boeckx, M. K. Miller, M. G. MacDonald, G. P. August, and S. I. Goodman. 1983. Hyperosmolality in small infants due to propylene glycol. *Pediatrics* 72 (3):353–355.

Golightly, L. K., S. S. Smolinske, M. L. Bennett, E. W. Sutherland III, and B. H. Rumack. 1988. Pharmaceutical excipients: Adverse effects associated with inactive ingredients in drug products (Part I). *Med. Toxicol.* 3:128–165.

González de la Riva Lamana, J. M. 1987. Medicaniemtos con alcohol bencilico en neonatologia. *Farm. Clin.* 4 (6):474–478.

Gorman, W. G., and G. D. Hall. 1964. Dielectric constant correlations with solubility and solubility parameters. *J. Pharm. Sci.* 53:1017–1020.

Greenblatt, D. J., R. I. Shader, and J. Koch-Weser. 1976. Serum creatinine phosphokinase concentrations after intramuscular chlordiazepoxide and its solvent. *J. Clin. Pharmacol.* 16:118–121.

Grisson, C. B., A. M. Chagovetz, and Z. Wang. 1993. Use of viscosigens to stabilize vitamin B12 solutions against photolysis. *J. Pharm. Sci.* 82 (6):641–643.

Grosicki, T. S., and W. J. Husa. 1954. Isotonic solutions. III. Amino acids and sugars. *J. Am. Pharm. Assoc. Sci. Ed.* 43 (10):632–635.

Gross, D. R., J. V. Kitzman, and H. R. Adams. 1979. Cardiovascular effects of intravenous administration of propylene glycol and oxytetracycline in propylene glycol in calves. *Am. J. Vet. Res.* 40 (6):783–791.

Guindon, B., J. Harvey, A. Peacocke, S. Shirley, and J. Valberg. 1981. Factors modifying vitreous pressure in cataract surgery. *Can. J. Ophthalmol.* 16:73–75.

Gupta, P. K., J. P. Patel, and K. R. Hahn. 1994. Evaluation of pain and irritation following local administration of parenteral formulations using the rat paw lick model. *J. Pharm. Sci. Tech.* 48 (3):159–166.

Hagnevik, K., E. Gordon, L-E. Lins, S. Wilhelmsson, and D. Forster. 1974. Glycerol-induced haemolysis with haemoglobinuria and acute renal failure. *Lancet* i:75–77.

Hammarlund, E. R., and K. Pedersen-Bjergaard. 1958. A simplified graphic method for the preparation of isotonic solutions. *J. Amer. Pharm. Assoc. Sci. Ed.* 47:107–114.

Hammarlund, E. R., and K. Pedersen-Bjergaard. 1961. Hemolysis of erythrocytes in various iso-osmotic solutions. *J. Amer. Pharm. Assoc. Sci. Ed.* 50:24–30.

Hartman, C. W., and W. J. Husa. 1957. Isotonic solutions. V. The permeability of red corpuscles to various salts. *J. Am. Pharm. Soc. Sci. Ed.* 46:430–433.

Havel, M., M. Muller, W. Graninger, R. Kurz, and H. Lindemayr. 1987. Tolerability of a new vitamin K preparation for parenteral administration to adults: One case of anaphylactoid reaction. *Clin. Ther.* 9 (4):373–378.

Heilman, R. D., E. W. Bauer, and J. P. DaVanzo. 1972. Effect of polyethylene glycol on the cardiovascular response of the dog to autonomic agents. *Tox. Appl. Pharm.* 23:263–270.

Heine, D. L., P. F. Parker, and D. E. Francke. 1950. Propylene glycol. *Am. Soc. Hosp. Pharm.* 7:8–17.

Heistand, W. A., F. W. Stemler, and J. E. Wiebers. 1952. The relationship of dilution of ethyl alcohol to intraperitoneal toxicity in mice. *Quart. J. Alcohol Studies* 13:361–364.

Helbro-Hansen, S., V. Westergaard, B. L. Krogh, and H. P. Svendson. 1988. The reduction of pain on injection of propofol: The effect of addition of lidocaine. *Acta Anesthesiol. Scand.* 32:502–504.

Hem, S. L., D. R. Bright, G. S. Banker, and J. P. Pogue. 1974–1975. Tissue irritation evaluation of potential parenteral vehicles. *Drug Dev. Comm.* 1 (5):471–477.

Higuchi, T., M. Gupta, and L. W. Busse. 1953. Influence of electrolytes, pH, and alcohol concentration on the solubilities of acidic drugs. *J. Am. Pharm. Assoc. Sci. Ed.* 42:157–161.

Hildebrand, J. H. 1916. Solubility. *JACS*. 38:1452–1473.

Hildebrand, J. H. 1917. Solubility and internal pressure. *JACS*. 39:2297–2301.

Hildebrand, J. H. 1919. Solubility. III. Relative values of internal pressures and their practical application. *JACS*. 41:1067–1080.

Hildebrand, J. H., and R. L. Scott. 1950. Evaluation of solubility parameters. In *Solubility of non-electrolytes*, 3rd ed., New York: Reinhold Publishing Corp., pp. 424–439.

Hill, N. S., E. M. Antman, L. H. Green, and J. S. Alpert. 1981. Intravenous nitroglycerin: A review of the pharmacology, indications, therapeutic effects and complications. *Chest* 79 (1):69–76.

Hiller, J. L., G. I. Benda, M. Rahatzad, J. R. Allen, D. H. Culver, C. V. Carlson, and J. W. Reynolds. 1986. Benzyl alcohol toxicity: Impact on mortality and intraventricular hemorrhage among very low birth weight infants. *Pediatrics* 77 (4): 500–506.

Hitotosumatsu, T., T. Iwaki, M. Fukui, and J. Tateishi. 1995. Toxic myocardial damage due to intravenous phenytoin administration. *Histopath.* 26 (5):479–480.

Hopkins, C. S. 1988. Adverse reaction to a Cremophor-containing preparation of intravenous vitamin K. *Inten. Ther. Clin. Monit.* 9:254–255.

Huff, E. 1961. Metabolism of 1,2-propanediol. *Biochim. Biophys. Acta.* 48:506–517.

Huggon, I., I. James, and D. Macrae. 1990. Hyperosmolality related to propylene glycol in an infant treated with enoximone infusion. *Brit. Med. J.* 301:19–20.

Husa, W. J., and J. R. Adams. 1944. Isotonic solutions. II. The permeability of red corpuscles to various substances. *J. Am. Pharm. Assoc. Sci. Ed.* 33:329–332.

Husa, W. J., and O. A. Rossi. 1942. A study of isotonic solutions. *J. Am. Pharm. Assoc. Sci. Ed.* 31:270–277.

Hynynen, M., K. Kortilla, and T. Tammisto. 1985. Pain on IV injection of propofol (ICI 35 868) in emulsion formulation. *Acta Anesthesiol. Scand.* 29:651–652.

Jacobs, M. H., H. N. Glassman, and A. K. Parpart. 1935. Osmotic properties of the erythrocyte. *J. Cell. Comp. Physiol.* 7:197–225.

Jarvis, W. R., J. M. Hughes, J. L. Mosser, J. R. Allen, and R. W. Haley. 1983. Benzyl alcohol poisoning. *Am. J. Dis. Child.* 137:505.

Johnson, R. A., N. J. N. Harper, S. Chadwick, and A. Vohra. 1990. Pain on injection of propofol: Methods of alleviation. *Anesth.* 45:439–442.

Jones, A. R. 1982. Glycerol and propylene glycol in pharmacy. *Aust. J. Pharm.* (March):178–181.

Jung, A. L., Y. Roan, and A. R. Temple. 1980. Neonatal death associated with acute transplacental ethanol intoxication. *J. Dis. Child.* 134:419–420.

Jusko, W. J., M. Gretch, and R. Gassett. 1973. Precipitation of diazepam from intravenous preparations. *JAMA*. 225 (2):176.

Kawar, P., and J. W. Dundee. 1982. Frequency of pain on injection and venous sequelae following the IV administration of certain anaesthetics and sedatives. *Br. J. Anaesth.* 54:935–939.

Kelner, M. J., and D. N. Bailey. 1985. Propylene glycol as a cause of lactic acidosis. *J. Anal. Tox.* 9:40–42.

Kennedy, G. L. Jr., and R. D. Short Jr. 1986. Biological effects of acetamide, formamide and their monomethyl and dimethyl derivatives. *Crit. Rev. Toxicol.* 17 (2):129–182.

Kim, S-N. 1988. Preclinical toxicology and pharmacology of dimethylacetamide, with clinical notes. *Drug Metab. Rev.* 19:345–368.

Kimura, E. T., T. D. Darby, R. A. Krause, and H. D. Brondyk. 1971. Parenteral toxicity studies with benzyl alcohol. *Tox. Appl. Pharm.* 18:60–68.

King, S. Y., F. M. Davis, J. E. Wells, D. J. Murchison, and P. J. Pryor. 1992. Lidocaine for the prevention of pain due to injection of propofol. *Anesth. Analg.* 74:246–249.

Klugmann, F. B., G. Decorti, F. Mallardi, S. Klugmann, and L. Baldini. 1984. Effect of polyethylene glycol 400 on adriamycin toxicity in mice. *Eur. J. Can. Clin. Oncol.* 20 (3):405–410.

Kortilla, K., A. Sothman, and P. Andersson. 1976. Polyethylene glycol as a solvent for diazepam: Bioavailability and clinical effects after intramuscular administration, comparison of oral, intramuscular and rectal administration, and precipitation from intravenous solutions. *Acta Pharmacol. et Toxicol.* 39:104–117.

Krzyzaniak, J. F., F. A. Alvarez Nunez, D. M. Raymond, and S. H. Yalkowsky. 1997a. Lysis of human red blood cells. 4. Comparison of in vitro and in vivo hemolysis data. *J. Pharm. Sci.* 86 (11):1215–1217.

Krzyzaniak, J. F., D. M. Raymond, and S. H. Yalkowsky. 1997b. Lysis of human red blood cells 1: Effect of contact time on water induced hemolysis. *PDA J. Pharm. Sci. Tech.* 50 (4):223–226.

Krzyzaniak, J. F., D. M. Raymond, and S. H. Yalkowsky. 1997c. Lysis of human red blood cells 2: Effect of contact time on cosolvent induced hemolysis. *Int. J. Pharm.* 152:193–200.

Ku, S-H., and D. E. Cadwallader. 1975. Behavior of erythrocytes in ternary solvent systems. *J. Pharm. Sci.* 64 (11):1818–1821.

Ku, S-H., and D. E. Cadwallader. 1984. Behavior of erythrocytes in various solvent systems. VII. Water-monohydric alcohols. *J. Pharm. Sci.* 63:60–64.

Kutzsche, A. 1965. Zur toxikologie des dimethylformamids. *Arzneim.-Forsch.* 15:618–624.

Laine, G. A., S. M. H. Hossain, R. T. Solis, and S. C. Adams. 1995. Polyethylene glycol nephrotoxicity secondary to prolonged high-dose intravenous lorazepam. *Annals Pharmacother.* 29:1110–1114.

Lampe, K. F., and O. D. Easterday. 1953. A note on a contraindication to propylene glycol, as a solvent in toxicity studies. *J. Am. Pharm. Assoc. Sci. Ed.* 42 (7):455.

Langdon, D. E., J. R. Harlan, and R. L. Bailey. 1973. Thrombophlebitis with diazepam used intravenously. *JAMA.* 223:184–185.

Latven, A. R., and A. Molitor. 1939. Comparison of the toxic, hypnotic and irritating properties of eight organic solvents. *J. Pharm. Exp. Ther.* 65:89–93.

Lehman, A. J., and H. W. Newman. 1937a. Comparative intravenous toxicity of some monohydric saturated alcohols. *J. Pharm. Exp. Ther.* 26:103–106.

Lehman, A. J., and H. W. Newman. 1937b. Propylene glycol: Rate of metabolism, absorption, and excretion, with a method for estimation in body fluids. *J. Pharm. Exp. Ther.* 60:312–322.

Levy, M. L., M. Aranda, V. Zelman, and S. L. Giannotta. 1995. Propylene glycol toxicity following continuous etomidate infusion for the control of refractory cerebral edema. *Neurosurg.* 37 (2):363–369.

Lindgren, P., G. F. Saltzman, and G. Tornell. 1968. Vascular reaction to water-soluble contrast media. *Acta Radiologica Diag.* 7:152–160.

Lockard, J. S., R. H. Levy, W. C. Congdon, and L. L. DuCharme. 1979. Efficacy and toxicity of the solvent polyethylene glycol 400 in monkey model. *Epilepsia* 20:77–84.

Lockard, J. S., and R. H. Levy. 1978. Polyethylene glycol 400: Solvent and anticonvulsant? *Life Sci.* 23:2499–2502.

Lolin, Y., D. A. Francis, R. J. Flanagan, P. Little, and P. T. Lascellis. 1988. Cerebral depression due to propylene glycol in a patient with chronic epilepsy: The value of plasma osmolal gap in diagnosis. *Postgrad. Med. J.* 64:610–613.

Lorch, V., M. D. Murphy, L. R. Hoersten, E. Harris, J. Fitzgerald, and S. N. Sinha. 1985. Unusual syndrome among premature infants: Association with a new intravenous vitamin E product. *Pediatrics* 75 (3):598–602.

Lovelock, J. E., and M. W. H. Bishop. 1959. Prevention of freezing damage with dimethyl sulfoxide. *Nature* 183:1394–1395.

Lunsford, L. D. 1982. Treatment of Tic Douloureux by percutaneous retrogasserian glycerol injection. *JAMA.* 248 (4):449–453.

MacCannell, K. 1969. Hemodynamic responses to glycols and to hemolysis. *Can. J. Phys. Pharmacol.* 47:563–569.

MacDonald, J. T., and D. L. Uden. 1982. Intravenous glycerol and mannitol therapy in children with intracranial hypertension. *Neurology* 32:437–440.

MacDonald, M. G., A. B. Fletcher, E. L. Johnson, R. L. Boeckx, P. R. Getson, and M. K. Miller. 1987. The potential toxicity to neonates of multivitamin preparations used in parenteral nutrition. *J. Parent. Ent. Nutr.* 11 (2):169–171.

MacGregor, D. C., E. Schonbaum, and W. G. Bigelow. 1964. Acute toxicity studies on ethanol, propanol and butanol. *Can. J. Physiol. Pharm.* 42 (6):689–696.

Macht, D. I. 1920. A toxicological study of some alcohols, with special reference to isomers. *J. Pharm. Exp. Ther.* 16 (1):1–10.

Maling, H. M. 1970. Toxicology of single doses of ethyl alcohol. *Int. Encyc. Pharmacol. Ther.* 20:277–299.

Marcek, J. M., W. J. Seaman, and R. J. Weaver. 1992. A novel approach for the determination of the pain-producing potential of intravenously injected substances in the conscious rat. *Pharm. Res.* 9 (2):182–186.

Marcus, D., and W. J. Husa. 1959. Isotonic solutions. X. The permeability of red corpuscles to various local anesthetics. *J. Am. Pharm. Assoc. Sci. Ed.* 48 (10): 569–573.

Martin, A., and M. J. Miralles. 1982. Extended Hildebrand solubility approach: Solubility of tolbutamide, acetohexamide and sulfisomidine in binary solvent mixtures. *J. Pharm. Sci.* 71 (4):439–442.

Martin, A., J. Newburger, and A. Adjei. 1980. Extended Hildebrand solubility approach: Solubility of theophylline in polar binary solvents. *J. Pharm. Sci.* 69 (5): 487–491.

Martin, G., and L. Finberg. 1970. Propylene glycol: A potentially toxic vehicle in liquid dosage forms. *J. Pediatrics* 77 (5):877–878.

Massmann, W. 1956. Toxicological investigations on dimethylformamide. *Brit. J. Industr. Med.* 13:51–54.

McClish, A. 1966. Diazepam as an intravenous induction agent for general anesthesia. *Can. Anaesth. Soc. J.* 13:562–575.

McCloskey, S. E., J. J. Gershank, J. J. L. Lertora, L. White, and W. J. George. 1986. Toxicity of benzyl alcohol in adult and neonatal mice. *J. Pharm. Sci.* 75 (7): 702–705.

McCulloch, M. J., and N. W. Lees. 1985. Assessment and modification of pain on induction with propofol (Diprivan). *Anesth.* 40:91–92.

McOrmond, P., B. Gulck, H. E. Duggan, and J. Hopper. 1980. Hemolytic effect of benzyl alcohol. *Drug Intel. Clin. Pharm.* 14:549.

Meyer, J. S., J. Z. Charney, V. M. Rivera, and N. T. Mathew. 1971. Treatment with glycerol of cerebral oedema due to acute cerebral infarction. *Lancet* 2:993–997.

Mickell, J. J., D. H. Reigel, and D. R. Cook. 1977. Intracranial pressure monitoring and normalization therapy in children. *Pediatrics* 59:606–613.

Montaguti, P., E. Melloni, and E. Cavalletti. 1994. Acute intravenous toxicity of dimethyl sulfoxide, polyethylene glycol 400, dimethylformamide, absolute ethanol and benzyl alcohol in inbred mouse strains. *Arzneim.-Forsch.* 44:566–570.

Moon, P. F. 1994. Acute toxicosis in two dogs associated with etomidate-propylene glycol infusion. *Lab. Animal Sci.* 44 (6):590–594.

Moore, W. E. 1958. The use of an approximate dielectric constant to blend solvent systems. *J. Am. Pharm. Assoc. Sci. Ed.* 48 (12):855–857.

Morgan, M., J. Lumley, and J. G. Whitman. 1977. Respiratory effects of etomidate. *Br. J. Anaesth.* 49:233–236.

Morris, H. J, A. A. Nelson, and H. O. Calvery. 1942. Observations of the chronic toxicities of propylene glycol, ethylene glycol, diethylene glycol, ethylene glycol mono-ethyl-ether, and diethylene glycol mono-ethyl-ether. *J. Pharm. Exp. Ther.* 74:266–273.

Napke, E., and D. G. H. Stevens. 1990. Excipients and additives: Hidden hazards in drug products and in product substitution. *Vet. Hum. Toxicol.* 32 (3):253–256.

Nishio, T., S. Hirota, J. Yamashita, K. Kobayashi, Y. Motohashi, and Y. Kato. 1982. Erythrocyte changes in aqueous polyethylene glycol solutions containing sodium chloride. *J. Pharm Sci.* 71 (9):977–979.

Norred, W. P., H. C. Ansel, I. L. Roth, and J. J. Peifer. 1970. Mechanism of dimethyl sulfoxide-induced hemolysis. *J. Pharm. Sci.* 59:618–622.

Novak, E., S. S. Stubbs, E. C. Sanborn, and R. M. Eustice. 1972. The tolerance and safety of intravenously administered benzyl alcohol in methylprednisolone sodium succinate formulations in normal human subjects. *Tox. Appl. Pharm.* 23:54–61.

Obeng, E. K., and D. E. Cadwallader. 1989. In vitro method for evaluating the hemolytic potential of intravenous solutions. *J. Parent. Sci. Tech.* 43 (4):167–173.

Ohmiya, Y., and K. Nakai. 1978. Interaction of benzyl alcohol with human erythrocytes. *Japan. J. Pharmacol.* 28:367–373.

Ohnhaus, E. E., and R. Adler. 1975. Methodological problems in the measurement of pain: A comparison between the verbal rating scale and the visual analogue scale. *Pain* 1:379–384.

Oshida, S., K. Degawa, Y. Takahashi, and S. Akaishi. 1979. Physico-chemical properties and local toxic effects of injectables. *Tnhoku J. Exp. Med.* 127:301–316.

Paruta, A., B. J. Sciarrone, and N. G. Lordi. 1962. Correlation between solubility parameters and dielectric constants. *J. Pharm. Sci.* 51 (7):704–705.

Paruta, A. N., B. J. Sciarrone, and N. G. Lordi. 1964. Solubility of salicylic acid as a function of dielectric constant. *J. Pharm. Sci.* 53:1349–1353.

PDR. 1994. *Physicians desk reference*, 48th ed. Montvale, N.J., USA: Medical Economics Data Production Company.

Pesola, G. R., H. P. Sauerwein, N. A. Vydelingum, G. Carlon, and M. F. Brennan. 1990. Intravenous glycerol infusions: Effect on free fatty acid metabolism. *J. Parent. Ent. Nutr.* 14 (2):162–164.

Porterfield, J. S., and M. J. Ashwood-Smith. 1962. Preservation of cells in tissue culture by glycerol and dimethyl sulphoxide. *Nature* 193:548–550.

Potter, B. J. 1958. Haemoglobinuria caused by propylene glycol in sheep. *Brit. J. Pharmacol.* 13:385–389.

Pyle, H. M., and H. Boyer. 1962. The use of dimethyl sulfoxide in the preservation of human bone marrow. *Fed. Proc.* 21:164.

Rajagopalan, N., C. M. Dicken, L. J. Ravin, and L. A. Sternson. 1988. A study of the solubility of amphotericin B in nonaqueous solvent systems. *J. Parent. Sci. Tech.* 42(3):97–102.

Randolph, T. G., and O. T. Mallery. 1944. The effect in vitro of propylene glycol on erythrocytes. *J. Lab. Clin. Med.* 29:197–202.

Rasmussen, F., and O. Svendson. 1976. Tissue damage and concentration at the injection site after intramuscular injection of chemotherapeutics and vehicles in pigs. *Res. Vet. Sci.* 20:55–60.

Reed, K. W., and S. H. Yalkowsky. 1985. Lysis of human red blood cells in the presence of various cosolvents. *J. Parent. Sci. Tech.* 39 (2):64–68.

Reed, K. W., and S. H. Yalkowsky. 1986. Lysis of human red blood cells in the presence of various cosolvents. II. The effect of differing NaCl concentrations. *Bull. Parent. Drug Assoc.* 40 (3):88–94.

Reed, K. W., and S. H. Yalkowsky. 1987. Lysis of human red blood cells in the presence of various cosolvents. III. The relationship between hemolytic potential and structure. *J. Parent. Sci. Tech. Assoc.* 41 (1):37–39.

Reynolds, D. J., and J. K. Aronson. 1992. Selected side-effects: 8. Anaphylactoid reactions to intravenous vitamin K. *Prescrib. J.* 32 (4):167–170.

Rhodes, A., J. B. Eastwood, and S. A. Smith. 1993. Early acute hepatitis with parenteral amiodarone: A toxic effect of the vehicle. *Gut* 34:565–566.

Rosenkrantz, H., Z. Hadidian, H. Seay, and M. M. Mason. 1963. Dimethyl sulfoxide: Its steroid solubility and endocrinologic and pharmacologic-Toxicologic characteristics. *Cancer Chemother. Rep.* 31:7–24.

Ross, S., and A. M. Silverstein. 1954. Hemolysis by colloidal electrolytes. *J. Coll. Sci.* 9:157–165.

Rowe, V. K., and M. A. Wolf. 1982. Glycols. In *Patty's industrial hygiene and toxicology*, 3rd ed., vol. IIC, New York: John Wiley & Sons, pp. 3817–3908.

Rubino, J. T. 1987. Effect of cosolvents on the action of pharmaceutical buffers. *Bull. Parent. Drug Assoc.* 41:45–49.

Rubino, J. T. 1990. Cosolvents and cosolvency. *Encyclopedia of pharmaceutical technology*, vol 3., edited by J. Swarbrick and J. C. Boylan. New York: Marcel Dekker, Inc., pp. 375–398.

Rubino, J. T., and W. S. Berryhill. 1986. Effect of solvent polarity on the acid dissociation constants of benzoic acids. *J. Pharm. Sci.* 75 (2):182–186.

Rubino, J. T., and S. H. Yalkowsky. 1985. Solubilization by cosolvents III. Diazepam and benzocaine in binary solvents. *J. Parent. Sci. Tech.* 39 (3):106–111.

Rubino, J. T., and S. H. Yalkowsky. 1987. Cosolvency and cosolvent polarity. *Pharm. Res.* 4:220–230.

Rubino, J. T., J. Blanchard, and S. H. Yalkowsky. 1984. Solubilization by cosolvents II: Phenytoin in binary and ternary systems. *J. Parent. Sci. Tech.* 38 (6):215–221.

Ruddick, J. A. 1972. Toxicology, metabolism and biochemistry of 1,2-propanediol. *Tox. Appl. Pharmacol.* 21:102–111.

Santeiro, M. L. 1989. Benzyl alcohol toxicity in newborn infants. *Fl. J. Hosp. Pharm.* 9:17–18.

Savege, T. M., E. I. Foley, and B. R. Simpson. 1973. Some cardiorespiratory effects of Cremophor EL in man. *Brit. J. Anaesth.* 45:515–517.

Schnell, L. A., and W. J. Husa. 1962. Isotonic solutions. XII. Permeability of red corpuscles to various water-soluble organic iodine compounds. *J. Pharm. Sci.* 51 (9):904–905.

Scott, R. P. F., D. A. Saunders, and J. Norman. 1988. Propofol: Clinical strategies for preventing the pain on injection. *Anesth.* 43:492–494.

Sebel, P. S. 1989. Propofol: A new intravenous anesthetic. *Anesth.* 71:260–277.

Seidenfeld, M. A., and P. J. Hanzlik. 1932. The general properties, actions and toxicity of propylene glycol. *J. Pharmacol.* 44:109–121.

Sherman, G. P., L. Gatlin, and P. P. DeLuca. 1978. A note on the acute toxicity of substituted amide solvents. *Drug Dev. Indus. Pharm.* 4 (5):485–489.

Shook, T. L., J. M. Kirshenbaum, R. F. Hundley, J. M. Shorey, and G. Lamas. 1984. Ethanol intoxication complicating intravenous nitroglycerin therapy. *Ann. Intern. Med.* 101 (4):498–499.

Singh, P. P., A. Y. Junnarkar, C. Seshagirirao, R. Kaushal, M. U. R. Naidu, R. K. Varma, R. M. Tripathi, and D. R. Shridhar. 1982. A pharmacological study of propane-1,2-Diol. *Arzneim.-Forsch.* 32 (11):1443–1146.

Smith, A. U. 1950. Prevention of haemolysis during freezing and thawing of red blood cells. *Lancet* 2:910–911.

Smith, B. L., and D. E. Cadwallader. 1967. Behavior of erythrocytes in various solvent systems. III. Water-polyethylene glycols. *J. Pharm. Sci.* 56 (3):351–355.

Smith, J. M., and T. R. P. Dodd. 1982. Adverse reactions to pharmaceutical excipients. *Adv. Drug React. Ac. Pois. Rev.* 1:93–142.

Smyth, H. F. Jr., C. P. Carpenter, and C. S. Weil. 1950. The toxicity of polyethylene glycols. *J. Am. Pharm. Assoc. Sci. Ed.* 39:349–353.

Speth, P. A. J., T. B. Vree, N. F. M. Neilen, P. H. M. de Mulder, D. R. Newell, M. E. Gore, and B. E. de Pauw. 1987. Propylene glycol pharmacokinetics and effects after intravenous infusion in humans. *Ther. Drug Monitoring* 9:255–258.

Spiegel, A. J., and M. M. Noseworthy. 1963. Use of nonaqueous solvents in parenteral products. *J. Pharm. Sci.* 52 (10):917–926.

Stark, R. D., S. M. Binks, V. N. Dutka, K. M. O'Connor, M. J. A. Arnstein, and J. B. Glen. 1986. A review of the safety and tolerance of propofol (Diprivan). *Postgrad. Med. J.* 61 (Supp):152–156.

Steiness, E., F. Rasmussen, O. Svendson, and P. Nielsen. 1978. A comparative study of serum creatinine phosphokinase (CPK) activity in rabbits, pigs and humans after intramuscular injection of local damaging drugs. *Acta Pharmacol. et Toxicol.* 42:357–364.

Steiness, E., O. Svendson, and F. Rasmussen. 1974. Plasma digoxin after parenteral administration: Local reaction after intramuscular injection. *Clin. Pharm. Ther.* 16 (3):430–434.

Stokes, D. N., N. Robson, and P. Hutton. 1989. Effect of diluting propofol on the incidence of pain on injection and venous sequelae. *Br. J. Anesth.* 62:202–203.

Svedson, O. 1983. Local muscle damage and oily vehicles: A study on local reactions in rabbits after intramuscular injection of neuroleptic drugs in aqueous or oily vehicles. *Acta Pharm. Toxicol.* 52:298–304.

Svendsen, O., F. Rasmussen, P. Neilsen, and E. Steiness. 1979. The loss of creatinine phosphokinase (CK) from intramuscular injection sites in rabbits. A predictive tool for local toxicity. *Acta Pharm. Toxicol.* 44:324–328.

Svendson, O., F. Hojelse, and R. E. Bagdon. 1985. Tests for local toxicity of intramuscular drug preparations: Comparison of in vivo and in vitro methods. *Acta Pharmacol. et Toxicol.* 56:183–190.

Sweet, A. Y. 1958. Fatality from intravenous nitrofurantoin. *Pediatrics* 22:1204.

Tao, R. C., R. E. Kelley, N. N. Yoshimura, and F. Benjamin. 1983. Glycerol: Its metabolism and use as an intravenous energy source. *J. Parent. Ent. Nutr.* 7 (5): 479–488.

Thiersch, J. B. 1962. Effects of acetamides and formamides on the rat litter in utero. *J. Rep. Fert.* 4:219–220.

Thomasson, C. L., and W. J. Husa. 1958. Isotonic solutions. VII. The permeability of red corpuscles to various alkaloid salts. *J. Am. Pharm. Assoc. Sci. Ed.* 43:711–714.

Tillmann, U., R. Adler, and W. A. Fuchs. 1979. Pain in peripheral arteriography—A comparison of a low osmolality contrast medium with a conventional compound. *Br. J. Radiol.* 52:102–104.

Tourtellotte, W. W., J. L. Reinglass, and T. A. Newkirk. 1972. Cerebral dehydration action of glycerol. *Clin. Pharmacol. Ther.* 13:159–171.

Trissel, L. A. 1996. *Handbook of injectable drugs*, 9th ed. Bethesda, Md., USA: American Society of Health-System Pharmacists, Inc.

Trèmolières, J., and R. Lowy. 1964. Données actuelles sur la toxicité de l'alcool. *Actual Pharmacologiques* 17:191–211.

Turitto, V. T., and H. L. Goldsmith. 1996. Rheology, transport and thrombosis in the circulation. In *Vascular medicine*, 2nd ed., edited by J. Loscalzo, M. A. Creager, and V. A. Dzau. Boston: Little Brown.

Uche, E. M., R. O. A. Arowolo, and J. O. Akinyemi. 1987. Toxic effects of glycerol in swiss albino rats. *Res. Comm. Chem. Path. Pharmacol.* 56:125–128.

Van de Wiele, B., E. Rubinstein, W. Peacock, and N. Martin. 1995. Propylene glycol toxicity caused by prolonged infusion of etomidate. *J. Neurosurg. Anesth.* 7 (4): 259–262.

Van Metre, T. E. Jr., G. L. Rosenberg, S. K. Vaswani, S. R. Ziegler, and N. F. Adkinson. 1996. Pain and dermal reaction caused by injected glycerin in immunotherapy solutions. *J. Allergy Clin. Immunol.* 97 (5):1033–1039.

Vierck, C. J. Jr., and B. Y. Cooper. 1984. Guidelines for assessing pain reactions and pain modulation in laboratory animal subjects. *Adv. Pain Res. Ther.* 6:305–322.

Vitkova, Z., K. Gardavska, and J. Cizmarik. 1995. Influence of glycerol, propylene glycol and sorbitol on the surface tension, partition coefficient and diffusion of N-(2-(2-pentyloxyphenylcarbamoyloxy)ethyl) piperidinium chloride (Drug XIII). *Pharmazie* 50:199–200.

WADC. 1955. Technical Report 55-16. Springfield, Ohio, USA: Carpenter Litho & Prtg Co.

Wade, A., and P. J. Weller. 1994. *Handbook of pharmaceutical excipients*, 2nd ed. Washington, D.C.: American Pharmaceutical Association; and London: The Pharmaceutical Press, Royal Pharmaceutical Society of Great Britain.

Wald, S. L., and R. L. McLaurin. 1982. Oral glycerol for the treatment of traumatic intracranial hypertension. *J. Neurosurg.* 56:323–331.

Wang, Y-C. J., and R. R. Kowal. 1980. Review of excipients and pH's for parenteral products used in the United States. *J. P. D. A.* 34 (6):452–462.

Ward, G. H., and S. H. Yalkowsky. 1992. The role of the effective concentration in interpreting hemolysis data. *J. Parent. Sci. Tech.* 46 (5):161–162.

Watkins, J. 1979. Anaphylactoid reactions to IV substances. *Br. J. Anesth.* 51:51–60.

Watkins, J., A. M. Ward, and J. A. Thornton. 1978. Adverse reactions to intravenous induction agents. *Br. Med. J.* 2:1431.

Watkins, J., A. Clark, T. N. Apleyard, and A. Padfield. 1976. Immune-mediated reactions to althesin (Alphaxalone). *Br. J. Anesth.* 48:881–886.

Weast, R. C., and G. L. Tuve, eds. 1967. *Handbook of chemistry and physics,* 48th ed. Cleveland, Ohio, USA: The Chemical Rubber Company.

Weatherby, J. H., and H. B. Haag. 1938. Toxicity of propylene glycol. *J. Am. Pharm. Assoc. Sci. Ed.* 27:466–471.

Weiss, A. J., L. G. Jackson, R. A. Carabasi, E. L. Mancall, and J. C. White. 1962. A phase I study of dimethylacetamide. *Canc. Chemo. Rep.* 16:477–485.

Welch, K. M. A., J. S. Meyer, S. Okamoto, N. T. Mathew, V. M. Rivera, and J. Bond. 1974. Glycerol-induced haemolysis. *Lancet* i:416–417.

Wiberg, G. S., H. T. Trenholm, and B. B. Coldwell. 1970. Increased ethanol toxicity in old rats: Changes in LD_{50}, in vivo and in vitro metabolism and liver alcohol dehydrogenase activity. *Tox. Appl. Pharm.* 16:718–727.

Wickliffe, B. W., D. E. Cadwallader, and H. C. Ansel. 1968. Radioisotope analysis of in vivo hemolysis following intravenous injections. *Bull. Parent. Drug Assoc.* 22 (3):105–124.

Wiles, J. S., and J. K. Narcisse Jr. 1971. The acute toxicity of dimethylamides in several animal species. *Am. Ind. Hyg. Assoc. J.* 32 (8):539–545.

Willson, J. E., D. E. Brown, and E. K. Timmens. 1965. A toxicologic study of dimethyl sulfoxide. *Tox. Appl. Pharm.* 7:104–112.

Wilson, J. P., D. A. Solimando, and M. S. Edwards. 1986. Parenteral benzyl alcohol-induced hypersensitivity reaction. *Drug Intel. Clin. Pharm.* 20:689–691.

Windebank, A. J., M. D. Blexrud, and P. C. de Groen. 1994. Potential neurotoxicity of the solvent vehicle for cyclosporine. *J. Pharm. Exp. Ther.* 268 (2):1051–1056.

Winters, E. P., and W. J. Husa. 1960. Isotonic solutions. XI. The permeability of red corpuscles to various sympathomimetic amine salts and phenothiazine derivatives. *J. Am. Pharm. Assoc. Sci. Ed.* 49 (11):709–713.

Woodforde, J. M., and H. Merskey. 1972. Some relationships between subjective measures of pain. *J. Psychosomat. Res.* 16:173–178.

Yalkowsky, S. H., and J. T. Rubino. 1985. Solubilization by cosolvents I. Organic solutes in propylene glycol-water mixtures. *J. Pharm. Sci.* 74 (4):416–421.

Yalkowsky, S. H., and T. J. Roseman. 1981. Solubilization of drugs by cosolvents. In *Techniques of solubilization of drugs,* edited by S. H. Yalkowsky. New York: Marcel Dekker, Inc., pp. 91–134.

Yalkowsky, S. H., S. C. Valvani, and G. L. Amidon. 1976. Solubility of nonelectrolytes in polar solvents. IV. Nonpolar drugs in mixed solvents. *J. Pharm. Sci.* 65 (10):1488–1494.

Zanowiak, P., and W. J. Husa. 1959. Isotonic solutions. IX. The permeability of red corpuscles to some monohydric and polyhydric alcohols. *J. Am. Pharm. Assoc. Sci. Ed.* 48:565–569.

Zaroslinski, J. F., R. K. Browne, and L. H. Possley. 1971. Propylene glycol as a drug solvent in pharmacologic studies. *Tox. Appl. Pharm.* 19:573–578.

12

Prodrugs

Laszlo Prokai
Katalin Prokai-Tatrai

College of Pharmacy
University of Florida
Gainesville, Florida

The physicochemical properties of a drug often impel its formulation for intramuscular (IM), intravenous (IV) and other parenteral uses. There are several drugs currently available that have limited water solubility and, therefore, are commonly formulated for administration in solutions that include organic cosolvents or detergents. These excipients may impair the safety of the injectable products by causing muscle or vein irritation and other toxic systemic effects, as well as a decrease in patient tolerance by inflicting pain and distress upon or after administration. Such adverse effects may also be caused by the drug itself. In order to omit unwanted organic cosolvents and detergents and/or to attenuate the drug's harmful effects in the formulated products, the prodrug approach has been utilized for various therapeutic agents. In essence, a water-soluble and bioreversible derivative of the drug is used to overcome the limitations imposed by the physicochemical properties of a sparingly aqueous-soluble agent in order to develop safe and tolerable injectable dosage forms.

DESIGN OF PRODRUGS

Prodrugs are, by definition, inactive but bioreversible derivatives of known therapeutic agents that are enzymatically or chemically converted to the parent drug in vivo (Bundgaard 1985), as shown schematically in Figure 12.1. The modification of the physicochemical properties of a given drug is carried out via transient chemical derivatization (pro-moiety). The goal in this approach concerning safe and tolerable injectable dosage forms has been to synthesize water-soluble derivatives with more favorable physicochemical characteristics than those of the parent drugs (Stella 1975), which

267

Figure 12.1. The prodrug approach.

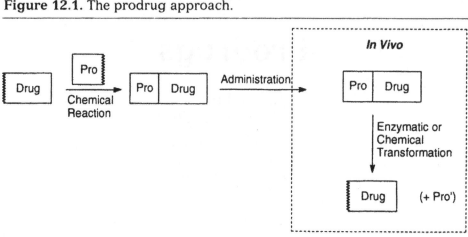

permits a "kinder and gentler" dosage form. Ideally, prodrugs produce activity equal to that of the parent drug in vivo without enhancing toxicity. However, the most important requirement of a prodrug candidate is that it must undergo rapid and quantitative cleavage to regenerate the target compound in vivo by either an enzymatic mechanism or chemical reaction (usually hydrolysis) under physiological conditions, once the barrier to delivery has been averted (Jensen and Bundgaard 1992; Oliyai and Stella 1993). Thus, the original drug should be chemically manipulated so that the obtained molecule (a prodrug candidate), as a precursor of the parent drug, is chemically and/or enzymatically unstable in vivo. In general, an enzymatic conversion is preferred, because chemical conversion rates under physiological conditions may be difficult to optimize (e.g., Venuti et al. 1988).

Low water solubility may be due to the hydrophobic character of the drug and/or because of strong intermolecular interactions in the solid state (crystal lattice). Therefore, water soluble prodrug forms can be developed based on two different approaches. The first is to prepare a derivative considerably more hydrophilic than the parent drug, where the increase in solubility is achieved through enhanced solvent-solute interactions. The second approach is to increase solubility due to the perturbation of the geometry of the crystal and/or because of a decrease in the capacity to engage in intermolecular interactions.

The rational development of prodrugs with increased water solubility compared to the parent compound based on the above principles can be illustrated by the cytotoxic nucleoside arabinosyladenine (**1**), an epimer of adenosine (**2**). This compound has been shown to be effective in the inhibition of the growth of viruses and tumors in vitro and in vivo. However, the low water solubility (0.5 mg/mL, 1.8 mM) hampered its clinical testing due to the intended large (2.5 g) parenteral doses, requiring the IV infusion of several liters of drug solution. The about 10-times lower solubility of arabinosyladenine compared to adenosine may be explained by its stronger intermolecular hydrogen bonding in the crystal lattice because of different geometry (Repta et al. 1975). Prodrugs with improved solubility in the IV vehicle were developed based on these specific structural and physicochemical considerations (Figure 12.2). An example for an arabinosyladenine prodrug more hydrophilic than the parent drug is the 5'-phosphate derivative (3) (LePage et al. 1972). Representatives for the second approach, where increased solubility is due to perturbation of the crystal geometry and/or decrease in the capacity for intramolecular interactions, include the N^6-(dimethylamino)methylene derivative (4, Hanessian 1973) and the 5'-formate (5, Repta et al. 1975) of arabinosyladenine. The majority of prodrugs designed to increase water solubility have relied on obtaining products more hydrophilic than the parent drug.

In general, ester-type prodrugs (Figure 12.3a, b) have been applied most frequently when the parent drug contains a hydroxyl group, due to the significant esterase activity in the body. Esters may be obtained by condensation between an alcohol and an acid, a reaction based on an equilibrium (Figure 12.3a). The condensation is commonly carried out by using coupling agents, such as 1,3-dicyclohexylcarbodiimide (DCC), and in the

---

Figure 12.2. Arabinosyladenine (1), an epimer of adenosine (2), and its prodrugs (3–5). (Abbreviations: S = solubility, ++ = very soluble, n.d. = not determined quantitatively)

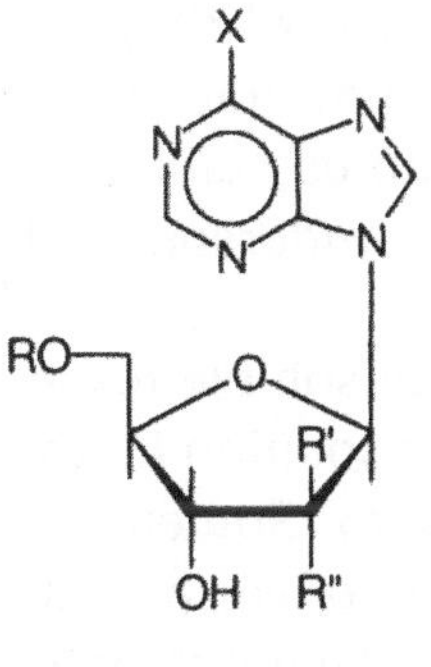

					$S(H_2O)$
1	R = R" = H	R' = OH	X = -NH$_2$		1.8×10^{-3} M
2	R = R' = H	R" = OH	X = -NH$_2$		2.0×10^{-2} M
3	R = OPO$_3^-$	R' = OH	X = -NH$_2$		++ (n.d.)
	R' = H				
4	R = R" = H	R' = OH	X = -N = CHNMe$_2$		7.2×10^{-2} M
5	R = HCO	R' = OH	X = -NH$_2$		1.2×10^{-1} M
	R" = H				

Figure 12.3. General methods to obtain ester- and amide-type prodrugs.

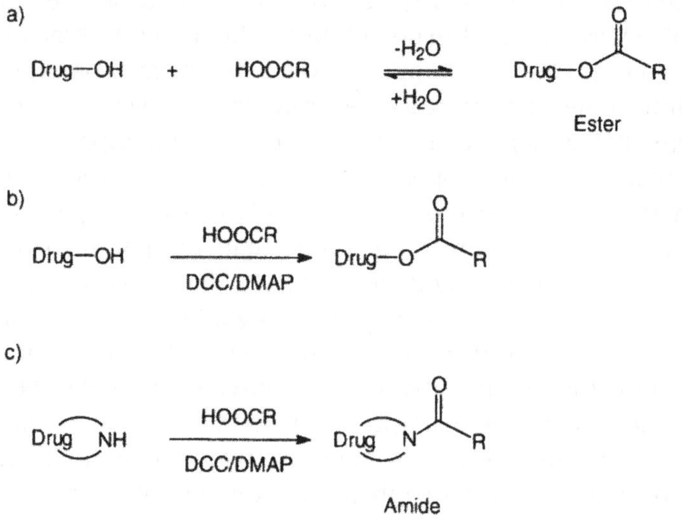

a)

Drug—OH   +   HOOCR $\underset{+H_2O}{\overset{-H_2O}{\rightleftharpoons}}$ Drug—O—C(=O)R

Ester

b)

Drug—OH $\xrightarrow[\text{DCC/DMAP}]{\text{HOOCR}}$ Drug—O—C(=O)R

c)

Drug NH $\xrightarrow[\text{DCC/DMAP}]{\text{HOOCR}}$ Drug N—C(=O)R

Amide

presence of a catalyst such as 4-(dimethylamino)pyridine (DMAP) (Figure 12.3b). A similar reaction can be used to derivatize free amino groups of drugs to obtain amides (Figure 12.3c).

However, not all esters can be considered prodrugs. It is expected that an ester prodrug possesses the suitable physicochemical characteristics (i.e., sufficient solubility) and chemical stability allowing long-term storage in ready-to-use solutions (> 2 years), and it should be rapidly and quantitatively converted to the parent drug in vivo. Sulfate esters, for example, are very water soluble compounds, but their enzymatic hydrolysis is very slow in vivo (Miyabo et al. 1981; Williams et al. 1983). Succinate esters of corticosteroids, (Melby and St. Cyr 1961; Derendorf et al. 1985; Mollmann et al. 1988), chloramphenicol (Nahata and Powell 1981; Ambrose 1984) or metronidazole (Bundgaard et al. 1984; Larsen et al. 1988) not only slowly and incompletely hydrolyze in vivo, but they also have limited stability in solution (Rattie et al. 1970; Anderson and Taphouse 1981; Anderson et al. 1984).

Phosphate esters are, on the other hand, freely water soluble (especially as sodium salts), stable toward hydrolysis in aqueous solution (in the injectable product), and generally easily hydrolyzed in vivo. Sometimes, even the formulation in an aqueous solution yields an acceptable shelf life (Poos et al. 1958; Flynn and Lamb 1970; Varia et al. 1984b). General methods for their preparation are summarized in Figure 12.4.

Esters of α-amino acids are usually unstable in aqueous solution at pH 3 to 5 (where the solubility is the highest) because the amino group is

Figure 12.4. General methods for the preparation of phosphate ester prodrugs.

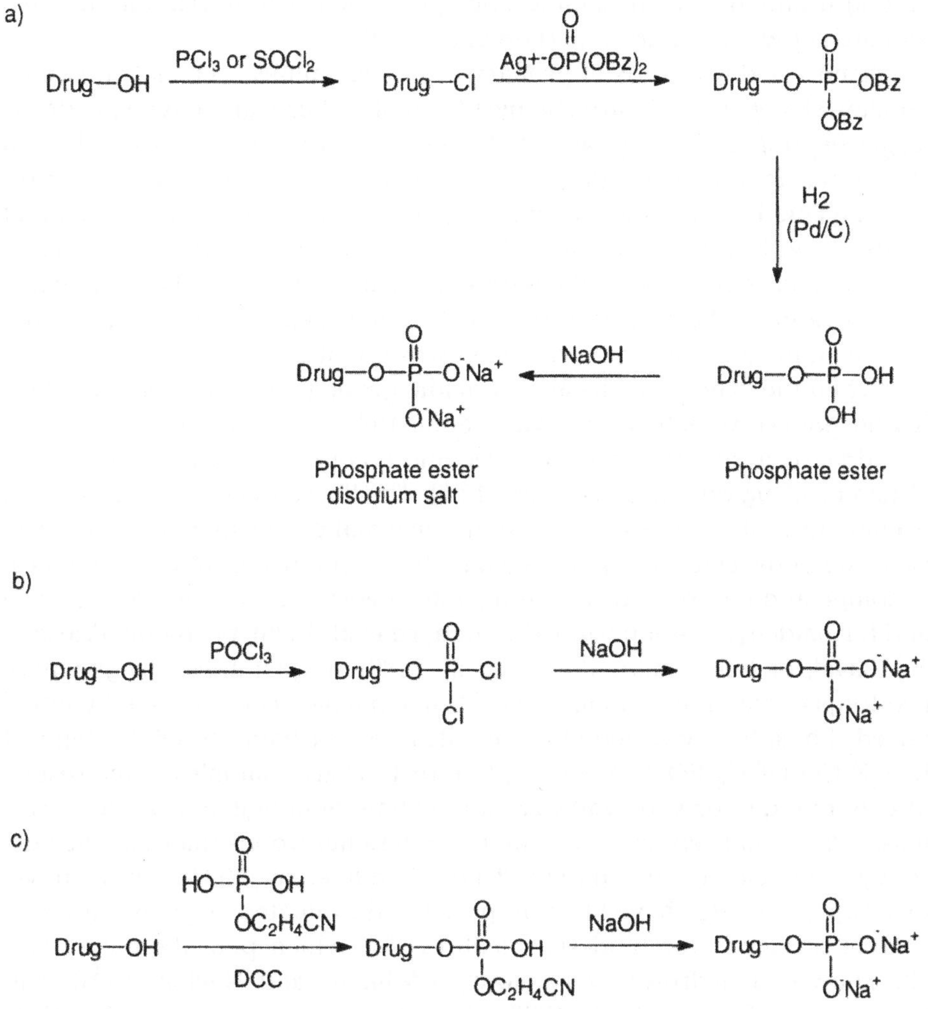

a)

$$Drug-OH \xrightarrow{PCl_3\ or\ SOCl_2} Drug-Cl \xrightarrow{Ag^+\ {}^-OP(OBz)_2} Drug-O-\overset{O}{\underset{OBz}{\overset{\|}{P}}}-OBz$$

$$\downarrow \begin{array}{c} H_2 \\ (Pd/C) \end{array}$$

$$Drug-O-\overset{O}{\underset{O^-Na^+}{\overset{\|}{P}}}-O^-Na^+ \xleftarrow{NaOH} Drug-O-\overset{O}{\underset{OH}{\overset{\|}{P}}}-OH$$

Phosphate ester
disodium salt

Phosphate ester

b)

$$Drug-OH \xrightarrow{POCl_3} Drug-O-\overset{O}{\underset{Cl}{\overset{\|}{P}}}-Cl \xrightarrow{NaOH} Drug-O-\overset{O}{\underset{O^-Na^+}{\overset{\|}{P}}}-O^-Na^+$$

c)

$$Drug-OH \xrightarrow[DCC]{\overset{HO-\overset{O}{\overset{\|}{P}}-OH}{\underset{OC_2H_4CN}{}}} Drug-O-\overset{O}{\underset{OC_2H_4CN}{\overset{\|}{P}}}-OH \xrightarrow{NaOH} Drug-O-\overset{O}{\underset{O^-Na^+}{\overset{\|}{P}}}-O^-Na^+$$

protonated at this condition, and, therefore, it has a strong electron withdrawing effect that activates the ester bond toward hydroxide ion (OH⁻) attack, and to the intramolecular catalysis that is assisted by the neighboring effect of the amino group (Bruice and Benkovic 1966; Kirby and Lloyd 1976). If the solubilizing amino group is more distant from the ester linkage such as for a 6-aminocaproic acid esters for methylprednisolone (Anderson et al. 1985), the stability is somewhat enhanced. The amino group's hydrolysis-facilitating effect was reportedly blocked without the loss of the rapid enzymatic hydrolysis on incorporating a phenyl group between the amino group and the ester moiety. This was due to steric reasons believed to play an important role (Bundgaard et al. 1989). General methods for obtaining α-amino, α-dialkylamino and quaternary α-trialkylamino acid esters are shown in Figure 12.5 (Pop et al. 1996a).

Amino acid prodrugs of primary aromatic amines such as benzocaine (Slojkowska et al. 1982), are chemically stable. These amide type prodrugs target peptidases for cleavage to the parent drug in vivo. Various L- and D-amino acid amides for dapsone, a model aromatic amine, exhibited reversible kinetics and established a pseudoequilibrium in vivo (Pochopin et al. 1994). While the L-amino acid derivatives were rapidly ($t_{1/2} < 2$ min) and quantitatively converted to the parent aromatic amine after IV administration to rabbits, the half-lives for the D-amino acid amides ranged from 30 to 60 min, although the conversion was quantitative.

When the drug contains an NH-acidic group (e.g., imidazoles, imides), N-phosphoryloxymethylation (Varia et al. 1984a) or N-acyloxymethylation (Bundgaard et al. 1989) has also become a commonly used approach to obtain prodrug derivatives (Figure 12.6). The liberation of the parent drug occurs through a two-step reaction—enzymatic (phosphatase, esterase) cleavage of the ester group followed by the spontaneous and fast chemical decomposition of the hydroxymethyl intermediate to the original molecule and formaldehyde. Allopurinol (Bundgaard et al. 1985), phenytoin (Varia et al. 1984a), or fetindomide (Sendo et al. 1988) are just a few drugs where prodrugs containing an ionizable acyl-group have been successfully introduced. Phosphoryloxymethyl carbonates and carbamates of the type of $R_1R_2X\text{-CO-OCH}_2\text{-PO}_3^{2-}$ (X = O, N, Figure 12.7) are examples of the results of continuing efforts to synthesize a new type of potential prodrug candidates that would represent a formulation less hazardous than the one currently available for the parent drug (Safadi et al. 1993). These novel prodrug candidates have been prepared and evaluated as plausible water soluble prodrugs for hindered alcohols (for which phosphomonoesters are known to hydrolyze very slowly [Williams and Naylor 1971]), and for amines (Safadi et al. 1993). Benzocaine, 2-indanol, and β-(3,4-dimethoxyphenyl)ethyl amine were derivatized to the corresponding phosphoryloxymethycarbonyl compounds, and the aqueous stability of the prodrugs was studied. It was found that the alcohol derivatives were chemically too unstable to be considered for further investigation. However, the amine derivatives might have more potential for additional investigation.

For the safer formulation of the specific drugs discussed below, numerous approaches have been considered, but prodrugs have been used successfully to overcome the obstacles posed by the poor water solubility of the parent drugs.

Figure 12.5. Synthetic scheme to obtain amino acid esters and related prodrugs.

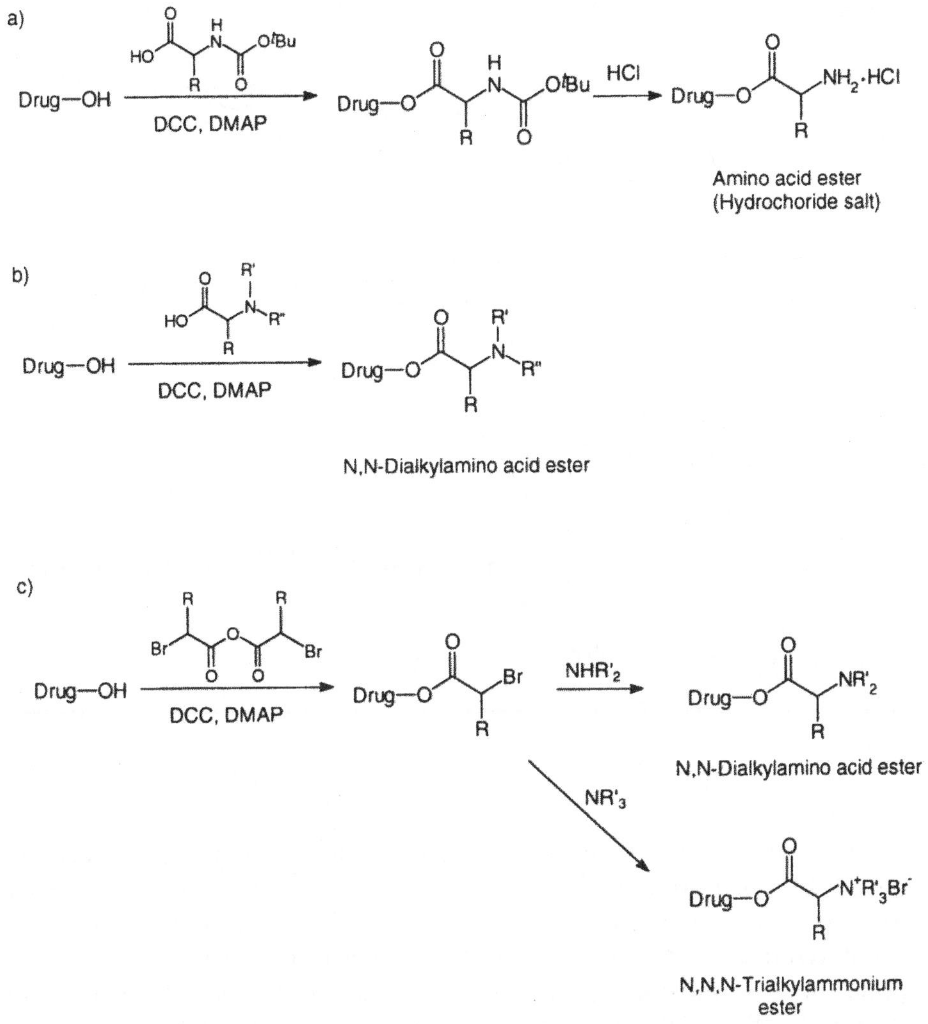

a)

Amino acid ester
(Hydrochoride salt)

b)

N,N-Dialkylamino acid ester

c)

N,N-Dialkylamino acid ester

N,N,N-Trialkylammonium
ester

SPECIFIC EXAMPLES OF PRODRUGS DEVELOPED TO IMPROVE WATER SOLUBILITY OF INJECTABLES

Anticancer Agents

Semisynthetic glycosides of podophyllotoxin, extracted from *Phodophyllum emodi* grown in the Himalayas and Kashmir, are ancient medicinal agents (Doyle 1984; Schachter 1996). Structural modification of the

Figure 12.6. General methods for the preparation of N-acyloxy/ phosphoryloxymethyl prodrugs.

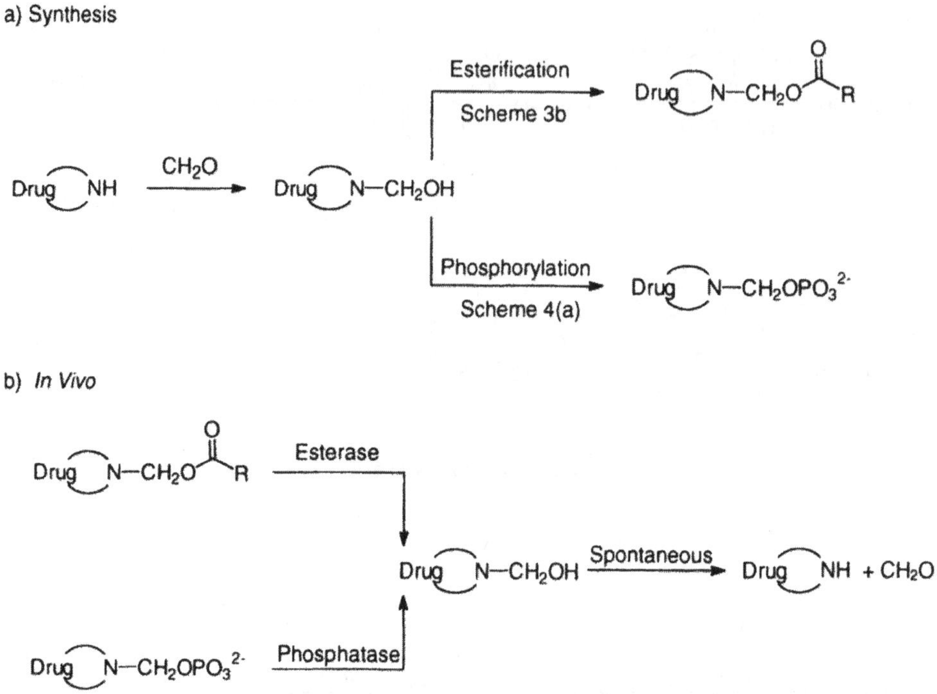

a) Synthesis

b) *In Vivo*

original toxin was necessary after numerous tests for antitumor activity showed in disappointing results, mainly due to nonspecific toxicity (Greenspan et al. 1954). Researchers at Sandoz Pharmaceutical prepared several synthetic derivatives of the toxin (Keller-Juslen et al. 1971) and, among those, etoposide (6) emerged as a drug with a broad spectrum of anticancer activity, alone or in combination with other cytotoxins (Rose and Bradner 1984; O'Dwyer at al. 1985; Bender et al. 1990; Schacter 1996). Nevertheless, the toxin has little efficacy in several important tumors (colon and breast cancer). In addition, the drug, as is apparent from its chemical structure, is not water soluble. Therefore, it must be formulated in propylene glycol (PG), ethanol, and polysorbate 80 (Tween, ICA Americas, Wilmington, Del.). For administration, only a 0.4 mg/mL solution is prepared to avoid the risk of precipitation (Schacter 1996) or a large volume must be infused to give higher doses (Linker et al. 1993). When infused rapidly, significant orthostatic hypotension occurs, possibly due to the polysorbate 80 (Brooks and Alberts 1996). Despite these limitations, etoposide continues to generate significant interest (Doyle and Vyas 1990).

Figure 12.7. Synthesis of phosphoryloxymethyl carbonates and carbamates.

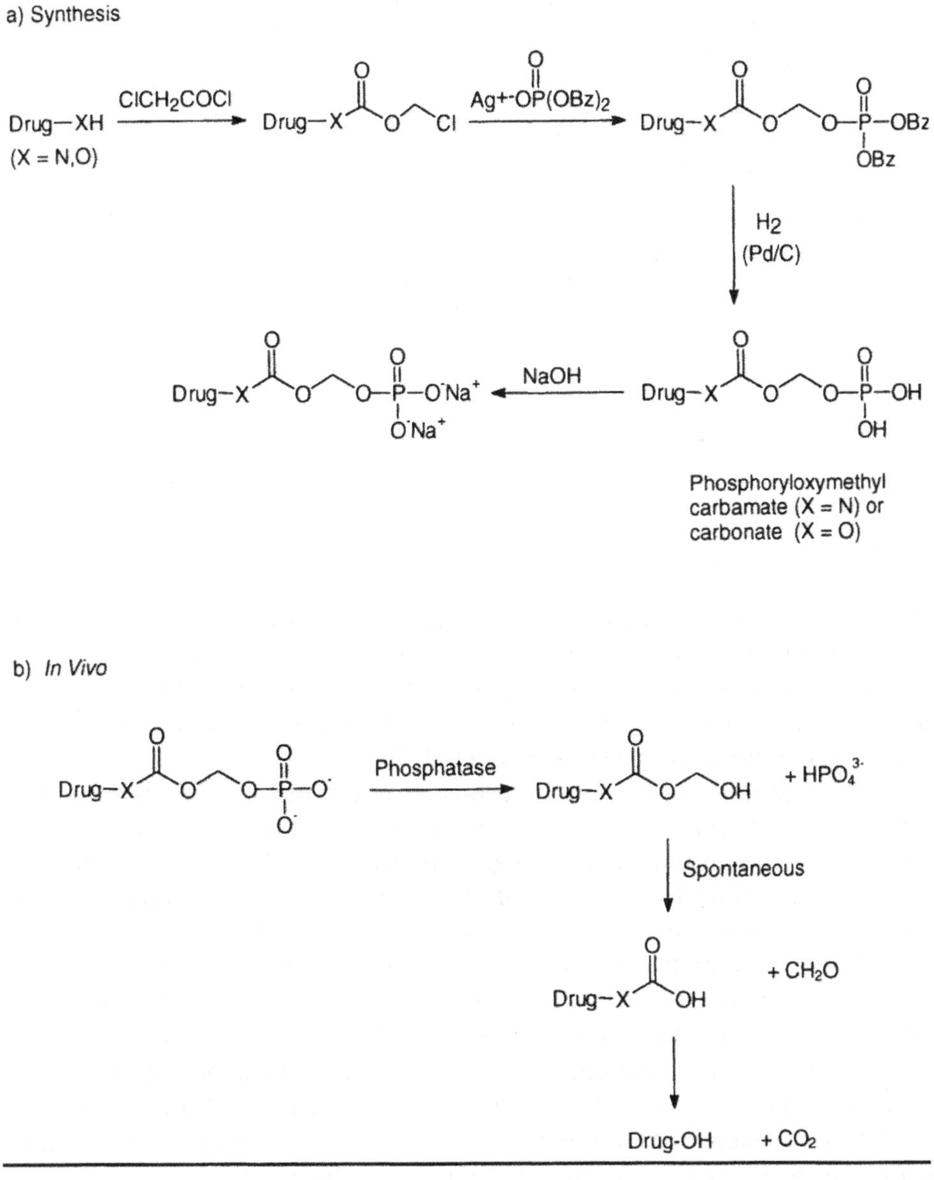

a) Synthesis

b) *In Vivo*

Conversion of etoposide to its 4'-phosphate ester (**7**, Figure 12.8) in a two-step reaction (Senter et al. 1988) was a succesful approach to improve the parenteral administration of the drug. The phosphate ester is a proddrug that renders the compound water soluble; it can be formulated at a

Figure 12.8. Etoposide (6) and its phosphate ester prodrug (7).

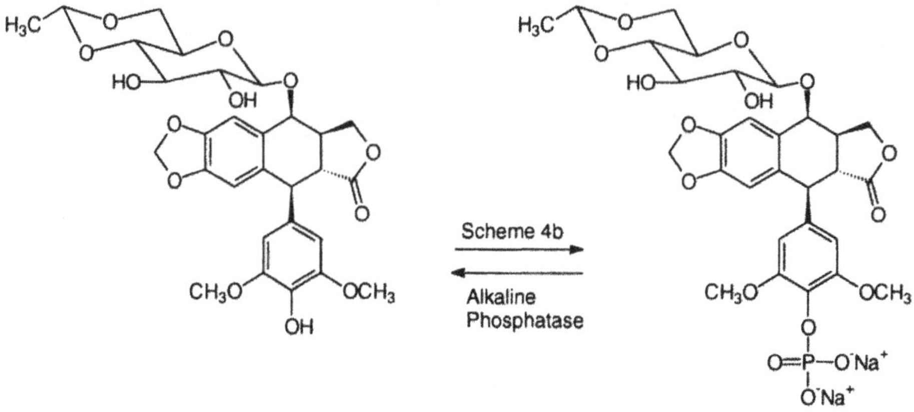

Scheme 4b →
← Alkaline Phosphatase

5   6

concentration of up to 20 mg/mL (Schacter 1996). Thus, the prodrug of the cytotoxic agent can be used much easier in high doses and continuous as well as bolus infusion. Unlike etoposide itself, the 4'-phosphate ester can be given as a 5 min bolus injection without the risk of hypotension or acute toxicity (Budman et al. 1994; Brooks et al. 1995).

Clinical studies have been undertaken to examine, among other factors related to the 4'-phosphate ester, the rate of conversion of the prodrug to the parent drug (etoposide), the maximum tolerated dose, and its pharmacokinetics compared with those of etoposide. It has been concluded that the 4'-phosphate ester rapidly and completely converted in vivo to etoposide after IV administration (over 5 or 30 min) regardless of the duration of the administration, the dose, or treatment schedule used (Millward et al. 1995; Brooks et al. 1995). The feasibility of chronic infusion has also been proven. The pharmacokinetics of the phosphate ester prodrug are identical to those of the etoposide (Rose et al. 1990; Schacter et al. 1994; Millward et al. 1995; Schacter 1996). Furthermore, the biological effect of the ester is proven to be equivalent to that of etoposide (Schacter 1994).

Paclitaxel (8, taxol), a natural product, is a diterpenoid taxane derivative isolated from *Taxus brevifolia* (Wani et al. 1971). The compound is one of the most potent chemotherapeutic agents used in the treatment of breast and ovarian cancers. The drug acts by promoting tubulin assembly into microtubules (Schiff et al. 1979; Schiff and Horowitz 1980). The formulation of taxol for antitumor testing has been difficult due to its essential water insolubility and the lack of functional groups that would allow salt formation.

Taxol is formulated in a Cremophor® EL/ethanol mixture diluted with saline or 5 percent dextrose in water to the desired concentration. However, because large doses of taxol are needed, the patients receive large doses of Cremophor® EL, resulting in frequent idiosyncratic histamine release (Huttel et al. 1980; Rowinsky et al. 1990). Although this side effect can be ameliorated by antihistamines, this additional medication adds discomfort and cost to the patient treated. Evaluations are also hampered by the low availability and structural complexity of taxol.

Therefore, attempts to produce water soluble taxol prodrugs and derivatives have been reported (Figure 12.9). The chemical modifications target the 2' and/or 7 position. The sodium salts of 2'-succinyl and 2'-glutaryl (**9**) derivatives of taxol (Deutsch et al. 1989) showed improved water solubility, and other amino acid derivatives (**10–15**) have also been prepared and studied (Zhao et al. 1991; Mathew et al. 1992). Water soluble 2'-taxol polyethylene glycol (PEG) esters that function in vitro as prodrug (**16–18**) by virtue of the facile enzymatic cleavage of PEG have also been reported (Greenwald et al. 1994, 1996). Esters with PEG as an electron-withdrawing group in the α-position seem to be effective linkers. In vivo testing showed that the molecular weight of the PEG must be ≥ 30 kDa in order to prevent rapid elimination of the PEGylated species. Prodrugs containing phosphate groups have also been reported (Vyas et al. 1993; Mamber et al. 1995). While phosphate esters were unable to hydrolyze enzymatically (by alkaline phosphatase), promising results have been obtained upon evaluation of the 2'- and especially of the 7-phosphonoxyphenylpropionate prodrugs (**19**), demonstrating that these water soluble prodrugs could be metabolized to produce effective tubulin assembly activity.

The potential therapeutic application of the naturally occurring, cytotoxic pseudoguaianolide sesquiterpene lactone ambrosin (**20**) has also been limited by its aqueous insolubility. As shown in Figure 12.10, Michael addition of several secondary amines to both the α,β-unsaturated ketone and α-methylene lactone moieties of ambrosin afforded water soluble tertiary amine diadducts when converted to hydrochloride salts (**21–25**, Hejchmann et al. 1995). Diaddition of bisulfite (HSO_3^-) and sulfoxylate (HSO_2^-) anion to the drug to yield the corresponding water soluble sodium salts (**26–27**) was also applied. These products might be converted back to ambrosin after administration by a retro-Michael mechanism, and the tertiary amine Michael adducts might be activated through metabolic N-oxidation of the amines followed by Cope elimination. The sodium salt of the bis-sulfonic acid (**26**) derivative was inactive upon testing its cytotoxicity in various types of human cancer cells in vitro; thus, it cannot be considered a prodrug for pseudoguaianolide sesquiterpene lactone ambrosin, possibly because of the lack of conversion to the cytotoxic agent. The sodium salt of the bis-sulfinic acid analog (**27**) also had low activity. The bis-piperidine adduct (**21**) proved to be the most potent, producing

Figure 12.9. Taxol (8) and its water-soluble derivatives (9–19).

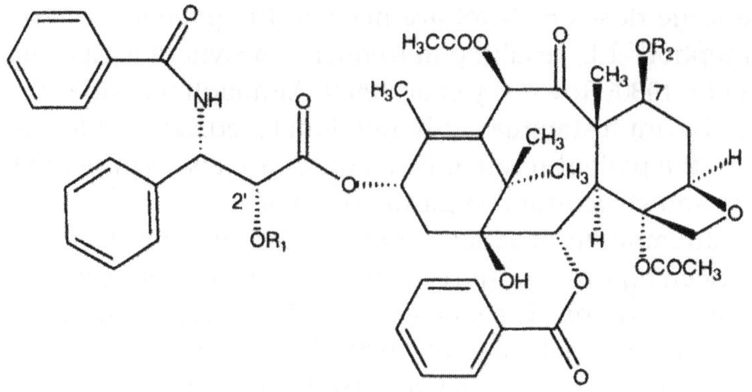

	R_1	R_2	S (mg/mL)
8	H	H	0.03^a
9	$CO(CH_2)_3COONa$	H	3^b
10	$CO(CH_2)_3CONH(CH_2)_3N(CH_3)_2 \cdot HCl$	H	10^b
11	$COCH_2N(CH_3)_2 \cdot CH_3SO_3H$	H	5^a
12	$COCH_2CH_2N(C_2H_5)_2 \cdot CH_3SO_3H$	H	$>10^a$
13	$COCH_2N(CH_3)_2 \cdot CH_3SO_3H$	$COCH_2N(CH_3)_2 \cdot CH_3SO_3H$	$>10^a$
14	H	$COCH_2N(CH_3)_2 \cdot CH_3SO_3H$	$>2^a$
15	H	$COCH(CH_3)N(CH_3)_2 \cdot CH_3SO_3H$	$>2^a$
16	$COCH_2O\text{-}PEG_{Mw5000}$	H	$96 \cdot ^c$
17	$COCH_2O\text{-}PEG_{Mw20000}\text{-}OCH_2CON(iPr)CONHiPr$	H	$15 \cdot ^c$
18	$COCH_2O\text{-}PEG_{Mw40000}\text{-}OCH_2CON(iPr)CONHiPr$	H	$5 \cdot ^c$
19	H	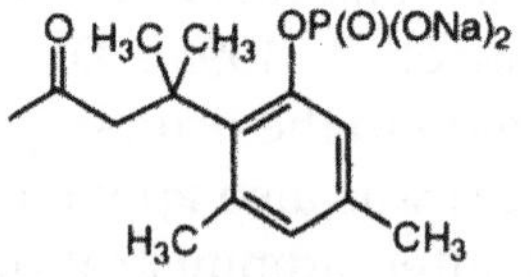	6^d

*Expressed in taxol equivalent, mg/mL; a. Swindell and Krauss (1991); b. Deutsch et al. (1989); c. Greenwald et al. (1995); d. Vyas et al. (1993)

Figure 12.10. Ambrosin (20) and its water-soluble derivatives (21–25).

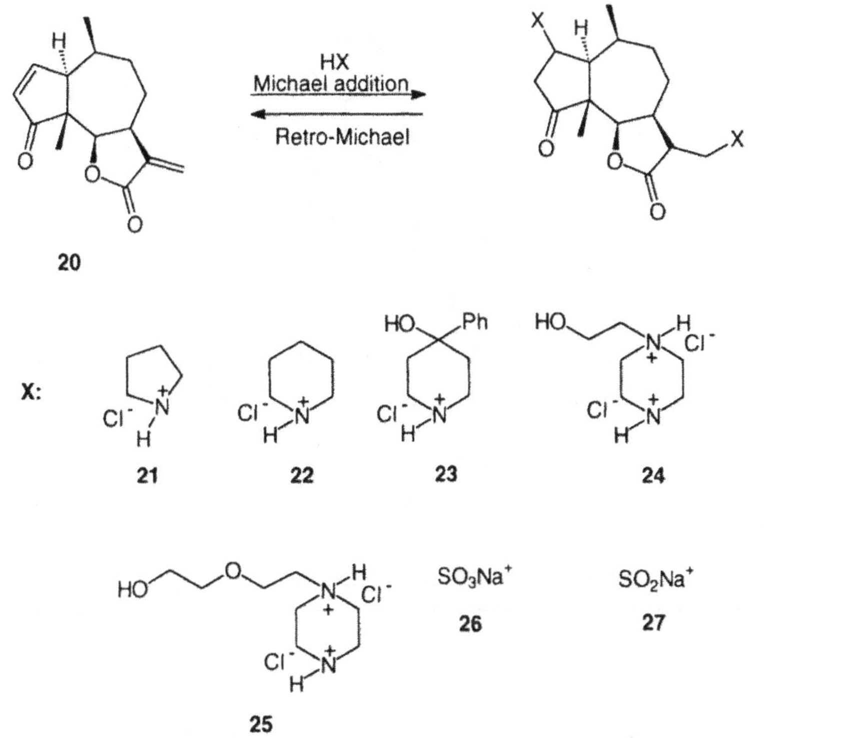

cytotoxic activity only slightly less than ambrosin itself. However, no evidence has been provided as to whether these derivatives act as prodrugs or active analogs.

Rapamycin (**28**) was identified as the antifungal constituent in organic extracts of the bacterium *Streptomyces hygroscopicus* indigenous to Easter Island (Vezina et al. 1975); the compound is effective against a broad spectrum of ascites and transplantable solid tumors in mice (Eng et al. 1984). However, its solubility in water and mixed aqueous solvent systems is limited, and parenteral formulation involving surfactants was accompanied by toxicity. Rapamycin-28-N,N-dimethylglycinate methanesulfonate salt (**29**), synthesized as a potential water soluble prodrug to facilitate parenteral administration (Figure 12.11), exhibited dose-dependent pharmacokinetics, and conversion to rapamycin appeared to represent a prominent route of rapamycin elimination (Supko and Malspeis 1994). The prodrug effectively served as a slow release delivery system for the active agent, which raised the possibility of maintaining therapeutic plasma levels of rapamycin by a more convenient dosing regimen than a continuous infusion schedule.

Figure 12.11. Rapamycin (**28**) and rapamycin-28-N,N-dimethylglycinate methanesulfonate salt (**29**).

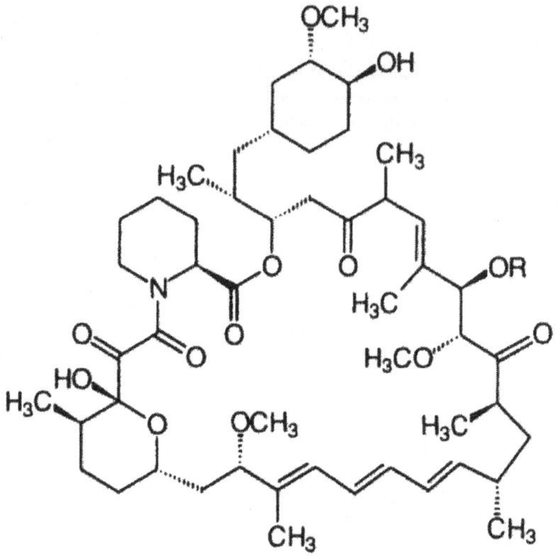

28, R = H   **29**, R = COCH$_2$N(CH$_3$)$_2$·CH$_3$SO$_3$H

Oxysterols (**30, 31**), a family of naturally occurring compounds, possess a broad range of biological activity, including cytotoxicity toward tumor cells in vitro (Luu 1986). Besides low water solubility, the efficacy of oxysterols is attenuated by rapid metabolism in the liver (Pajewski et al. 1989). Therefore, prodrug development for oxysterols may serve a dual purpose by improving their aqueous solubility and also overcoming a metabolic barrier that limits the intended therapeutic effects. Sodium salts of phosphodiesters of 7β-hydroxycholesterol or 7,25-dihydroxycholesterol and 2'-deoxyuridine or 5-fluoro-2'-deoxyuridine (**32–34**, Figure 12.12) have been evaluated as water-soluble prodrugs (Ji et al. 1990; Christ et al. 1991). They have a similar toxicity to their parent compound under in vitro conditions; have been shown to release free oxysterols in the blood, liver, and kidney after intraperitoneal (IP) or IV administration (Moog et al. 1983); and prevented or delayed tumor development in transgenic mice when injected before the onset of adenoma (Allemand et al. 1993).

The dose-limiting toxicities, limited spectrum of antitumor activity, and the acquisition of resistance to the transition metal complex *cis*-[PtCl$_2$(NH$_3$)$_2$] (cisplatin) has prompted the development of its analogs (Hydes and Russel 1988). A common approach has been the replacement of the NH$_3$ ligands with amines or chelating diamines. The drawback of neutral Pt complexes with lipophilic amine ligands is their poor water

Figure 12.12. Oxysterols (**30–31**) and their water-soluble prodrugs (**32–34**).

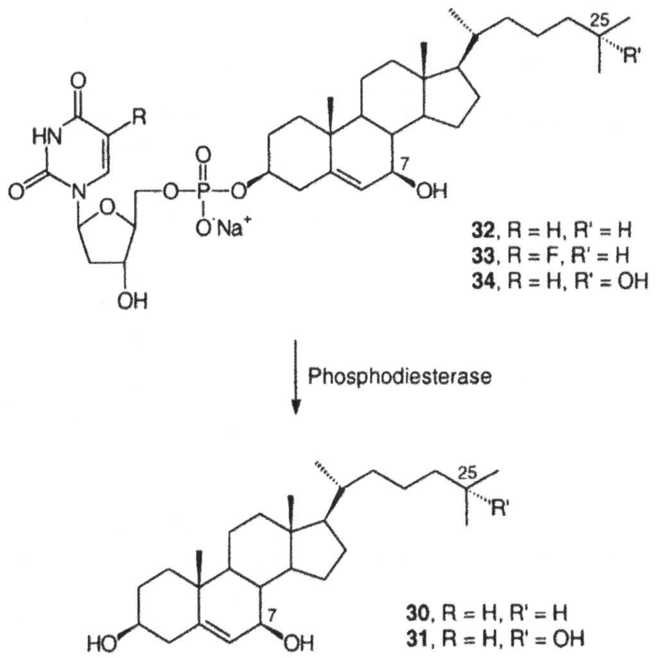

O
HN
R
O
N
O
O
O-P-O
O⁻Na⁺
25
R'
7
OH
OH
32, R = H, R' = H
33, R = F, R' = H
34, R = H, R' = OH
Phosphodiesterase
25
R'
HO
7
OH
30, R = H, R' = H
31, R = H, R' = OH

solubility (Cleare et al. 1978). Water soluble prodrugs of cisplatin analogs bearing chelating diamines (**35**) have also been introduced (Köckerbauer and Bednarski 1995), as shown in Figure 12.13. The zwitterionic, "open-ring" form (**36**) of the chelated complex [2-(aminomethyl)aniline]dichloroplatinum(II) (**35**) prepared under acidic conditions (pH 3), where only the aniline nitrogen is coordinated to Pt, rapidly converts to the neutral form at physiologic pH. This prodrug had a solubility of 10 mM in aqueous acidic medium—about 20 times greater than that of **35** (0.4 mM). Both [2-(aminomethyl)aniline]dichloroplatinum(II) and **36** were equally effective in aborting the growth of different human cancer cell lines in vitro, indicating a quantitative conversion of the prodrug to the active neutral complex in a biological medium. The prodrug form (at a dose of 25 μmol/kg 3 times a week for 6 weeks) also significantly inhibited the growth of MXT (M3.2) mammary tumor in animals (BDF mice), while the cisplatin analog (**35**) had no antitumor activity at the same dose.

Combretastatin A-4 (**37**), the principal cancer cell growth-inhibitory constituent of the Zulu medicinal plant *Combretum caffrum*, has been undergoing preclinical development. However, the very limited water

Figure 12.13. A cisplatin analog-bearing chelating diamine (**35**) and its precursor (**36**) with improved water solubility.

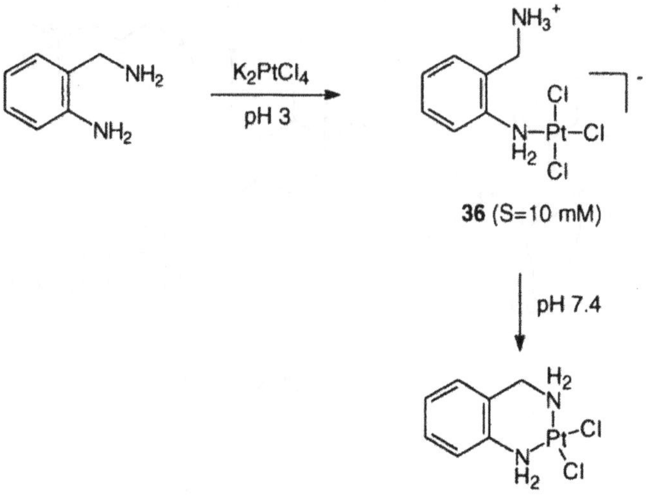

36 (S=10 mM)

pH 7.4

35 (S=0.4 mM)

solubility of this phenol has complicated drug formulation. Hence, derivatives based on the 3'-phenol group of combretastatin A-4 were prepared for evaluation as possible water soluble prodrugs (Pettit et al. 1995b). The most soluble derivatives evaluated included the ammonium, potassium and sodium phosphate salts (**38**, Figure 12.14); the latter two proved most stable and suitable. Both the potassium and sodium phosphate derivatives of combretastatin A-4 were also found to exhibit the requisite biological properties necessary for a useful prodrug. The sodium salt was selected for drug formulation and further preclinical development. The disodium phosphate of pancratistatin to be used as a water soluble prodrug of the potential anticancer agent has also been synthesized (Pettit et al. 1995a).

A very interesting class of prodrugs has been designed as hypoxia-selective agents that release diffusible cytotoxins upon bioreduction (Tercel et al. 1993; Denny et al. 1994), as shown in Figure 12.15. The prodrug N,N-bis (2-chloroethyl)-N-methyl-N-(2-nitrobenzyl)ammonium chloride (**39**) (Denny et al. 1994) is a water soluble (> 400 mM at 20°C) compound designed to produce (via one-electron reduction on the nitro group by specific reductases in the hypoxic environment of the solid tumor) a radical anion that fragments to the aliphatic nitrogen mustard cytotoxin mechlorethamine (**40**), which can back-diffuse to kill the majority of the surrounding oxygenated cells. This pro-moiety may, therefore, serve not only as a water solubility enhancer for anticancer drugs with a tertiary amine group, but also as a tumor targeter.

Figure 12.14. Combrestatin A-4 **(37)** and the phosphate ester prodrug **(38)**.

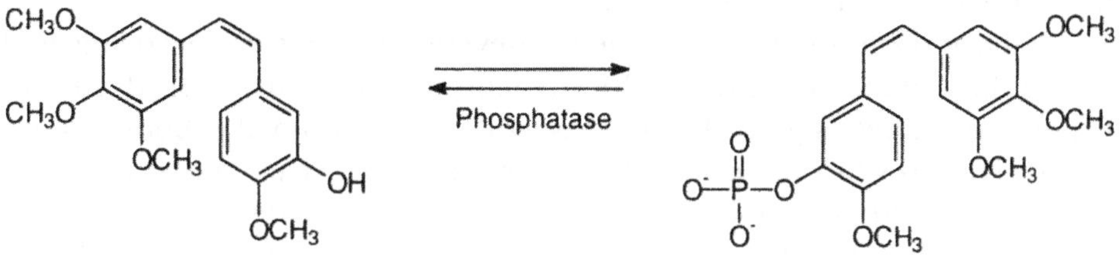

Figure 12.15. A hypoxia-selective, water-soluble prodrug **(39)** for mechlorethamine **(40)**.

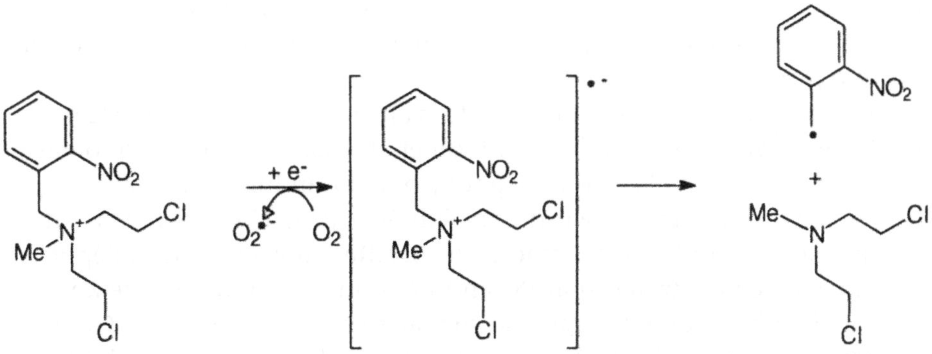

Central Nervous System Agents

Parenteral administration, where rapid onset of action is usually granted, is the preferred route of administration for various drugs acting on the central nervous system (CNS). A number of hydantoins, including phenytoin **(41)**, are widely used drugs. Parenteral phenytoin is, for example, used to treat status epilepticus and sometimes is given after neurosurgical procedures (Cranford et al. 1979; Newton and Kluza 1980; Paulson et al. 1982; Leppik 1986). It is a weak acid with limited water solubility (0.02 mg/mL at pH 7, according to Varia et al. 1984b). Although the formulation in propylene glycol (PG) (40 percent) and ethanol (10 percent) at pH 12 enhances the solubility to 50 mg/mL, it also produces various disadvantages (Cloyd et al. 1978; Varia et al. 1984b). Undiluted solution can cause pain and irritation to the vein (Earnest et al. 1983) and cardiac arrest, mainly due to the PG content (Louis et al. 1967). Improperly diluted solution can result in precipitation. IM administration is characterized by a slow and erratic absorption (Serrano and Wilder 1974; Perrier et al. 1976).

Stella and Higutchi (1973) aimed at developing transient prodrugs with acceptable aqueous solubility for hydantoins, and these prodrugs are capable of converting to the desired structure within the body (Figure 12.16). Their results suggested that esters (**42–43**) or carbonates (**44**) were potential candidates for prodrugs of the respective hydantoins. However, only the disodium phosphate ester of 3-hydroxymethyl-5,5-diphenylhydantoin (**45**), fosphenytoin sodium (ACC-9653, Cerebyx, Parke-Davis), ended up with practical usability (Varia and Stella 1984a, b; Varia et al. 1984a, b). As shown in Figure 12.16, these phenytoin prodrugs are first converted enzymatically to 3-hydroxymethyl-phenytoin (**46**), which breaks down to the parent drug and formaldehyde with a half-life of about 2 sec at 37°C and pH 7.4 (spontaneous). In vivo, fosphenytoin was reported to yield phenytoin rapidly and completely (Browne et al. 1989). A comparative evaluation of water solubility, shelf life in a vehicle solution, and bioavailability in dogs after IV administration of phenytoin and its prodrugs (**42–45**) is given in Table 12.1.

In humans, the conversion half-life is approximately 8–15 min (Boucher et al. 1989; Jamerson et al. 1990; Eldon et al. 1993). The absolute bioavailability of phenytoin (**41**) from fosphenytoin (**45**) in humans is 99 ± 11 percent when given in equimolar doses with phenytoin (Jamerson et al. 1990). Animal studies and human studies in healthy subjects and epileptic patients have demonstrated that IM and IV administration are safe and well tolerated with a side effect profile similar to that of phenytoin (Gerber et al. 1988; Eldon et al. 1993; Boucher et al. 1996). The safety, tolerability, and pharmacokinetics of the prodrug offer distinct advantages over the conventional USP (U. S. Pharmacopeia) phenytoin sodium in neurosurgery patients requiring parenteral anticonvulsant therapy. Fosphenytoin is safe up to 14 days and well received by acutely ill neurosurgical patients. The therapeutic drug concentration can be rapidly attained and maintained by either administration over the duration of the therapy. Based on the studies conducted by Jamerson et al. (1994), fosphenytoin also offers a significant advantage over phenytoin in the frequency and severity of infusion-site reactions, with special emphasis on venous irritation. Although it does not deliver the active drug at a more rapid rate then the present IV formulation, fosphenytoin can be given both intravenously and intramuscularly. No doubt, fosphenytoin represents a clinically significant advance in the formulation for parenteral phenytoin (Leppik et al. 1990).

Alprazolam (**47**), one of the most commonly prescribed minor tranquilizers, is insoluble in aqueous media; thus, formulation for rapid onset parenteral administration represents a significant problem. This 1,4-

Figure 12.16. Selected acyloxymethyl derivatives (**42–44**) and fosphenytoin sodium (**45**) as prodrugs for phenytoin (**41**).

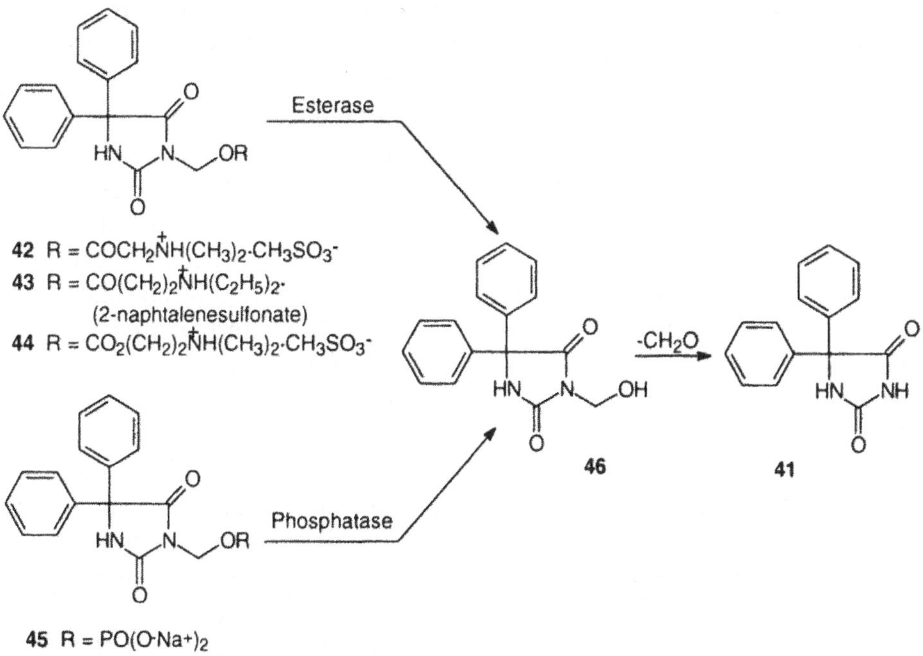

42 R = COCH$_2$$\overset{+}{N}$H(CH$_3$)$_2$·CH$_3SO_3$$^-$
43 R = CO(CH$_2$)$_2$$\overset{+}{N}$H(C$_2H_5$)$_2$·
     (2-naphtalenesulfonate)
44 R = CO$_2$(CH$_2$)$_2$$\overset{+}{N}$H(CH$_3$)$_2$·CH$_3SO_3$$^-$

45 R = PO(O·Na$^+$)$_2$

Table 12.1. Aqueous Solubility, Shelf Life, and Bioavailability of Phenytoin Prodrugs

Compound	Aqueous Solubility (mM)	Shelf Life (t$_{90}$, days)[a]	IV Bioavailability in Dogs[b]
41	0.08	n/a	100
42	302	17.4 (pH 3.2)	78 (83)[c]
43	3.1	138.7 (pH 3.2)	not determined
44	375	107.3 (pH 4.0)	75[d]
45	350	24,769 (pH 7.4)	75 (97)[c]

a. Time for 10 percent hydrolysis, μ = 0.25, 25°C (Varia et al. 1984b).

b. Percentage, relative to **41** (Varia and Stella 1984a).

c. Value corrected for enzyme saturation (Varia and Stella 1984a) given in parentheses.

d. Excessive pain detected upon IV administration (Varia and Stella 1984a).

benzodiazepine analog seemingly does not offer a functional group for a convenient attachment of a pro-moiety. However, alprazolam undergoes ring-opening hydrolysis under acidic conditions to form a triazolobenzophenon (**48**), which cyclizes back to the 1,4-benzodiazepine structure at a neutral pH rapidly and quantitatively, as illustrated in Figure 12.17 (Cho et al. 1983). The open-ring triazolobenzophenon was utilized in developing water soluble prodrugs of alprazolam by attaching solubilizing acyl pro-moieties (formyl, acetyl, succinyl, glycyl, leucyl and γ-aminobutyryl groups) to form amides (Cho et al. 1986). Although the solubility of these derivatives was reported to exceed the concentration required for parenteral formulation in aqueous media, only the glycyl (**49**) and leucyl amides (**50**) were able to regenerate the 1,4-benzodiazepine analog in human plasma within a reasonable amount of time. An ex vivo competitive binding study against tritium-labeled flurnitrazepam in mice also revealed that the in vivo hydrolytic lability of the acyl moiety governed the extent of binding to the cognate receptor of alprazolam.

The amphipatic nature of dexanabinol (**51**) (a nonpsychotic cannabinoid with potential use in the treatment of brain damage associated with stroke, cardiac arrest, and trauma due to its neuroprotective effects [Feigenbaum et al. 1989]), enables its access to the CNS because it readily passes the blood-brain barrier. The lipophilic character of dexanabinol results in a very poor solubility in water, which has made the development of safe formulations suitable for IV administration problematic. Water soluble prodrugs of dexanabinol have been designed (**52–58**, Figure 12.18) to overcome the obstacle hampering its development and clinical application (Pop et al. 1996a, b). Glycinate (**52**) and N,N-dialkylglycinate salts (**53**),

Figure 12.17. The alprazolam (**47**) ↔ triazolobenzophenon (**48**) equilibrium and two amide type prodrugs (**49–50**) developed based on the open-ring form.

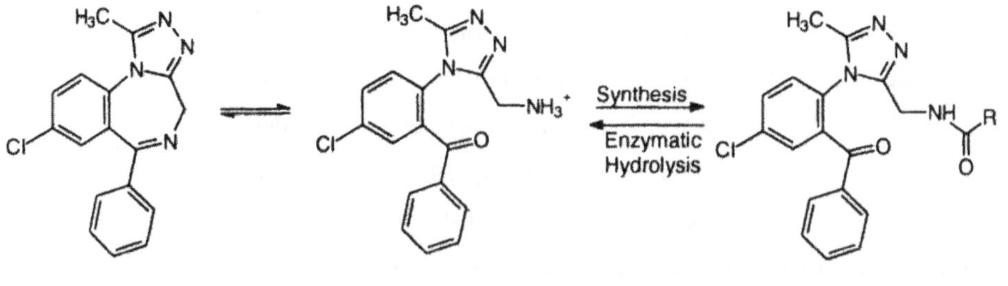

47

48

49 R = CH$_2$NH$_2$

50 R = CH(iBu)NH$_2$

Figure 12.18. Dexanabinol (51) and its prodrugs (52–58).

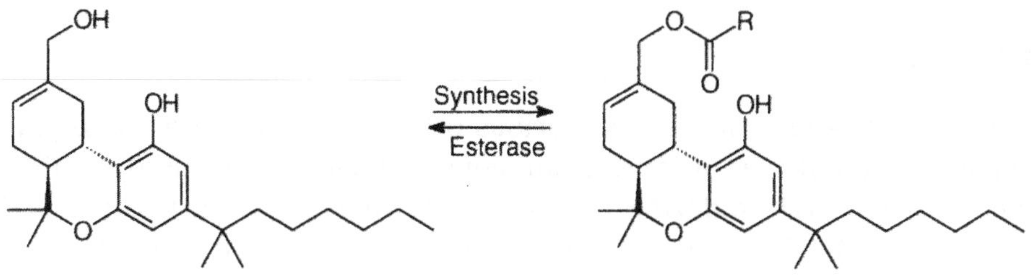

51

52 R = CH$_2$NH$_2$·HCl
53 R = CH$_2$NR'$_2$·HCl (**a** R' = CH$_3$, **b** R' = C$_2$H$_5$)
54 R = CH$_2$N$^+$R'$_3$Cl$^-$ (**a** R' = CH$_3$, **b** R' = C$_2$H$_5$)

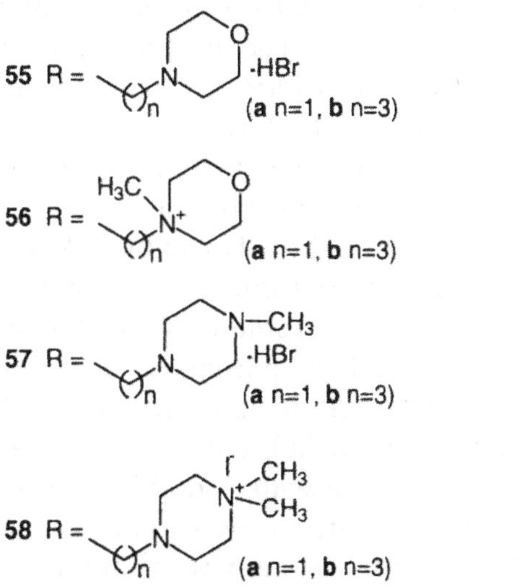

55 R = (**a** n=1, **b** n=3) ·HBr

56 R = (**a** n=1, **b** n=3)

57 R = (**a** n=1, **b** n=3) ·HBr

58 R = (**a** n=1, **b** n=3)

quaternary N,N,N-trialkylglycinates (**54**), as well as salts of amino acid esters containing tertiary (**55, 57**) and quaternary heterocyclic nitrogen (**56,
58**) were synthesized (Figure 12.18) and evaluated as potential prodrugs.
These derivatives exhibited improved solubility (2 to 7 mg/mL). A purely
aqueous vehicle could be used for the glycinate (**52**) and the quaternary
ammonium derivatives (**54, 56, 58**). The tertiary amine salts (**53, 55**) were
solubilized in a medium of 10 percent (v/v) ethanol in water (were also reasonably stable in the medium). However, quaternary derivatives of dexanabinol (**54, 56, 58**) were found to hydrolyze faster in vivo. All examined
compounds inhibited binding of an appropriate radioligand ([^{3}H]MK-801)
to the N-methyl-D-aspartate (NMDA) receptor and protected neurons
against NMDA–induced toxicity, and neuroprotection could be attributed

mostly to the parent dexanabinol (**51**) released by hydrolysis during the assay.

Other Drugs

The parenteral administration of various other drugs is hampered by inadequate solubility in a purely aqueous vehicle. Metronidazole (**59**, 2-methyl-5-nitro-1H-imidazole-1-ethanol) is often used for the treatment of anaerobic infections, but IV administration may require infusion of about 100 mL when formulated in an aqueous vehicle. To develop a parenteral solution of relatively water-insoluble (~ 10 mg/mL at 25°C) metronidazole, its phosphate ester (**60**, Figure 12.19) was synthesized as a prodrug (Cho et al. 1982). Being a zwitterionic compound, its solubility at pH 7 was approximately 50 times that of metronidazole. In human serum, the hydrolysis of the prodrug followed zero-order kinetics at an initial concentration of 0.25 mg/mL or higher, presumably due to enzyme saturation (0.035 mg/mL/h at 37°C), but its subcutaneous administration to rats produced a blood level and bioactivity comparable to those observed after administration of metronidazole.

Tosufloxacin (**61**) has been found to be extremely effective in treating several bacterial infections. However, due to its inherent low water solubility, the development of an IV formulation will be extremely difficult and may preclude its parenteral use. In search of a more water-soluble analog of tosufloxacin for parenteral use, the 3-formyl derivative of tosufloxacin (**62**, Figure 12.20), has been synthesized for evaluation (Chu et al. 1990). The improved water solubility of this analog was probably due to its reduced capacity for intermolecular interactions compared to tosufloxacin. The 3-formyl analog was found to produce high plasma levels of tosufloxacin upon both oral and subcutaneous administration to mice, which indicates an oxidative conversion of the analog to tosufloxacin; high plasma levels of tosufloxacin were also obtained when the 3-formyl analog was administered both orally and intravenously to dogs. Accordingly, the 3-formyl derivative functioned as a prodrug for tosufloxacin.

Figure 12.19. Metronidazole (**59**) and its phosphate ester prodrug (**60**).

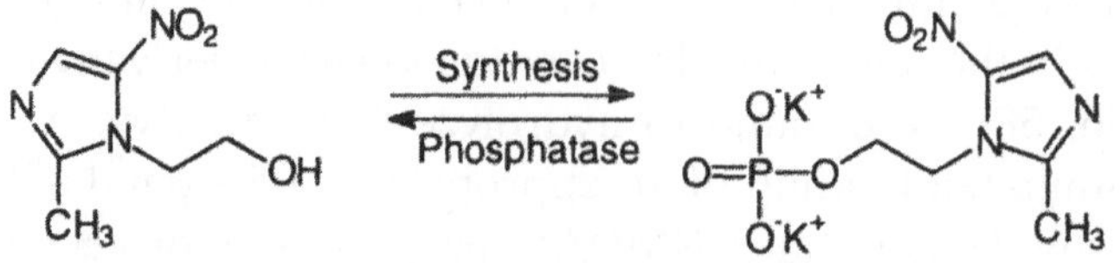

59   60

Figure 12.20. Tosufloxacin (**61**) and the 3-formyl derivative (**62**).

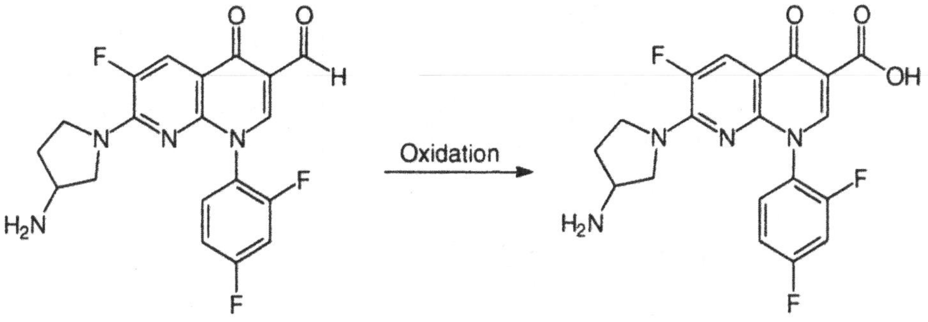

62
(Prodrug)

61

Cyclic hexapeptides related to echinocandin B have received attention as antifungal agents, especially in treating opportunistic infections affecting immunocompromised individuals (Debono 1995). These peptides exhibit poor oral absorption and, thus, require parenteral administration. Echinocandin lipopeptides lack appreciable water solubility (< 0.1 mg/mL), and potential prodrugs with improved solubility have been reported (Balkovec et al. 1992). Although several derivatives (ester, carbamate, carbonate, glycinate, etc.) of the semisynthetic echinocandin L-688,786 (**63**) showed acceptable efficacy comparable to the parent compound in vivo in both the rat *Pneumocystis carinii* pneumonia and in the mice target organ kidney assays; only the phosphate prodrug (**64**, Figure 12.21) showed high activity in both assays and exhibited superior solution stability, thus, warranting further pharmaceutical development.

The efficacy of vitamin E [α-tocopherol, (**65**), a biological antioxidant] in preventing or reducing oxidative stresses (Massey et al. 1989; Grisar et al. 1991) and other disorders (hematologic, malabsorption, etc.) has been investigated. The vitamin is practically insoluble in water and readily oxidized by air. For clinical use, the acetate (**66**) or the succinate ester is commonly used because of their stability to oxidation. Parenteral application, however, raises problems because these esters are also insoluble in aqueous media. The acetate (**66**) is solubilized by a large amount of surfactant that causes toxicity, such as anaphylactoid reactions. Furthermore, it has been established that the rate-limiting step in the bioavailability of the vitamin is the hydrolysis of the ester group (Pedraz et al. 1989). Nine aminoalkanecarboxylic acid esters of the α-tocopherol derivatized on the phenolic functional group have been reported (Takata et al. 1994). The hydrochloride salts of the esters are water soluble (greater than 20 mM at

Figure 12.21. The semisynthetic echinocandin L-688,786 (**63**), an antifungal agent, and its prodrug (**64**).

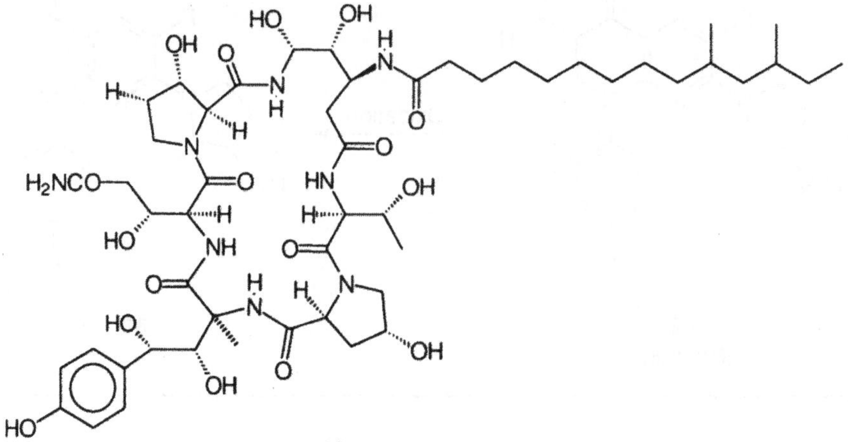

63

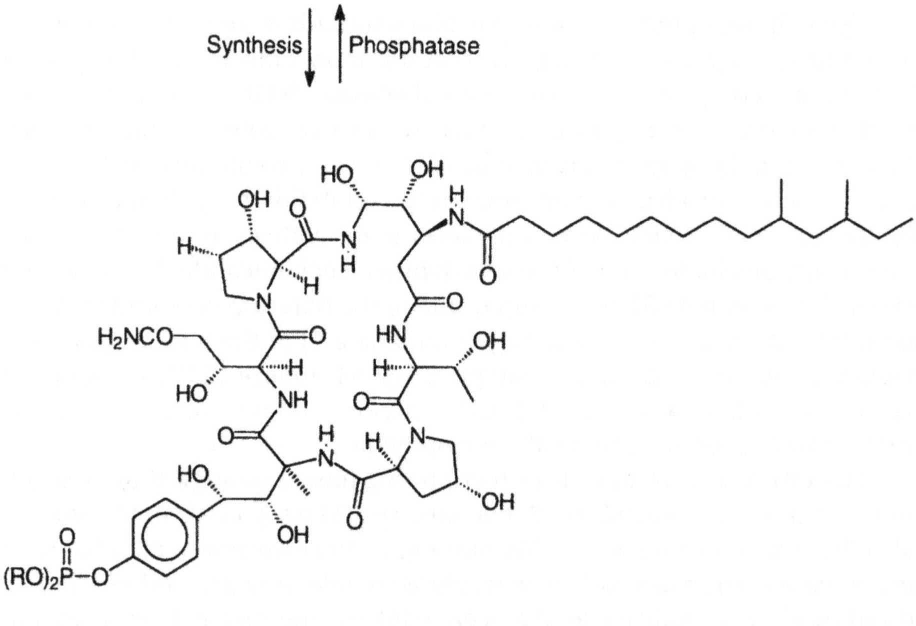

R = (H, Na)

64

25°C) and consequently suitable for parenteral administration. The N-methylaminoacetyl (**67**) and N,N-dimethylaminoacetyl (**68**) esters (Figure 12.22) were found to hydrolyze more rapidly than the acetate, the commercially available d-α-tocopheryl ester. Based on these findings N-methylaminoacetyl and N,N-dimethylaminoacetyl esters are promising prodrug candidates.

A similar approach was applied to another lipid-soluble vitamin—vitamin K. The efficacy and toxicity of vitamin K (MK-4, **69**) depends on the pathway and the extent of enzymatic reductive activation to vitamin K hydroquinone (MHK, **70**), which is an essential cofactor for the synthesis of clotting factors. Parenteral use of the vitamin has been impaired by its water insolubility. IV application often produces an anaphylactoid reaction, presumably due to the polyoxyethylene hydrogenated castor oil (HCO-60) used in the IV dosage form (Reynolds 1989). N,N-Dimethylglycine esters (1-mono, 4-mono and 1,4-bis) of MHK (**71–73**, Figure 12.23) were synthesized and assessed as potential water soluble prodrugs (Takata et al. 1995a, b). The esters can deliver the hydroquinone to the site of action without the quinone reductive activation step. They are rapidly and selectively taken up by the liver, and quantitatively hydrolyzed by esterases to MHK in the rat liver and plasma. They also possess high water solubility; therefore, they are aspiring prodrug candidates for systemic, site-specific delivery of MHK with enhanced pharmacological efficacy, without a toxicity induced by the solubilizing agent used in the current IV formulation.

Acyclovir (**74**) is a widely used agent to treat herpes virus infections, and IV, oral, and topical formulations are available. Acyclovir is given by infusion or by bolus injection IV in a strongly alkaline (pH 10–11) solution of its sodium salt, but it cannot be given as an IM injection (O'Brien and Campoli-Richards 1989). The properties of acyclovir following administration are, however, far from being optimal due to poor aqueous solubility

Figure 12.22. Vitamin E (**65**) and its prodrugs (**66–68**).

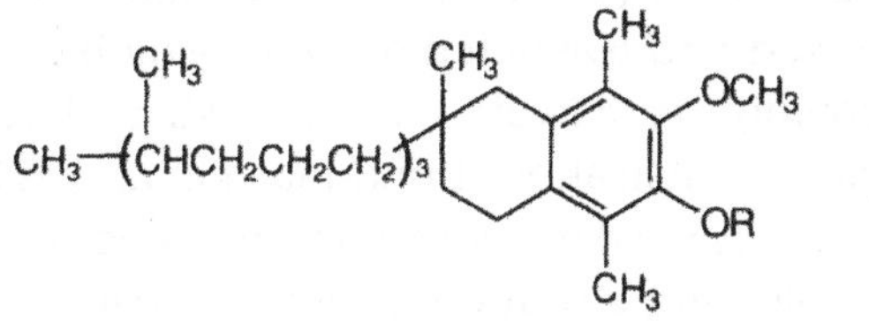

65 R = H   **67** R = COCH$_2$NHCH$_3$·HCl

66 R = COCH$_3$ **68** R = COCH$_2$N(CH$_3$)$_2$·HCl

Figure 12.23. Systemic site-specific delivery of vitamin K hydroquinone (70) via water-soluble prodrugs (71–73) of vitamin K (69).

71 R_1 = H, R_2 = $COCH_2N(CH_3)_3$
72 R_1 = $COCH_2N(CH_3)_3$, R_2 = H
73 R_1 = $COCH_2N(CH_3)_3$, R_2 = $COCH_2N(CH_3)_3$

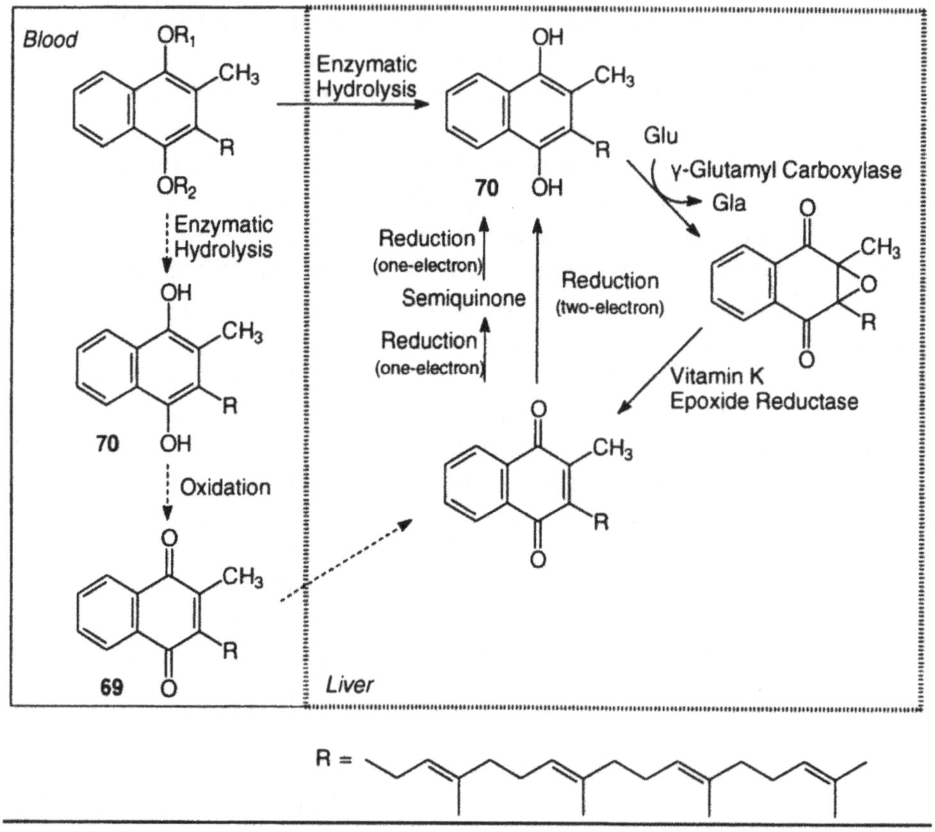

(1.4 mg/mL) and/or low lipophilicity of the drug. As shown in Figure 12.24, various N-substituted 3- or 4-(aminomethyl)benzoate esters of acyclovir (75, 76) were synthesized and evaluated as water-soluble prodrugs forms with the aim of improving the delivery characteristics of acyclovir, particularly after parenteral administration (Bundgaard et al. 1991). These esters showed a high solubility in weakly acidic solutions and also a high stability in such solutions, allowing storage for several years. The esters combined these properties with a high susceptibility (half-lives of 0.8 to 57 min) to undergo enzymatic hydrolysis in 80 percent human plasma, the rate being highly dependent on the position of the aminomethyl group relative to the ester moiety. In addition, all esters were more lipophilic than acyclovir

Figure 12.24. Acyclovir (74) and its ester prodrugs (75–76).

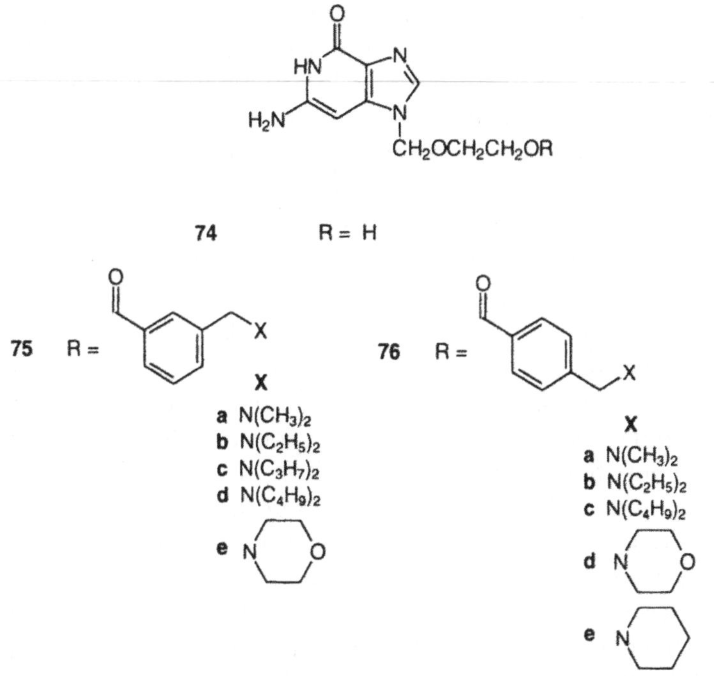

74   R = H

75   R =

X
a N(CH₃)₂
b N(C₂H₅)₂
c N(C₃H₇)₂
d N(C₄H₉)₂
e

76   R =

X
a N(CH₃)₂
b N(C₂H₅)₂
c N(C₄H₉)₂
d
e

in terms of octanol-buffer (pH 7.4) partition coefficients. These properties make the N-substituted benzoate esters promising new prodrugs for acyclovir to enhance its delivery characteristics. Such N-substituted 3- or 4-(aminomethyl)benzoate esters have also been prepared with various other drugs containing a hydroxy group, including ganciclovir (Jensen and Bundgaard 1991a), metronidazole (Jensen et al. 1990), chloramphenicol (Jensen and Bundgaard 1991b), paracetamol (Jensen et al. 1991), and corticosteroids (Jensen and Bundgaard 1992).

Platelet-activating factor (PAF) is a potent, endogenous phospholipid mediator of inflammation (Page 1988). While its precise function in the specific diseases remains ambiguous, in vivo studies with PAF and PAF antagonists in animal models suggest pathophysiological roles in life-threatening conditions having inflammatory components, such as septic shock (Sanchez-Crespo 1993), nephritis (Schlondorff and Neuworth 1986), and asthma (Parsons 1991). In animal models of allergic asthma, PAF-receptor antagonists have been shown to block PAF-induced late-phase bronchoconstriction and delayed hyperresponsiveness (Parsons 1991). The structurally diverse classes of PAF antagonists include pyrrolothiazole (Davidsen et al. 1994; Sheppard et al. 1995) and diaryltetrahydrofuran derivatives (Girotra et al. 1992). This latter class was discovered via the natural products veraguensin (Bitfu et al. 1986) and kadsurenone (Ponpipom et al. 1987). Chemical modifications on the structure of veraguensin led to a third generation of tetrahydrofuran derivative, (-)-trans-(2S,5S)-2-[3-(2-oxypropyl)sulfonyl]-4-N-propoxy-5-(3-hydroxypropoxy)phenyl]-5-(3,4,5-trimethoxyphenyl)tetrahydrofuran (**77**), which is one of the most potent PAF antagonists (Girotra et al. 1992). This compound inhibits the binding of [^{3}H]-C_{18}-PAF to human platelet membranes (K_i = 1.85 nM). However, the antagonist has poor water solubility, less than 100 μg/mL.

To boost the aqueous solubility and retain bioequivalence to the parent drug, only the prodrug obtained by preparation of the phosphate ester on the 5' position of the hydroxylpropyl group (**78**, Figure 12.25) was satisfactory. The phosphate ester produced a greater than 30 mg/mL water solubility making it suitable for IV administration. Furthermore, in vivo rat and guinea pig models employing an exogenously administered PAF showed the phosphate ester to be equipotent to the parent drug (**77**), exhibiting ED_{50} values of 6.5 μg/kg IV and 13 μg/kg IV, respectively.

A unique type of prodrug was designed for another class of potent PAF agonists—pyrrolothiazole. Pyrrolothiazole, also lacking water solubility, precludes IV administration (Davidsen et al. 1994; Alberth et al. 1995). Albeit highly effective in a variety of in vitro and in vivo assays (Sheppard et al. 1994, 1995), the indole pyrrolothiazole derivative, A-85783 (**79**), is essentially a water insoluble molecule (<1 μg/mL at pH 7, Alberth et al. 1995). Attempts to enhance the solubility by designing analogs having a solubilizing handle, such as polar or charged groups attached to the indole nitrogen, fluorophenyl ring, or other parts of the molecule, usually resulted in a decreased intrinsic and/or in vivo potency.

Bodor (1977) described a general strategy for improving aqueous solubility of tertiary or unsaturated nitrogen-containing drugs by converting them to biolabile quaternary prodrugs. The essence of this method is that the nitrogen in question is reacted with an α-haloester resulting in an (acyloxyalkyl)ammonium salt (having a charged/ionic character) that results in an enhanced water solubility compared to that of the parent drug. The "solubilizing modification" (charge) is on the actual parent drug moiety in this prodrug design (as opposed to the previous examples), where the solubilizing property is provided by an attached moiety.

By using this approach, several pyridinium prodrugs of A-85783 (**80–86**, Figure 12.26) have been reported (Davidsen et al. 1994), all of which had aqueous solubility of greater than 20 mg/mL. The prodrug (R)-1-[[(acetyloxycarbonyl)oxy]methyl]-3-[7-[1-(N,N-dimethylcarbamoyl)-6-(4-fluorophenyl)indol-3-oyl]-1H,3H-pyrrolo[1,2-c]thiazol-3-yl]pyridinium chloride (**82**) [the N-(acetyloxymethyl)pyridinium analog of A-85783 obtained upon reacting the drug with bromomethylacetate (Davidsen et al. 1994; Alberth et al. 1995)], is currently undergoing clinical evaluation for

Figure 12.25. A PAF antagonist, (-)-trans-(2S,5S)-2-[3-(2-oxypropyl)sul-
fonyl]-4-N-propoxy-5-(3-hydroxypropoxy)phenyl]-5-(3,4,5-trimethoxy-
phenyl)tetrahydrofuran (77), and its phosphate ester prodrug (78).

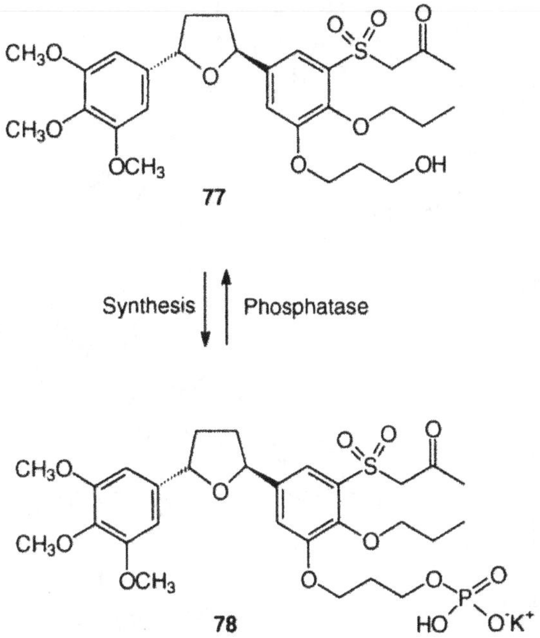

the treatment of sepsis. It is rapidly converted in blood to the parent drug; thus, the acetyloxymethyl side chain is hydrolyzed enzymatically, and the prodrug (82) is bioequivalent in vivo to A-85783. When administered intravenously, the ED_{50} value of 82 was between 6 and 10 μg/kg in the rat and mouse and 100 μg/kg in the guinea pig. A dose of 100 μg/kg in the rat provides greater than 60 percent protection for 8 to 16 h against cutaneous and systemic PAF challenge. Therefore, the prodrug approach proved to be suitable for a potent, long-acting, and selective PAF agonist for IV administration essential for acute therapeutic treatment of sepsis.

CONCLUSIONS

Various examples for improving the water solubility of pharmaceutical agents by developing prodrugs were discussed in this review. This approach represents probably one of the most studied methods and offers a viable route to safer and less irritating parenteral formulations for a

Figure 12.26. The PAF agonist A-385783 (**79**) and its pyridinium prodrugs (**80–86**).

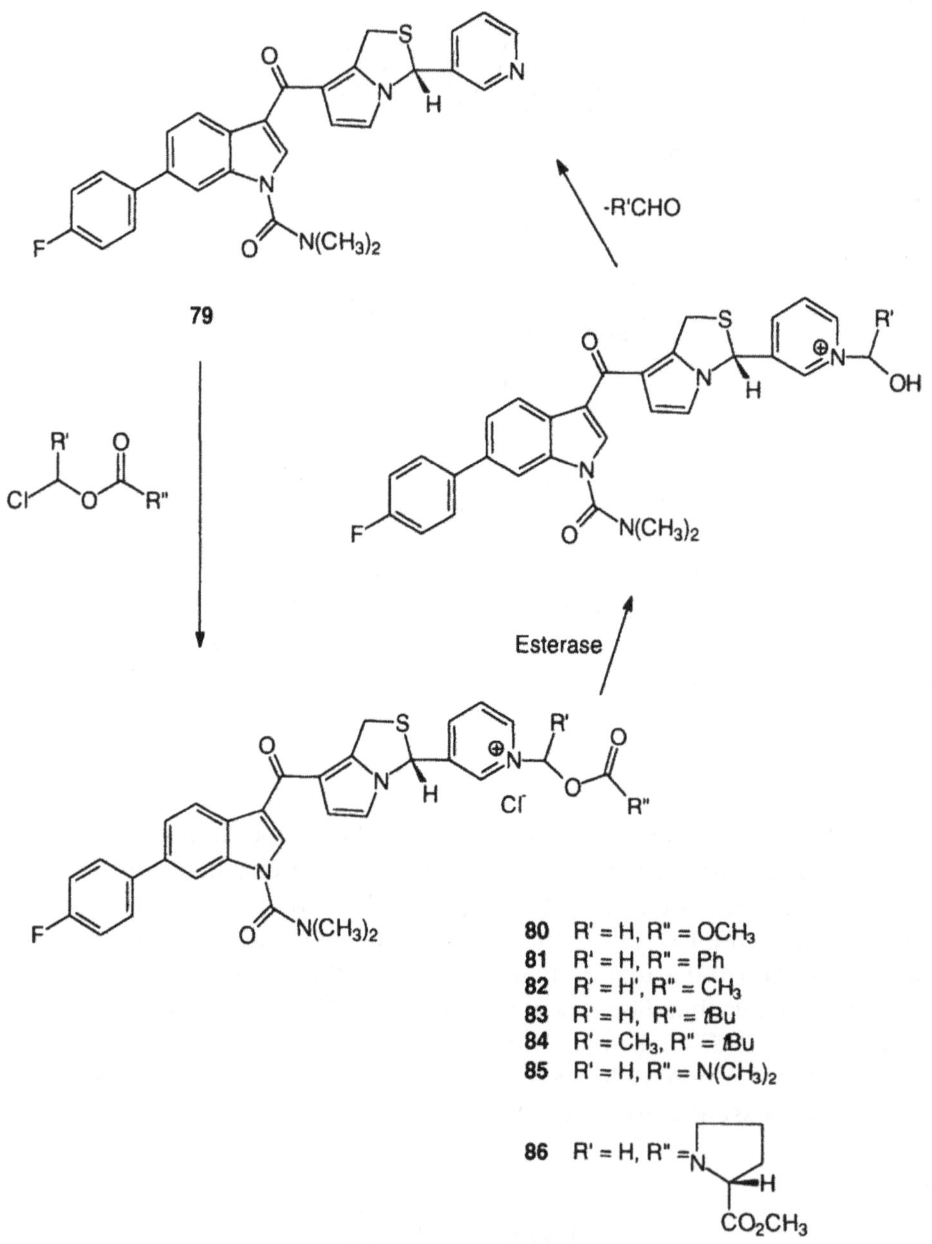

80 R' = H, R" = OCH₃
81 R' = H, R" = Ph
82 R' = H', R" = CH₃
83 R' = H, R" = tBu
84 R' = CH₃, R" = tBu
85 R' = H, R" = N(CH₃)₂

86 R' = H, R" =

variety of drugs that manifest problems due to their lack of adequate solubility in aqueous vehicles. Many prodrug candidates developed to improve water solubility warranted further studies, various prodrugs discussed here advanced to clinical trials, and a few have been under consideration for, or already have received, approval. No recommendations can be given about the preferred prodrug types for any application. The chemical structure of the drug should dictate the design of appropriate derivatives to be considered as potential prodrugs, and thorough in vitro and in vivo evaluation should be conducted to ascertain their safety and efficacy. Prodrugs are considered new drug entities and, thus, they are subject to approval by regulatory agencies.

REFERENCES

Alberth, D. H., R. G. Conway, T. J. Magoc, P. Tapang, D. A. Rhein, G. Luo, J. Holms, S. K. Davidsen, J. B. Summers, and G. W. Carter. 1995. Properties of ABT-299, a prodrug of A-85783, a highly potent platelet activating factor receptor antagonist. *J. Pharmacol. Exp. Ther.* 277:1595–1606.

Allemand, I., M. Christ, X. Pannecoucke, T. Molina, B. Luu, and P. Briand. 1993. Effect of oxysterol derivatives on the time course development of hepatocarcinoma in transgenic mice. *Anticancer Res.* 13:1097–1101.

Anderson, B. D., and V. Taphouse. 1981. Initial rate studies of hydrolysis and acyl migration in methylprednisolone 21-hemiacetate and 17-hemisuccinate. *J. Pharm. Sci.* 70:181–186.

Anderson, B. D., R. A. Conradi, and J. W. Lambert. 1984. Carboxyl group catalysis of acyl transfer reactions in corticosteroid 17-and 21-monoesters. *J. Pharm. Sci.* 73:604–611.

Anderson, B. D., R. A. Conradi, and K. E. Knuth. 1985. Strategies in the design of solution-stable, water-soluble prodrugs II: properties of micellar prodrug of methylprednisolone. *J. Pharm. Sci.* 74:375–381.

Ambrose, P. J. 1984. Clinical pharmacokinetics of chloramphenicol and chloramphenicol succinate, *Clin. Pharmacokin.* 9:222–238.

Balkovec, J. M., M. Black, M. L. Hammond, J. V. Heck, R. A. Zambias, G. Abruzzo, K. Bartizal, H. Kropp, C. Trainor, R. E. Schwartz, D. C. McFadden, K. H. Nollstack, L. A. Pittarelli, M. A Powles, and D. M. Schmatz. 1992. Synthesis, stability, and biological evaluation of water-soluble prodrug of a new echinocandin lipopeptide. Discovery of a potential clinical agent for the treatment of systemic candidiasis and pneumocystis carinii pneumonia (PCP). *J. Med. Chem.* 35:194–198.

Bender, R. A., E. Hamel, and K. R. Hande. 1990. *Cancer chemotherapy: Principles and practice.* Philadelphia: Lippincott, pp. 253–275.

Bitfu, T., N. F. Gamble, T. Doebber, S. B. Hwang, T. Y. Shen, J. Sneyder, J. P. Springer, and R. Stevenson. 1986. Conformation and activity of tetrahydrofuran lignans and analogues as specific platelet activating factor antagonists. *J. Med. Chem.* 29:1917–1921.

Bodor, N. 1977. Novel approaches for the design of membranes transport properties of drugs. In *Design of biopharmaceutical properties through prodrugs and analogs*, edited by E. B. Roche. Washington D.C.: Academy of Pharm. Sci., pp. 96–135.

Boucher, B. A., A. M. Bombassaro, S. N. Rasmussen, C. B. Watridge, R. Achari, and P. Turlapaty. 1989. Phenytoin prodrug 3-phosphoryloxymethyl phenytoin (ACC-9653): Pharmacokinetics in patients following intravenous and intramuscular administration. *J. Pharm. Sci.* 78:929–932.

Boucher, B. A., C. Feler, C. Dean, D. D. Michie, B. K. Tipton, K. R. Schmith, R. E. Kramer, B. Young, B. R. Parks, and A. R. Kugler. 1996. The safety, tolerability and pharmacokinetics of fosphenytoin after intramuscular and intravenous administration in neurosurgical patients. *Pharmacotherapy* 16:638–645.

Brooks, D. J., and D. S. Alberts. 1996. A phase I study of etoposide plus paclitaxel. *Sem. Oncol.* 23:30–33.

Brooks, D. J., N. Srinivas, D. S. Alberts, T. Thomas, L. M. Igwemzie, L. M. McKinney, J. Randolph, L. Schacter, S. Kaul, and R. H. Barbhaiya. 1995. Phase I and pharmacokinetic study of etoposide phosphate. *Anticancer Drugs* 6:637–644.

Browne, T. R., H. Davoudi, K. H. Donn, C. L. Dougherty, G. E. Dukes, B. Evans, J. E. Evans, B. Jamerson, J. Kres, C. M. McEntegart, J. A. Messenheimer, Jr., J. R. Powell, C. Y. Quon, and G. K. Szabo. 1989. Bioavailability of ACC-9653 (phenytoin prodrug). *Epilepsia* 30:S27–32.

Bruice, T. C., and S. J. Benkovic. 1966. Acyl transfer reactions involving carboxylic acid esters and amides. In *Bioorganic mechanism*, vol. 1, edited by T. C. Bruice and S. J. Benkovic. New York: W.A. Benjamin, pp. 134–145.

Budman, D. R., L. N. Igwemezie, S. Kaul, J. Behr, S. Lichtman, P. Schulman, V. Vinciguerra, S. L. Allen, J. Kolitz, K. Hock, K. O'Neil, L. Schacter, and R. H. Barbhaiya. 1994. Phase I evaluation of a water-soluble etoposide prodrug, etoposide phosphate, given as a 5-minutes infusion on days 1, 3, and 5 in patients with solid tumors. *J. Clin. Oncol.* 12:1902–1909.

Bugianesi, R. L., W. H. Parson, J. C. Chabala, P. Davies, T. W. Doebber, J. Doherty, D. W. Graham, S. B. Hwang, C. H. Kuo, M. H. Lam, D. E. MacInture, R. Meurer, C. D. Roberts, S. P. Sahoo, and M. S. Wu. 1992. Development, synthesis, and biological evaluation of (-)-trans-(2S,5S)-2-[3-(2-oxypropyl)sulfonyl]-4-N-propoxy-5-(3-hydroxypropoxy)phenyl]-5-(3,4,5-trimethoxyphenyl)tetrahydrofuran, a potent orally active platelet-activating factor (PAF) antagonist and its water-soluble prodrug phosphate ester. *J. Med. Chem.* 35:3474–3482.

Bundgaard, H. 1985. *Design of prodrugs*. Amsterdam: Elsevier, pp. 1–92.

Bundgaard, H., and E. Falch. 1985. Allopurinol prodrug. II. Water-soluble N-acyloxymethyl allopurinol derivatives for rectal and parenteral use. *Int. J. Pharm.* 25:27–39.

Bundgaard, H., E. Falch, and E. Jensen. 1989. A novel solution-stable, water-soluble prodrug type for drugs containing a hydroxyl or an NH-acidic group. *J. Med. Chem.* 32:2503–2507.

Bundgaard, H., E. Jensen, and E. Falch. 1991. Water-soluble, solution-stable, and biolabile N-substituted (aminomethyl)benzoate ester prodrug of acyclovir. *Pharm Res.* 8:1087–1093.

Bundgaard, H., C. Larsen, and P. Thorbek. 1984. Prodrug as drug delivery systems XXVI. Peparation and enzymatic hydrolysis of various water-soluble amino acid esters of metronidazole. *Int. J. Pharm.* 18:67–77.

Cho, M. J., T. A. Scahill, and J. B. Hester, Jr. 1983. Kinetics and equilibrium of the reversible alprazolam ring-opening reaction. *J. Pharm. Sci.* 72:356–362.

Cho, M. J., V. H. Sethy, and L. C. Haynes. 1986. Sequentially labile water-soluble prodrug of alprazolam. *J. Med. Chem.* 29:1346–1350.

Christ, M., Y. H. Ji, C. Moog, X. Pannecoucke, G. Schmitt, P. Bischoff, and B. Luu. 1991. Antitumor activity of oxysterols. Effect of two water-soluble monophosphoric acid diesters of 7β-hydroxycholesterol on Mastocytoma P815 in Vivo. *Anticancer Res.* 11:359–364.

Chu, D. T., I. M. Lico, R. N. Swanson, K. C. Marsh, J. J. Plattner, and A. G. Pernet. 1990. Synthesis and biological properties of A-71497: A prodrug of tosufloxacin. *Drugs Exp. Clin. Res.* 16:435–443.

Cleare, M. J., P. C., Hydes, B. W. Malerbi, and D. M. Watkins. 1978. Anti-tumor platinum complexes—relationship between chemical properties and activity. *Biochemie* 60:835–850.

Cloyd, J. C., D. E. Bosch, and R. J. Sawchuk. 1978. Concentration-time profile of phenytoin after admixture with small volumes of intravenous fluids. *Am. J. Hosp. Pharm.* 35:45–48.

Cranford, R. E., I. E. Leppik, B. Patrick, C. B. Anderson, and B. Kostick. 1979. Intravenous phenytoin in acute seizure disorders. *Neurology* 29:1474–1479.

Davidsen, S. K., J. B. Summers, D. H. Albert, J. H. Holms, R. Heyman, T. J. Magoc, R. G. Conway, D. A. Rhein, and G. W. Carter. 1994. N-(acyloxyalkyl)pyridinium salts as soluble prodrug of a potent platelet activating factor antagonist. *J. Med. Chem.* 37:4421–4429.

Debono, M. 1995. Echinocandin lipopeptide antifungal agents: new agents and recent chemical modification studies. *Exp. Opin. Ther. Patents* 5:771–786.

Denny, W. A., W. R. Wilson, M. Tercel, P. Van Zijl, and S. Pullen. 1994. Nitrobenzyl mustard quaternary salts: A new class of hypoxia-selective cytotoxins capable of releasing diffusible cytotoxins on bioreduction. *Int. J. Radiation Biol. Phys.* 29:317–321.

Derendorf, H., H. Mollmann, P. Rohdewald, J. Rehder, and E. W. Schmidt. 1985. Kinetics of methylprednisolone and its hemisuccinate ester. *Clin. Pharmacol. Ther.* 37:502–507.

Deutsh, H. M., J. A. Glinski, M. Hernandez, R. D. Hauwitz, V. L. Narayanan, M. Suffness, and L. H. Zalkow. 1989. Synthesis of congeners and prodrug. 3. Water-soluble prodrug of taxol with potent antitumor activity. *J. Med. Chem.* 32:788–972.

Doyle, T. W. 1984. The Chemistry of etoposide. In *Etoposide (VP-16): Current status and new developments*, edited by B. F. Issel, F. M. Muggia, and S. K. Carter. New York: Academic Press Inc., pp. 15–32.

Doyle, T. W., and D. M. Vyas. 1990. Second generation of etoposide and mitomycin C. *Cancer Treatment Reviews* 17:127–131.

Earnest, M. P., J. A. Marx, and L. R. Drury. 1983. Complications of intravenous phenytoin for acute treatment of seizures. *JAMA* 249:762–765.

Eldon, M. A., G. R. Loewen, R. E. Voightman, G. B. Holmes, T. L. Hunt, and A. J. Sedman. 1993. Safety, tolerance and pharmacokinetics of intravenous fosphenytoin. *Clin. Pharmacol. Ther.* 53:212.

Eng, C. P., S. N. Sehgal, and C. Vezina. 1984. Activity of rapamycin (AY-22,989) against transplanted tumors. *J. Antibiot. (Tokyo)* 37:1231–1233.

Feigenbaum, J. J., F. Bergmann, S. A. Richmond, R. Mechoulam, V. Nadler, Y. Kloog, and M. Sokolovky. 1989. Nonpsychotropic cannabinoid acts as a functional N-methyl-D-aspartate blocker. *Proc. Natl. Acad. Sci. U.S.A.* 86:9584–9587.

Flynn, G., and D. J. Lamb. 1970. Factors influencing solvolysis of corticosteroid-21-phosphate esters. *J. Pharm. Sci.* 59:433–1438.

Gerber, N., D. C. Mays, K. H. Donn, A. Laddu, R. M. Guthrie, P. Turlapathy, C. Y. Quou, and W. K. Rivenburg. 1988. Safety, tolerance and pharmacokinetics of intravenous doses of the phosphate ester of 3-hydroxymethy-5,5'-diphenylhidantoin: A new prodrug of phenytoin. *J. Clin. Pharmacol.* 28:1023–1032.

Girotra, N. N., T. Biftu, M. M. Ponpipom, J. J. Acton, A. W. Alberts, T. N. Bach, R. G. Ball, R. L. Bugianesi, W. H. Parsons, J. C. Chabala, P. Davis, T. W. Doebber, J. Doherty, D. W. Graham, S. B. Hwang, C. H. Kuo, M. H. Lam, S. Luell, D. E. MacIntyre, R. Meure, C. D. Roberts, S. P. Sahoo, and M. S. Wu. 1992. Development, synthesis, and biological evaluation of (-)-trans-(2S,5S)-2-[3-[(2-oxopropyl)sulfonyl]-4-n-propoxy-5-(3-hydroxypropoxy)-phenyl]-5-(3,4,5-trimethoxyphenyl)tetrahydrofuran, a potent orally active platelet-activating factor (PAF) antagonist and its water-soluble prodrug phosphate ester. *J. Med. Chem.* 35: 3474–82.

Girotra, N. N., T. Bitfu, M. M. Ponpipom, J. J. Acton, A. W. Alberts, T. N. Bach, R. G. Ball, R. B. Greenwald, C. W. Gilbert, A. Pendri, C. D. Conover, J. Xia, and A. Martinez. 1996. Drug delivery systems: water soluble taxol 2'-poly(ethylene glycol) ester prodrug—design and in vivo effectiveness. *J. Med. Chem.* 39: 424–431.

Greenspan, E. M., J. Colsky, E. B. Schoenbach, and M. J. Shear. 1954. Response of patients with advanced neoplasia to the intravenous administration of alpha-peltatin. *J. Natl. Cancer Inst.* 14:1257–1275.

Greenwald, R. B., A. Pendri, and D. Bolikal. 1984. Highly water-soluble taxol derivatives: 2'-polyethylene glycol esters as potential prodrug. *Bioorg. Med. Chem. Lett.* 4: 465–2470.

Greenwald, R. B., W. C. Gilbert, A. Pendri, C. D. Conover, J. Xia, and A. Martinez. 1996. Water soluble taxol 2'-poly(ethylene glycol) ester prodrug-design and in vivo effectiveness. *J. Med. Chem.* 39:424–431.

Grisar, J. M., M. A. Petty, F. N. Bolkenius, J. Dow, J. Wagner, E. R. Wagner, K. D. Haegele, and W. D. Jong. 1991. A cardioselective, hydrophilic N,N,N-trimethylethaminium alpha-tocopherol analogue that reduces myocardial infarct size. *J. Med. Chem.* 34:257–260.

Hanessian, S. 1973. The N^6-(dimethylamino)methylene derivative of 9-β-d-arabinofuranosyladenine as an antiviral agent. *J. Med. Chem.* 16:290–292.

Hejchmann, E., R. D. Haugwitz, and M. Cushman. 1996. Synthesis and cytotoxicity of water-soluble ambrosin prodrug candidates. *J. Med. Chem.* 38:3407–3410.

Huttel, M. S., A. S. Olesen, and E. Stoffersen. 1980. Complement-mediated reactions to diazepam with cremophor as solvent (Stesolic MR). *Br. J. Anaesth.* 52:77–79.

Hydes, P. C., and J. H. Russell. 1988. Advances in platinum cancer chemotherapy. Advances in the design of cisplatin analogues. *Cancer Metast. Rev.* 7:67–89.

Jamerson, B. D., K. H. Donn, G. E. Dukes, J. A. Messenheimer, K. L. Brouwer, and J. R. Powell. 1990. Absolute bioavailability of phenytoin after 3-phosphoryloxymethyl-phenytoin disodium (Acc-9643) administration in humans. *Epilepsia* 31:592–597.

Jamerson, B. D., G. E. Dukes, K. L. Brouwer, K. H. Donn, J. A. Messenheimer, and J. R. Powell. 1994. Venous irritation related to intravenous administration of phenytoin versus fosphenytoin. *Pharmacotherapy* 14:47–52.

Jensen, E., and H. Bundgaard. 1991a. Synthesis, enzymatic hydrolysis and physicochemical properties of N-substituted 4-(aminomethyl)benzoate diester prodrug of ganciclovir. *Acta Pharm. Nord.* 3:243–247.

Jensen, E., and H. Bundgaard. 1991b. Aminomethylbenzoate esters of chloramphenicol as a novel prodrug type for parenteral administration. *Int. J. Pharm.* 70:137–146.

Jensen, E., and H. Bundgaard. 1992. N-substituted (aminomethyl)benzoate 21-esters of corticosteroids as water-soluble, solution-stable and biolabile prodrug. *Acta Pharm. Nord.* 4:35–42.

Jensen, E., H. Bundgaard, and E. Falch. 1990. Design of a water-soluble, solution-stable and biolabile prodrug of metronidazole for parenteral administration. *Int. J. Pharm.* 58:143–153.

Jensen, E., E. Falch, and H. Bundgaard. 1991. Water-soluble aminoalkylbenzoate esters of phenols as prodrug. Synthesis, enzymatic hydrolysis and chemical stability of paracetamol esters. *Acta Pharm. Nord.* 3:31–40.

Ji, J.-H., C. Moog, G. Schmitt, P. Bischoff, and B. Luu. 1990. Monophosphoric Acid diesters of 7β-hydroxycholesterol and of pyrimidine nucleosides as potential antitumor agents: Synthesis and preliminary evaluation of antitumor activity. *J. Med. Chem.* 33:2264–2270.

Keller-Juslen, C., M. Kuhn, A. von Wartburg, and H. Stahelin. 1971. Synthesis and antimitotic activity of glycosidic lignan derivatives related to podophyllotoxin. *J. Med.Chem.* 14:936–940.

Kirby, A. J., and G. J. Lloyd. 1976. Intramolecular general base catalysis in hydrolysis of 3-dimethylaminopropionates. *J. Chem. Soc. Perkin Trans.* 2:1748–1752.

Köckerbauer, R., and P. J. Bednarski. 1995. A novel approach to preparing water soluble prodrug forms of cisplatin analogues bearing chelating diamines. *J. Pharm. Sci.* 84:819–823.

Larsen, C., P. Kurtzhals, and M. Johansen. 1988. Kinetics of regeneration of metronidazole from hemiesters of maleic acid, succinic acid and glutamic acid in aqueous buffer, human plasma and pig liver homogenate. *Int. J. Pharm.* 41:121–129.

LePage, G. A., Y. T. Lin, R. E. Orth, and J. A. Gottlieb. 1972. 5'-Nucleotides as potential formulations for administering nucleoside analogs in man. *Cancer Res.* 32:2441–2444.

Leppik, I. E. 1986. Status epilepticus. *Neurol. Clin.* 4:633–643.

Leppik, I. E., B. A. Boucher, B. J. Wilder, V. S. Murthy, C. Watridge, N. M. Graves, R. J. Rangel, C. A. Rask, and P. Turlapathy. 1990. Pharmacokinetics and safety of a phenytoin prodrug given i. v. or i. m. in patients. *Neurology* 40:456–460.

Linker, C. A., C. A. Ries, L. E. Damon, H. S. Rugo, and J. L. Wolf. 1993. Autologous bone marrow transplantation for acute myeloid leukemia using busulfan plus etoposide as a preparative regimen. *Blood* 81:319–323.

Louis, S., H. Kutt, and F. McDowell. 1967. The cardiocirculatory changes caused by intravenous dilantin and its solvent. *Am. Heart J.* 74:523–529.

Luu, B. 1986. Use of in vitro cell cultures to study cytotoxic properties of natural products. In *Advances in Medical Phytochemistry I*, edited by D. Barton and W. D. Ellis. London: John Libbey, pp. 97–101.

Mamber, S. W., A. B. Mikkilineni, E. J. Pack, M. P. Rosser, H. Wong, Y. Ueda, and S. Forenza. 1995. Tubulin polymerization by paclitaxel (taxol) phosphate prodrug after metabolic activation with alkaline phosphatase. *J. Pharmacol. Exp. Ther.* 274:877–883.

Massey, K. D., and K. P. Burton. 1989. α-Tocopherol attenuates myocardial membrane-related alterations resulting from ischemia and reperfusion. *Am. J. Physiol.* 256:H1192–1199.

Mathew, A. E., M. R. Mejillano, J. P. Nath, R. H. Himes, and V. J. Stella. 1992. Synthesis and evaluation of some water-soluble prorug and derivatives of taxol with antitumor activity. *J. Med. Chem.* 35:145–151.

Melby, J. C., and M. St. Cyr. 1961. Comparative studies on absorption and metabolic disposal of water-soluble corticosteroid esters. *Metab. Clin. Exp.* 10:75–82.

Millward, M. J., D. R. Newell, V. Mummaneni, L. N. Igwemezie, K. Balmanno, C. J. Charlton, L. Gumbrell, M. J. Lind, F. Chapman, M. Proctor, D. Simmonds, B. M. Cantwell, G. S. Taylor, C. McDaniel, B. Winograd, S. Kaul, R. H. Barbaiya, and A. H. Calvert. 1995. Phase I and pharmacokinetic study of a water-soluble etoposide prodrug, etoposide phosphate (BMY-40481). *Eur. J. Canc.* 31A:2409–2411.

Miyabo, S., T. Nakamura, S. Kuwazima, and S. Kishida. 1981. A comparison of the bioavailability and potency of dexamethasone phosphate and sulphate in human. *Eur. J. Clin. Pharmacol.* 20:277–282.

Mollmann, H., P. Rohdewald, J. Barth, C. Mollmann, M. Verso, and H. Derendorf. 1988. Comparative pharmacokinetics of methylprednisolone phosphate and hemisuccinate in high doses. *Pharm. Res.* 5:509–513.

Moog, C., N. Frank, B. Luu, and B. Bertram. 1993. Metabolism of new anticancer oxysterol derivatives in rats. *Anticancer Res.* 13:953–958.

Nahata, M. C., and D. A. Powell. 1981. Bioavailability and clearance of cloramphenicol after intravenous chloramphenicol succinate. *Clin. Pharmacol. Ther.* 30:368–372.

Newton, D. W., and R. B. Kluza. 1980. Prediction of phenythoin solubility in intravenous admixtures: Psychiochemical theory. *Am. J. Hosp. Pharm.* 37: 1647–1651.

O'Brien, J. J., and D. M. Campoli-Richards. 1989. Acyclovir. An updated rewiev of its antiviral activity, pharmacokinetic properties and therapeutics efficacy. *Drugs* 37:233–309.

O'Dwyer, P. J., B. Leyland-Jones, M. T. Alonso, S. Marsoni, and R. E. Wittes. 1985. Etoposide (VP-16-213): Current status of an active anticancer drug. *N. Eng. J. Med.* 312:692–700.

Oliyai, R., and V. J. Stella. 1993. Prodrug of peptides and proteins for improved formulation and delivery. *Annu. Rev. Pharmacol. Toxicol.* 32:521–544.

Page, C. P. 1988. Platelet-activating factor, In *Asthma: Basic mechanism and clinical management*, edited by P. J. Barnes, E. W. Rodger, and N. C. Thomson. London: Academic Press Ltd., pp. 283–304.

Pajewski, T. N., J. S. Brabson, A. Kisic, K.-S. Wang, M. D. Hylarides, E. M. Jackson, and G. J. Schoepfer. 1989. Inhibition of sterol synthesis. Metabolism of (2,3-^{3}H) 5α-cholest-8(14)-en-3β-ol-15-one after oral administration to a nonhuman primate. *Chem. Phys. Lipids* 49:243–262.

Parsons, W. H. (1991) Platelet-activating factor, hyperreactivity and asthma, In *Airways hyperresponsiveness: Is it really important for asthma?*, edited by C. P. Page and P. Gardiner. Oxford: Blackwell Scientific Publications, pp. xx.

Paulson, O. B., A. Gyori, and M. H. Hertz. 1982. Blood-brain barrier transfer and cerebral uptake of antiepileptic drugs. *Clin. Pharmacol. Ther.* 32:466–477.

Pedraz, J. L., B. Calvo, A. Bortolotti, A. Celardo, and M. Bonati. 1989. Bioavailability of intramuscular vitamin E acatate in rabbits. *J. Pharm. Pharmacol.* 41: 415–417.

Perrier, D., R. Rapp, B. Young, H. Kostenbauder, W. Cady, S. Pancorbo, and J. Hackman. 1976 Maintenance of therapeutic phenytoin plasma levels via intramuscular administration. *Ann. Intern. Med.* 85:318–321.

Pettit, G. R., S. Freeman, M. J. Simpson, M. A. Thompson, M. R. Boyd, M. D. Williams, G. R. Pettit III, and D. L. Doubek. 1995a. Antineoplastic agents 320: Synthesis of a practical pancratistatin prodrug. *Anticancer Drug Des.* 10: 243–250.

Pettit, G. R., C. Temple, Jr., V. L. Narayanan, R. Varma, M. J. Simpson, M. R. Boyd, G. A. Rener, and N. Bansal. 1995b. Antineoplastic agents 322. Synthesis of combretastatin A-4 prodrug. *Anticancer Drug Des.* 10:299–309.

Pochopin, N. L., W. N. Charman, and V. J. Stella. 1994. Pharmacokinetics of dapsone and amino acid prodrug of dapsone. *Drug Metab. Dispos.* 22:770–775.

Ponpipom, M. M., R. L. Bugianesi, D. R. Brooker, B. Z. Yue, S. B. Hwang, and T. Y. Shen. 1987. Structure-activity relationships of kadsurenone analogs. *J. Med. Chem.* 30:136–142.

Poos, G. I., R. Hirschmann, G. A. Bailey, F. A. Cutler, L. H. Sarett, and J. M. Chemerdra. 1958. Water-soluble steroid phosphates. *Chem. Ind.* 1260–1261.

Pop, E., Z. Z. Liu, M. E. Brewster, Y. Barenholz, V. Korablyov, R. Mechoulam, V. Nadler, and A. Biegon. 1996a. Derivatives of dexanabinol. I. Water-soluble salts of glycinate esters. *Pharm. Res.* 13:62–69.

Pop, E., F. Soti, M. E. Brewster, Y. Barenholz, V. Korablyov, R. Mechoulam, V. Nadler, and A. Biegon. 1996b. Derivatives of dexanabinol. II. Salts of amino acid esters containing tertiary and quaternary heterocyclic nitrogen with increased water-solubility. *Pharm. Res.* 13:469–475.

Rattie, E. S., E. G. Shami, L. W. Ditter, and J. V. Switosky. 1970. Acetaminophen prodrug. 3. Hydrolysis of carbonate and carboxylic acid esters in aqueous buffers. *J. Pharm. Sci.* 59:1738–1741.

Repta, A. J., B. J. Rawson, R. D. Shaffer, K. B. Sloan, N. Bodor, and T. Higuchi. 1975. Rational development of a soluble prodrug of a cytotoxic nucleoside: Preparation and properties of arabinosyladenine 5'-formate. *J. Pharm. Sci.* 64:392–396.

Reynolds, J. E. F., ed. 1989. *Martindale. The Extra Pharmacopeia*. London: The Pharm. Press, pp. 1285–1287.

Rose, W. C., G. A. Basler, P. A. Trail, M. Saulnier, A. R. Crosswell, and A. M. Casazza. 1990. Preclinical antitumor activity of a soluble etoposide analog, BMY-40481-30. *Invest. New Drugs* 8:S25–32.

Rose, W. C., and W. T. Bradner. 1984. In vivo experimental antitumor activity of etoposide. In *Etoposide (VP-16): Current status and new developments*, edited by B. F. Issel, F. M. Muggia, and S. K. Carter. New York: Academic Press Inc., pp. 33–47.

Rowinsky, E. K., L. A. Cazenave, and R. C. Donehower. 1990. Taxol: A novel investigational antimicrotubule agent. *J. Natl. Cancer Inst.* 82:1247–1259.

Safadi, M., R. Oliyai, and V. J. Stella. 1993. Phosphoryloxymethyl carbamates and carbonates-novel water-soluble prodrug for amines and hindered alcohols. *Pharm. Res.* 10:1350–1355.

Sanchez-Crespo, M. 1993. Potential of PAF receptor antagonists in the treatment of septic shock. *Drug News Perspect.* 6:78–87.

Schacter, L. 1996. Etoposide phosphate: What, why, where, and how. *Sem. Oncol.* 23:1–7.

Schacter, L., L. N. Igwemezie, M. Seyedsadr, E. Morgenthien, J. Randolph, E. Albert, and P. Santabarbara. 1994. Clinical and pharmacokinetics overview of parenteral etoposide phosphate. *Cancer Chemother. Pharmacol.* 34:S58–63.

Schiff, P. B., J. Fant, and S. B. Horowitz. 1979. Promotion of microtubule assembly in vitro by taxol. *Nature* 277:665–669.

Schiff, P. B., and S. B. Horowitz. 1980. Taxol stabilizes microtubules in mouse fibroblast cells. *Proc. Natl. Acad. Sci. U.S.A.* 77:1561–1565.

Schlondorff, D., and R. Neuworth. 1986. Platelet-activating factor and the kidney. *Am. J. Physiol.* 251:F1–F11.

Sheppard, G. S., S. K. Pireh, G. M. Carrera, M. G. Bures, H. R. Heyman, D. H. Steinman, S. K. Davidsen, J. G. Philips, D. E. Guinn, P. D. May, M. L. Curtin, R. G. Conway, D. A. Rhein, W. C. Calhoun, D. H. Alberth, T. J. Magoc, G. W. Carter, and J. B. Summers. 1994. 3-(2-(3-Pyridinyl)thiazolidin-4-oyl)indoles, a novel series of platelet activating factor antagonists. *J. Med. Chem.* 37:1–32.

Sheppard, G. S., S. K. Davidsen, G. M. Carrera, D. Pireh, J. Holms, H. R. Heyman, D. H. Steinman, M. L. Curtin, R. G. Conway, D. A. Rhein, D. H. Alberth, P. Tapang, T. J. Magoc, and J. B. Summers. 1995. Synthesis and evaluation of water-soluble indole pyrrolothiazlole PAF antagonists. *Bioorg. Med. Chem. Lett.* 5:2913–2918.

Sendo, F., C. M. Riley, and V. J. Stella. 1988. Kinetics of hydrolysis of fetindomide (NSC-373965), bis-N,N'-phenylalanyloxymethyl prodrug of mitindomide (NSC-284356): An unexpected catalytic effect of generated formaldehyde. *Int. J. Pharm.* 45:207–216.

Senter, P. D., M. G. Saulnier, G. J. Schreiber, D. L. Hirschberg, J. P. Brown, I. Hellstrom, and K. E. Hellstrom. 1988. Anti-tumor effects of antibody-alkaline phosphatase conjugates in combination with etoposide phosphate. *Proc. Natl. Acad. Sci. USA* 85:4842–4846.

Serrano, E. E., and B. J. Wilder. 1974. Intramuscular administration of diphenylhydantoin. Histologic follow-up studies. *Arch. Neurol.* 31:276–278.

Slojkowska, Z., H. J. Krasuska, and J. Packecka. 1982. Enzymatic hydrolysis of amino acid derivatives of benzocaine. *Xenobiotica* 12:359–364.

Stella, V. J. 1975. Prodrugs. An overview and definition. In *Prodrugs as novel drug delivery systems, ACS Symp. Ser., vol. 14,* edited by T. Higuchi and V. J. Stella. Washington, DC: American Chemical Society, pp. 1–115.

Stella, V. J., and T. Higuchi. 1973. Esters of hydantoic acids as prodrugs of hydantoins. *J. Pharm. Sci.* 62: 962–967.

Supko, J. G., and L. Malspeis. 1994. Dose-dependent pharmacokinetics of rapamycin-28-N,N-dimethylglycinate in the mouse. *Pharmacotherapy* 33: 325–330.

Takata, J., Y. Karube, M. Hanada, K. Matsunaga, Y. Matsushima, T. Sendo, and R. Oishi. 1995a. Vitamin K prodrug: 2. Water-soluble prodrug of menahydroquinone-4 for systemic site-specific delivery. *Pharm. Res.* 12:1973–1979.

Takata, J., Y. Karube, M. Hanada, K. Matsunaga, T. Sendo, and T. Aoyama. 1995b. Vitamin K prodrug: 1. Synthesis of amino acid esters of menahydroquinone-4 and enzymatic reconversion to an active form. *Pharm. Res.* 12:18–23.

Takata, J., Y. Karube, Y. Nagata, and K. Matsunaga. 1994. Prodrug of vitamin E. 1. Preparation and enzymatic hydrolysis of aminoalkanecarboxylic acid esters of d-α-tocopherol. *J. Pharm. Sci.* 84:96–100.

Tercel, M., W. R. Wilson, and W. A. Denny. 1993. Nitrobenzyl mustard quaternary salts: A new class of hypoxia-selective cytotoxins showing in vitro selectivity. *J. Med. Chem.* 36:2578–2580.

Varia, S. A., and V. J. Stella. 1984a. Phenytoin prodrug V: In vivo evaluations of some water-soluble prodrug in dogs. *J. Pharm. Sci.* 73:1080–1086.

Varia, S. A., and V. J. Stella. 1984b. Phenytoin prodrug VI: In vivo evaluation of a phosphate ester prodrug of phenytoin after parenteral administration to rats. *J. Pharm. Sci.* 73:1087–1090.

Varia, S. A., S. Schuller, K. B. Sloan, and V. J. Stella. 1984a. Phenytoin prodrug III: Water-soluble prodrug for oral and/or parenteral use. *J. Pharm. Sci.* 73: 1068–1073.

Varia, S. A., S. Schuller, and V. J. Stella. 1984b. Phenytoin prodrug IV: Hydrolysis of various 3-(hydroxymethyl)phenytoin esters. *J. Pharm. Sci.* 73:1074–1079.

Venuti, M. C., R. Alvarez, J. J. Bruno, A. M. Strosberg, L. Gu, H.-S. Chiang, I. J. Massey, N. Chu, and J. H. Fried. 1988. Inhibitors of cyclic AMP phosphodiesterase. 4. Synthesis and evaluation of potential prodrug of Lixazinone (N-cyclohexyl-N-methyl-4-[(1,2,3,5-tetrahydro-2-oxoimidazo[2,1-b]quinazolin-7-yl)-oxy]butyramide, RS-82856). *J. Med. Chem.* 31:2145–2152.

Vezina, C., A. Kudelski, and S. N. Sehgal. 1975. Rapamycyn (AY-22,989), a new antifungal antibiotic. I. Taxonomy of the producing streptomycete and isolation of the active principle. *J. Anibiot. (Tokyo)* 28:721–726.

Vyas, D. M., H. Wong, A. R. Crossweell, J. O. Knipe, S. W. Mamber, and T. W. Doyle. 1993. Synthesis and antitumor evaluation of water-soluble taxol phosphates. *BioMed. Chem. Lett.* 3:1357–1360.

Wani, M. C., H. L. Taylor, M. E. Wall, P. C. Coogan, and A. J. McPail. 1971. Plant antitumor agents. IV. The isolation and structure of taxol, a novel antileukemic and antitumor agent from *Taxus Brevifolia. J. Am. Chem. Soc.* 93:2325–2327.

Williams, A., and R. A. Naylor. 1971. Evidence for $S_N2(P)$ mechanism in phosphorylation of alkaline phosphatase by substrates. *J. Chem. Soc.* 1073–1079.

Williams, D. B., S. A. Varia, V. J. Stella, and I. H. Pitman. 1983. Evaluation of the prodrug potential of the sulfate esters of acetaminophen and 3-hydroxymethyl-phenytoin. *Int. J. Pharm.* 14:113–120.

Zhao, Z., D. G. Kingston, and A. R. Croswell. 1991. Modified taxols. 6. Preparation of water-soluble prodrug of taxol. *J. Nat. Prod.* 54:1607–1611.

13

Complexation—Use of Cyclodextrins to Improve Pharmaceutical Properties of Intramuscular Formulations

Marcus E. Brewster

Janssen Research Foundation/Janssen Pharmaceutica
Beerse, Belgium

Thorsteinn Loftsson

Department of Pharmacy, University of Iceland
Reykjavik, Iceland

Intramuscular (IM) and other parenteral approaches provide an important formulation option for many pharmaceuticals. In circumstances of poor oral bioavailability or when rapid drug action is required, these administration routes often provide the only practical means of efficiently delivering the agents of interest (Greenblatt and Allen 1978; Alper 1978). Unfortunately, physicochemical properties of the drug often conspire to limit the usefulness of these dosage forms. Poorly water-soluble drugs must be formulated in partially nonaqueous systems that may include organic cosolvents or electroneutral detergents. Both of the excipient types can be deleterious, causing pain on injection, muscle damage, and various systemic toxicities (Yalkowsky and Rubino 1985). In addition to problems associated with the excipients, the administered drugs themselves may contribute to local irritation through a variety of mechanisms including alteration of surface activity (Brazeau and Fung 1989a). Given these limitations, salient approaches for improving IM formulations would appear to be the elimination of undesirable excipients from otherwise useful dosage forms and the attenuation of various physicochemical properties that render drug molecules irritating. Both of these goals are potentially addressable using pharmaceutical complexation, especially with cyclodextrins.

Complexation involves the noncovalent interaction between the drug of interest and the complexing agent (Martin 1993). These processes are extensively used in the pharmaceutical area with salient examples including metal complexation (e.g., ethylenediaminetetraacetic acid [EDTA] chelates of various metal ions), organic complexes (e.g., complexes of caffeine or nicotinamide with various drugs), polymeric complexes (e.g., between various drugs and polyethylene glycol [PEG], polyvinyl pyrrolidinone, or carboxymethylcellulose), and inclusion complexes (e.g., cyclodextrin systems). It is the purpose of this chapter to explore the use of cyclodextrin as a formulation adjunct in the preparation of IM dosage forms. While cyclodextrins have been selected for a more in-depth examination, the fact that all complexations are equilibrium processes governed by an equilibrium constant K indicates that many of the points discussed herein are generalizable to other systems.

CYCLODEXTRINS

Cyclodextrins are cyclic oligomaltoses produced from corn or other starches through the action of the amylase, cyclodextrin transglucosylase (CTG) (Szejtli 1982). These compounds are named based on the number of α-1,4-linked glucose residues in the formed rings with α-cyclodextrin referring to the hexomer, β-cyclodextrin referring to the heptomer, and γ-cyclodextrin the glucose octomer (Figure 13.1) (Loftsson and Brewster 1996; Uekama 1981; Szejtli 1982). Given the C-1 chair conformation of the component sugar residues, cyclodextrins are not perfectly cylindrical; instead, they take the shape of a truncated cone or torus. In this assembly, the maltosyl hydroxyl functions are oriented to the cone exterior with the primary hydroxyl groups located at the narrower end of the cone and the secondary hydroxyl groups present on the wider face. The cavity formed by the torus is lined by the skeletal carbons and ethereal oxygens of the carbohydrate. This molecular architecture imparts to the cyclodextrins their unique properties: the exterior is hydrophilic, and the inner cavity is hydrophobic (Brewster et al. 1989b). The hydrophilic exterior exhibits some degree of water solubility, which varies for the cyclodextrins, with β-cyclodextrin (approximately 1.85 mg/mL at 25°C) being the least water soluble. This is due to crystal lattice stabilization via intramolecular hydrogen bond formation (Uekama and Otagiri 1987). The hydrophobic central cavity provides a microenvironment into which appropriately sized nonpolar compounds can include and form complexes.

The amphiphatic nature of cyclodextrins and their ability to form complexes has been exploited pharmaceutically to camouflage various

Figure 13.1. Structure and various physical properties of α-cyclodextrin (α-CD), β-cyclodextrin (β-CD) and γ-cyclodextrin (γ-CD).

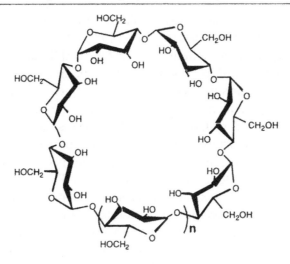

	α-CD (n = 0)	β-CD (n = 1)	γ-CD (n = 2)
Molecular Weight	972	1135	1297
Glucose Residues	6	7	8
Cavity Diameter (Å)	5	6	8
Sol. in Water (w/v %)	14.2	1.85	23.2
Surface Tension (mN/m)	71	71	71
Melting Range (°C)	255–260	255–265	240–245
Water of Crystallization	10.2	13–15	8–18
Water in Cavity	6	11	17

undesirable physicochemical properties (Szejtli 1994; Rajewski and Stella 1996; Brewster et al. 1989b; Froming and Szejtli 1994; Duchene 1987). Since cyclodextrins can interact with poorly water-soluble drugs giving rise to soluble inclusion complexes, these excipients make excellent solubilizers. In addition, starches find application in drug stabilization (both in aqueous solution and in the solid phase) and in lowering the vapor pressure of drugs, thereby masking unaesthetic tastes or smells (Loftsson 1995; Pagington 1987). Cyclodextrins can also be used to convert oils to free-flowing powders and to eliminate incompatibilities in various formulations (Szejtli 1982). Inclusion complexation has a number of other ramifications in terms of biopharmaceutics, as the process can increase drug availability and decrease gastric, ophthalmic and other irritation (Szejtli 1994). For these and other applications, β-cyclodextrin appears to be the most useful given its cavity size and efficiency of complexation, in addition to its availability in pure form and cost.

Unfortunately, β-cyclodextrin is limited in its water solubility, and this characteristic imparts several unwanted properties. First, the low aqueous solubility of the solubilizer generates technical difficulties, since large volumes of the solutions of interest must be used, and large volumes of water must be evaporated or sublimed if the solid complex is desired. Furthermore, complexes of β-cyclodextrin and various drugs may be of limited solubility (see "Characterization of Cyclodextrin Complexes" in this chapter) and, as such, may precipitate from solution (Uekama and Otagiri 1987). Finally, parenteral (intravenous [IV], IM, subcutaneous) administration of β-cyclodextrin leads to severe nephrotoxicity (Frank et al. 1976; Perrin et al., 1978; Hiasa et al. 1981). In rats, β-cyclodextrin increases the blood urea nitrogen (BUN), significantly increases the weight of the kidneys, and dramatically alters renal histology. These effects are thought to be associated with tubular reabsorption of β-cyclodextrin followed by precipitation of the compound in the formed vacuoles. The microcrystalline network then induces necrosis and other adverse effects.

These limitations have prompted a search for safer cyclodextrin derivatives. Since the limited water solubility of β-cyclodextrin is associated with intramolecular hydrogen bonding, derivatization of the secondary hydroxyl functions, even with lipophilic groups, may increase their water solubility (Uekama and Otagiri 1987). Methylation of β-cyclodextrin generates di- and trimethyl-β-cyclodextrin [i.e., heptakis(2,6-di-O-methyl)-β-cyclodextrin or DMβCD and heptakis(2,3,6-tri-O-methyl)-β-cyclodextrin or TMβCD)] (Figure 13.2) (Szejtli 1982). These compounds are significantly more soluble than β-cyclodextrin, and the extended length of the cavity, resulting from the added methyl groups, increases the stability of complexes formed. These compounds are, however, lipophilic and surface active. As a result, both their systemic and local toxicity are greater than that of β-cyclodextrin (Muller and Brauns 1985; Yoshida et al. 1988).

Other types of chemical modifications are also possible. Reaction of β-cyclodextrin with propylene oxide gives rise to a complex mixture of 2-hydroxypropyl isomers (i.e., 2-hydroxypropyl-β-cyclodextrin or HPβCD), similar in type to those produced in hydroxypropyl cellulose and other pharmaceutical starches (Figure 13.2) (Pitha et al. 1986a; Rao et al. 1990). The hydrophilicity of the substituent and the amorphous nature of the systems formed provide for very high water solubility (> 60 percent w/v).

Although these mixtures are complex, they can be well characterized by various analytical techniques, including mass spectrometry (Brewster et al. 1989b, 1990; Rao et al. 1990). Through analogous processes, hydroxyethyl-, 3-hydroxypropyl-, 2-hydroxyisobutyl-, and 2,3-dihydroxypropyl-β-cyclodextrin systems have been generated (Yoshida et al. 1989; Irie et al. 1988). Likewise, a family of randomly substituted sulfobutyl ethers has been

Figure 13.2. Chemically modified β-cyclodextrin derivatives.

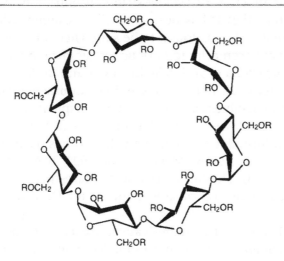

Cyclodextrin	Substituent
Dimethyl-β-cyclodextrin (DMβCD)	$-CH_3$ or -H
Trimethyl-β-cyclodextrin (TMβCD)	$-CH_3$
Hydroxyethyl-β-cyclodextrin (HEβCD)	$-CH_2CH_2OH$ or -H
2-Hydroxypropyl-β-cyclodextrin (HPβCD)	$-CH_2CHOHCH_3$ or -H
3-Hydroxypropyl-β-cyclodextrin (3HPβCD)	$-CH_2CH_2CH_2OH$ or -H
2,3-Dihydroxypropyl-β-cyclodextrin (DHPβCD)	$-CH_2CHOHCH_2OH$ or -H
2-Hydroxyisobutyl-β-cyclodextrin (HIBβCD)	$-CH_2C(CH_3)_2OH$ or -H
Sulfobutylether-β-cyclodextrin (SBEβCD)	$-(CH_2)_4SO_3Na$ or -H
Glucosyl-β-cyclodextrin (G_1βCD)	-glucosyl or -H
Maltosyl-β-cyclodextrin (G_2βCD)	-maltosyl or -H

prepared and characterized (Tait et al. 1992). Finally, branched cyclodextrins, such as glucosyl-β-cyclodextrin (G_1βCD) and maltosyl-β-cyclodextrin (G_2βCD), have been described as potential excipients (Koizumi et al. 1987; Yamamoto et al. 1989; Hashimoto 1991). These β-cyclodextrin derivatives are highly water soluble and manifest complexing potential similar to those of β-cyclodextrin.

Extensive testing and biological screening have suggested that several of these materials have the requisite characteristics to be useful as drug excipients (Irie and Uekama 1997). These include the HPβCD and sulfobutylether-β-cyclodextrin (SBEβCD). HPβCD is similar to β-cyclodextrin in its complexing efficiency but, as mentioned, is significantly more water soluble. As such, HPβCD tends to increase the solubility of drugs as a linear or curvilinear function of cyclodextrin concentration (Brewster et al. 1989b). In addition, HPβCD has been extensively examined in terms of its toxicological potential. It was found to be safe when administered acutely, subacutely, and subchronically to various test animals by a variety of administration routes (Pitha et al. 1986a; Brewster and Bodor 1990; Pitha and Pitha 1985; Brewster et al. 1990; Brewster 1991; Coussement et al. 1990; Pitha et al. 1988). Its usefulness as a solubilizing excipient and its low toxicological potential has allowed it to enter a number of human clinical trials, and the first drug formulation containing HPβCD has garnered regulatory approval in the United States (Mesens et al. 1991; Brewster 1991; Szejtli 1994; Estes et al. 1994). The SBEβCD system shares many of the solubilizing, stabilizing, and toxicological advantages of the HPβCD (Rajewski et al. 1995).

Finally, while β-cyclodextrin derivatives are usually most applicable to pharmaceutical complexation, many examples where γ-cyclodextrin may be optimal are available. Since this cyclodextrin has a central cavity larger than β-cyclodextrin, it lends itself more readily to the solubilization of large and bulky drugs, such as amphotericin B or tiamulin (Sato et al. 1982; Vikmon et al. 1985). In addition, γ-cyclodextrin is more water soluble than β-cyclodextrin (Table 13.1), although not as water soluble as HPβCD or SBEβCD. Thus, in certain circumstances, the naturally occurring γ-cyclodextrin may be the best choice for solubilization or stabilization.

PREPARATION OF CYCLODEXTRIN COMPLEXES

Various methods have been applied to the preparation of drug-cyclodextrin complexes (Duchene 1988; Loftsson and Brewster 1996). In solution, the

Table 13.1. Pharmacokinetics and Myotoxicity of Two IM Prednisolone Formulations Including a Cosolvent System (PEG 400: Ethanol:Water—40:10:50) and the SBEβCD in the Rabbit ($*p < 0.05$)

Parameter	Cosolvent	SBEβCD
Creatine Kinase AUC (Units·h/L)	$51,000 \pm 10,000$	$7,700 \pm 2,300*$
Prednisolone AUC (μg·h/mL)	14.6 ± 2.8	10.5 ± 0.6
Half-life ($t_{1/2}$, h)	2.5 ± 0.9	1.5 ± 0.2
T_{max} (h)	0.41 ± 0.09	0.47 ± 0.12
C_{max} (μg/mL)	4.58 ± 0.59	$6.45 \pm 0.35*$
Bioavailability (%)	100	87.0 ± 12.6

complexes are usually prepared by addition of an excess of the drug to an aqueous cyclodextrin solution. The suspension formed is equilibrated (which may require up to one week at the desired temperature) and then filtered or centrifuged to form a clear drug-cyclodextrin complex solution. Since the rate-determining step in complex formation is often the phase-to-phase transition of the drug molecule, it is sometimes possible to shorten this process through several manipulations.

Supersaturated drug solutions can be formed by sonication followed by precipitation (Loftsson and Brewster 1996). Likewise, the drug to be complexed can be taken up into a small volume of a water-miscible organic solvent and then added to the cyclodextrin solution (Brewster et al. 1995). Pitha et al. have also described an approach in which the drug and cyclodextrin were first solubilized in ethanol, after which the ethanol was removed, the residue dissolved in water, and the system filtered and further processed (Pitha et al. 1992; Pitha and Hoshino 1992). Aqueous ammonia was similarly suggested as a solvent in this regard, especially for drugs containing ionizable nitrogen moieties in their structures.

For preparation of the solid complexes, the water is removed from the aqueous drug-cyclodextrin solutions by evaporation or sublimation, e.g., spray-drying or freeze-drying. Other methods can also be applied to prepare solid drug-cyclodextrin complexes, including kneading, coprecipitation, neutralization, and grinding techniques (Duchene 1988). In the kneading method, the drug is added to an aqueous slurry of a poorly water-soluble cyclodextrin, such as β-cyclodextrin (Szjetli 1982). The mixture is thoroughly mixed, often at elevated temperatures, to yield a paste, which is then dried. Coprecipitation of cyclodextrin complex through addition of organic solvent is also possible. Unfortunately, the organic solvents used as precipitants can interfere with complexation, which makes this approach less attractive than the kneading method. Solid complexes of ionizable drugs can sometimes be prepared by the neutralization method, wherein the drug is dissolved in an acidic (for basic drugs) or basic (for acidic drugs) aqueous cyclodextrin solution. The solubility of the drug is then lowered through appropriate pH adjustments to force the complex out of solution. Finally, solid drug-cyclodextrin complexes can be formed by grinding a physical mixture of the drug and cyclodextrin and then heating the mixture in a sealed container to 60 to 90°C. Additional methodologies have been recently reviewed (Loftsson and Brewster 1996).

CHARACTERIZATION OF CYCLODEXTRIN COMPLEXES

Free drug molecules are in equilibrium with the molecules bound within the cyclodextrin cavity. Measurements of stability or equilibrium constants ($K_{1:1}$ or K_c) or the dissociation constants (K_d) of the drug-cyclodextrin complexes are important, since this value gives an index of changes in physicochemical properties of a compound upon inclusion (Hirayama and Uekama 1987). In all of the complexation processes of interest, the equilibrium (i.e., stability or association) constant (K_c or better expressed as $K_{m:n}$ in which the stoichiometric ratio of the complex is explicitly given) can be written:

$$mL + nS \xrightarrow{\;K_{m:n}\;} L_m S_n$$
$$[a - mx][b - nx] \qquad\qquad [x]$$

so that

$$K_{m:n} = \frac{[x]}{[a - mx]^m [b - nx]^n}$$

In addition, a dissociation constant can also be defined:

$$K_d = \frac{[a - mx]^m [b - nx]^n}{[x]} = \frac{1}{K_c} \text{ or } \frac{1}{K_{m:n}}$$

Most methods for determining the K values are based on titrating changes in the physicochemical properties of the guest molecule (i.e., the drug molecule), with the cyclodextrin and then analyzing the concentration dependencies (Szejtli 1982; Loftsson and Brewster 1996; Hirayama and Uekama 1987). Additive guest properties that can be titrated in this way include aqueous solubility, chemical reactivity, molar absorptivity and other optical properties (CD, ORD), phase solubility measurements, nuclear magnetic resonance (NMR) chemical shifts, pH-metric methods, calorimetric titration, freezing point depression, and liquid chromatography (LC) retention times (Loftsson and Brewster 1996).

One of the most useful and widely applied analytical approaches in this context is the phase-solubility method described by Higuchi and Connors (1965). Phase-solubility analysis involves an examination of the effect of a solubilizer (i.e., cyclodextrin or ligand) on the drug being solubilized (i.e., the substrate). Experimentally, the drug of interest is added to several vials, such that it is always in excess. The presence of solid drug in these systems is necessary to maximize the thermodynamic activity of the dissolved substrate. To the drug or substrate (S) is added a constant volume of water containing successively larger concentrations of the cyclodextrin or ligand (L). The vials are equilibrated at a constant temperature (a process that frequently takes about one week), the solid drug is removed, and the solution is assayed for the total concentration of S. A phase-solubility diagram is then constructed by plotting the total molar concentration of S on the y-axis and the total molar concentration of L added on the x-axis.

Phase-solubility diagrams prepared in this way fall into two main categories—A- and B-types (Figure 13.3) (Higuchi and Connors 1965). A-type curves are indicative of the formation of soluble inclusion complexes, while B-type behaviors are suggestive of the formation of inclusion complexes of

Figure 13.3. Phase-solubility relationships.

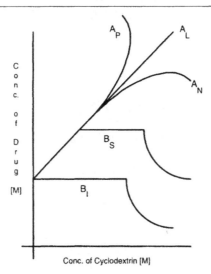

Conc. of Cyclodextrin [M]

poor solubility. A B_S-type response denotes complexes of limited solubility, and a B_I-curve is indicative of insoluble complexes. The A-curves are subdivided into A_L- (linear increases of drug solubility as a function of cyclodextrin concentration), A_P- (positively deviating isotherm), and A_N- (negatively deviating isotherms) subtypes (Brewster et al. 1989).

While β-cyclodextrin often gives rise to B-type curves due to the poor water solubility of L, the chemically modified cyclodextrins, including HPβCD and SBEβCD, usually produce soluble complexes (i.e., A-type systems). A_L-type diagrams are first order with respect to the L and may be first or higher order with respect to S, i.e., SL, S_2L, S_3L, . . . , S_mL. If the slope of an A_L-type system is greater than one, higher order complexes are indicated. A slope of less than one does not necessarily exclude higher order complexation, but 1:1 complexation is usually assumed in the absence of other information. A_P-type systems suggest the formation of higher order complexes with respect to the ligand at higher ligand concentrations, i.e., SL_2, SL_3, . . . , SL_n. A_N-type systems are problematic and difficult to interpret. The negative deviation from linearity may be associated with ligand-induced changes in the dielectric constant of the solvent or self-association of the ligands at high cyclodextrin concentrations.

These phase-solubility systems not only allow a qualitative assessment of the complexes formed but may also be used to derive equilibrium constants. The equilibrium constant (K) for the formation of S_mL_n can be represented by:

$$K = \frac{[S_m L_n]}{[S]^m [L]^n}$$

Given that:

$$[S] = S_o$$

$$S_t = S_o + m[S_m L_n]$$

$$L_t = L + n[S_m L_n]$$

then the values of $[S_m L_n]$, $[S]$, and $[L]$ can be obtained:

$$[S] = S_o$$

$$[S_m L_n] = \frac{S_t - S_o}{m}$$

$$[L] = L_t - n[S_m L_n]$$

where S_o is the equilibrium solubility of S (i.e., in the absence of solubilizer), S_t is the total concentration of S (complexed and uncomplexed), and L_t is the total concentration of L. For phase-solubility systems that are first order with respect to the cyclodextrin ($n = 1$), the following equation may be derived:

$$S_t = \frac{mKS_o^m L_t}{1 + KS_o^m} + S_o$$

A plot of S_t versus L_t for the formation of $S_m L$ should give a straight line with the y-intercept representing S_o and the slope being:

$$\text{slope} = \frac{mKS_o^m}{1 + KS_o^m}$$

Therefore, if m is known, then K can be calculated. If $m = 1$ (i.e., a 1:1 drug:cyclodextrin complex form), the following equation can be applied:

$$K_{1:1} = \frac{\text{slope}}{S_o(1 - \text{slope})}$$

If a series of complexes (i.e., SL, S_2L, . . . , $S_m L$) were present, an A_L-type system would still be observed and is indistinguishable from a simple 1:1 complex. Nevertheless, an apparent stability constant (K_c), assuming a 1:1 stoichiometry is often used to describe the system. Thus from the slope and intercept of the phase-solubility diagram, the apparent stability constant can be estimated.

For A_P-type systems, equilibrium constants can also be evaluated. For systems in which 1:1 and 1:2 (drug:cyclodextrin) complexes form:

$$K_{1:1} = \frac{[SL]}{[S][L]}$$

$$K_{1:2} = \frac{[SL_2]}{[SL][L]} \text{ or } \frac{[SL_2]}{[S][L]^2}$$

assuming that $S_o \ll [SL]$ or, in other words, that $[SL] \approx [S]$. The material balance equations are given by:

$$S_t = S + SL + SL_2$$

$$S = S_o$$

$$L_t = L + SL + 2(SL_2)$$

Combining these equations gives:

$$S_t = \frac{L_t[K_{1:1}S_o + K_{1:1}K_{1:2}S_o(L)]}{1 + K_{1:1}S_o + 2K_{1:1}K_{1:2}S_o(L)} + S_o$$

This equation indicates that a plot of S_t versus L_t will give a graph with intercept S_o and a slope that is a function of L, meaning that as L increases, the slope will increase, thus giving rise to the A_P-type system.

The above equation can be converted into the following linear form:

$$\frac{S_t - S_o}{L_t} = K_{1:1}S_o + K_{1:1}K_{1:2}S_oL_t$$

or the following curvilinear form:

$$S_t = S_o + K_{1:1}S_o[L] + K_{1:1}K_{1:2}S_o[L]^2$$

$$y = a + bx + cx^2$$

Thus, a plot of $[S_t]$ versus $[L_t]$ (which can be used in place of $[L]$ if the extent of complexation is low, i.e., $L \approx L_t$), fitted to a quadratic equation, will give a y-intercept equal to the equilibrium solubility of S and coefficients equal to $K_{1:1} \cdot S_o$ in the case of bx, and $K_{1:1} \cdot K_{1:2} \cdot S_o$ in the case of cx^2. Similarly, higher order complexation can be established through nonlinear curve fitting to higher order equations, i.e.,

$$y = a + bx + cx^2 + dx^3$$

$$y = a + bx + cx^2 + dx^3 + ex^4$$

$$y = a + bx + cx^2 + dx^3 + ex^4 + fx^5$$

would represent A_p-type systems involving 1:3, 1:4, and 1:5 complexes, respectively.

Various thermodynamic parameters (i.e., the standard free energy change [$\Delta G°$], the standard enthalpy change [$\Delta H°$], and the standard entropy change [$\Delta S°$]) can also be obtained in a straightforward manner (Loftsson and Brewster 1996; Martin 1993). The free energy of reaction is derived from the equilibrium constant using the relationship:

$$\Delta G = -RT \ln K_{1:1}$$

The enthalpies of reactions can likewise be determined from $K_{1:1}$ obtained at various temperatures using the van't Hoff equation. If two sets of data are available (i.e., two K_c values determined at two different temperatures in degrees K), then

$$\log\left(\frac{K_2}{K_1}\right) = \frac{\Delta H}{2.303R}\left(\frac{T_2 - T_1}{T_1 T_2}\right)$$

On the other hand, if a range of values are available, the ΔH values can be obtained from a plot of ln K versus $1/T$ using the following relationship:

$$\log K = -\frac{\Delta H}{2.303R} \times \frac{1}{T} + \text{constant}$$

where the slope will provide the enthalpy data.

The entropy for the complexation reaction can then be calculated using the expression

$$\Delta G = \Delta H - T\Delta S$$

The complex formation between cyclodextrin and various drugs is generally associated with a relatively large negative $\Delta H°$ and $\Delta S°$, which can either be positive or negative (Rekharsky et al. 1994, 1995). Also, complex formation is largely independent of the chemical properties of the guest (i.e., drug) molecules. The association of binding constants with substrate polarizability suggests that van der Waals forces are important in the complex formation (Saenger 1980). Furthermore, for a series of drugs there tends to be a linear relationship between enthalpy and entropy, with decreasing entropy related to less negative (higher positive) values of enthalpy (Szejtli 1982). This compensation is often correlated with water acting as a driving force in complex formation (Menard et al. 1990). The main driving force for the complex formation could be, therefore, the release of enthalpy-rich water from the cyclodextrin cavity. The water molecules located inside the cavity cannot satisfy their hydrogen bonding potentials and, therefore, they are of higher enthalpy. The energy of the system is lowered when these enthalpy-rich water molecules are replaced by suitable drug molecules that are less polar than water. To date, there is no simple explanation to describe the driving force for complexation. Although release of enthalpy-rich water molecules from the cyclodextrin cavity is probably an important driving force for the drug-cyclodextrin complex formation, other forces may be important (Loftsson and Brewster 1996). These forces include van der Waals interactions, hydrogen bonding, hydrophobic interactions, release of ring strain in the cyclodextrin molecule and changes in solvent-surface tensions.

Use of Cyclodextrins in IM Formulations

Methodologies

The poor aqueous solubility of various drugs intended for IM administration has necessitated the inclusion of organic cosolvents and various surfactants in the formulations. Examples of these solubilizers include propylene glycol, polyethylene glycol, glycerol, dimethylacetamide, and ethanol (in such products as hydralzine, lorazepam, phenytoin, diazepam, etc.) (Yalkowski and Rubino 1985). These organic cosolvents are problematic for several reasons. They are intrinsically irritating to muscle tissue, provoking pain on injection and subsequent muscle damage. In addition, the manner in which these excipients solubilize drugs can exacerbate their side-effect profile. Organic cosolvents generally affect solubility as a log function of their concentration (Martin et al. 1982; Pitha and Hoshino 1992). Thus, administration of an organic cosolvent–containing system into the aqueous environment of the circulation or skeletal muscles rapidly reduces their solubilizing power, often resulting in drug precipitation at the site of injection. Other solubilizing excipients, including electroneutral detergents such as Cremophor or Tween, can also be locally irritating. Additionally, these agents are systemically toxic—being associated with anaphylactoid reactions related to histamine release, hypotension, shock, and, in extreme cases, death (Watkins 1986; Tachon et al. 1983). Replacement of the solubilizing agents with nontoxic alternatives is clearly desirable. Cyclodextrins may help in this context.

As discussed elsewhere in this book, various models have been developed for assessing pain on injection and muscle damage subsequent to IM and other parenteral injections (Comereski et al. 1986; Chellman et al. 1990; Svendsen et al. 1985; Gray 1981). In vivo models for muscle damage include direct histological examination (both gross and microscopic) of muscle groups subsequent to formulation treatments. Of these methods, the system described by Shintani et al. (1967) has been widely applied. This method involves IM injection of 1.0 mL of the test solution into the hind leg of rabbits in the center of the vastus lateralis muscle using a 22-gauge needle at a 30° angle. At various times after drug administration, the animals are sacrificed by pentobarbital overdose, and the skin covering the injection site is removed. The tensor fasciae latae is then resected together with a portion of the rectus femoralis to expose the vastus lateralis. The muscle is removed via severing of the common tendon to the knee and the muscle origin. The muscle is then bisected with a scalpel to expose the injection site. Local tissue irritation is scored on a scale from 0 to 5 (highest irritation). A score of 0 indicates no discernible reaction; 1, slight hyperemia and discoloration; 2, moderate hyperemia and discoloration; 3, distinct discoloration; 4, brown area with some necrosis; and 5, widespread necrosis or abscess and a muscle appearance approximating "cooked meat." A range of 0–0.4 is defined as no irritation; 0.5–1.4, slight irritation; 1.5–2.4, mild irritation; 2.5–3.4, moderate irritation; 3.5–4.4 marked irritation; and > 4.5, severe irritation.

The use of surrogate marker for muscle damage, i.e., creatine kinase (CK—an intracellular sarcoplasmic enzyme) can also be indicative of muscle damage (Steiness et al. 1978). Studies have examined both depletion of muscle stores of the enzyme or release of the protein into the blood. In vitro approaches include assessments of formulations in various cell cultures (MRC-5 fibroblasts [Svendsen et al. 1985] and the L6 rat muscle cell line [Williams et al. 1987]), as well as evaluation of hemolytic potential. Hemolysis has been highly correlated with muscle irritation.

Finally, a recently developed isolated rat muscle model has been described and validated (Brazeau and Fung 1989a, b). The model gives excellent results in line with those determined in vivo using the standard rabbit model. In assessing the action of cyclodextrins and their inclusion complexes on muscle integrity, several of these techniques have been applied, most notably, direct muscle examination, assessment of changes in blood CK, and evaluation of hemolytic potential.

IM Toxicity of Cyclodextrins and Their Derivatives

The myotoxic potential of the cyclodextrins themselves has been examined by injecting 100 mg/mL solutions of various derivatives into the vastus lateralis muscle of rabbits and then histologically scoring the lesions 48 h after administration, as described by Shintani (Uekama et al. 1991; Yoshida et al. 1989). Results are given in Figure 13.4. In these evaluations, the poor aqueous solubility of β-cyclodextrin required that it be administered as a suspension which, no doubt, added to the irritation of this formulation. At the limit of its solubility (18–19 mg/mL), β-cyclodextrin demonstrated only

Figure 13.4. Muscle irritation scores of intramuscular cyclodextrin injections. Compounds were administered at a dose of 100 mg/mL into the vastus lateralis muscle of rabbits and scored, 48 h later, using the method of Shintani et al. (1967).

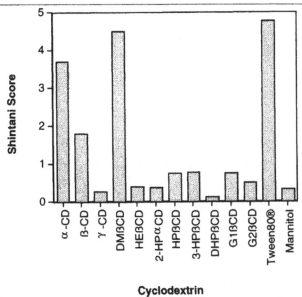

very slight irritation (Yamamoto et al. 1991). Mannitol is given as a control, and the surfactant, Tween 80®, is given for comparison.

As illustrated, several cyclodextrins, including α-cyclodextrin and DMβCD, are corrosive to muscles manifesting an irritation score similar to the nonionic detergent, Tween 80®. (Uekama and Otagiri 1987). The lipophilicity and surface activity of DMβCD cause it to be irritating not only to skeletal muscles but to other biological membranes, including the eye. By contrast, hydrophilic cyclodextrin systems, including HPβCD and the branched cyclodextrins $G_1βCD$ and $G_2βCD$, are similar in their irritation score to the control (mannitol) (Hashimoto 1991; Yamamoto et al. 1990; Uekama et al. 1992). The least myotoxic cyclodextrin appears to be 2,3-dihydroxypropyl-β-cyclodextrin (DHPβCD), but the complexing potential of this material is less than that of HPβCD (Yoshida et al. 1989). In a separate study, daily IM administration of a 10 percent w/v solution of HPβCD to rats over a 2-week time course revealed no substance-related irritation at the injection site (Mesens et al. 1991).

The hemolytic potential of these cyclodextrins is highly correlated with histological damage, with the notable exception of α-cyclodextrin, which is much less destructive to red blood cells than its myotoxicity would indicate (Figure 13.5) (Uekama et al. 1991; Leroy-Lechat et al. 1992). The low

Figure 13.5. Correlation between muscle irritation (as defined by Shin-tani et al. 1967) and hemolytic potential (defined as the reciprocal of the concentration (w/v percent) which induced 50 percent hemolysis).

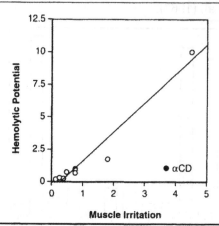

hemolytic potential of SBEβCD would suggest that, like HPβCD, this deriv-ative also manifests little, if any, myotoxicity (Shiotani et al. 1994). This was specifically examined through the use of a CK model (Stella et al. 1994, 1995). Saline, SBEβCD (15.3 percent w/v), or a cosolvent system consisting of polyethylene glycol:ethanol:water (40:10:50), was injected intramuscu-larly into rabbits. Blood was collected prior to and at various times after ve-hicle administration, and CK levels were determined. The area under the normalized CK curve was almost six times higher after organic cosolvent administration, while the SBEβCD gave results comparable to normal saline (Figure 13.6).

These data suggest that several of the hydrophilic chemically modified cyclodextrins may be useful in IM formulations based on their ability to sol-ubilize drugs and their safety when administered intramuscularly. In addi-tion to their intrinsic safety, cyclodextrins are also less likely to produce injection site precipitation of the administered drug. This is a consequence of the nature of the solubilization profiles produced by these starches. Cy-clodextrins, as would be suggested by their phase-solubility profiles, in-crease the solubility of guests as a linear function of their concentration. For A_L-type systems, precipitation should not, theoretically, occur since di-lution of the cyclodextrin results in an equivalent dilution of the drug (Pitha and Hohino 1992; Pitha et al. 1992). In the case of nonlinear isotherms (i.e., A_P-type systems), precipitation is theoretically possible depending on the concentrations examined (i.e., whether the dilution takes place in a linear or nonlinear portion of the phase-solubility diagram).

Figure 13.6. Effect of IM administration of saline, SBEβCD (15.3 percent w/v) or a cosolvent system (polyethylene glycol:ethanol:water [40:10:50]) on creatine kinase (CK) area under the curve (AUC) (*$p < 0.05$).

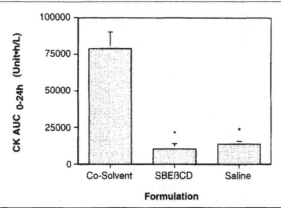

Use of Cyclodextrins to Replace Toxic Excipients in IM Formulations

Given the intrinsic IM safety of various cyclodextrins and other potential advantages, several examples of their use to replace unwanted excipients in IM formulations have been published. Alfaxalone (3α-hydroxy-5α-pregnan-11,20-dione) is a short-acting, injectable steroid anesthetic with an excellent profile of action including a rapid induction, high safety margin, and rapid deinduction with little emergence dysphoria (Morgan and Whitwar 1985; Campbell et al. 1971; Wright and Dundee 1982). The dosage forms intended for human use (Athesin®) and for veterinary use (Saffan®) contain the surfactant Cremophor to solubilize the poorly water-soluble steroid (Campbell et al. 1971). Unfortunately, these formulations are associated with severe side effects in sensitive individuals (e.g., anaphylactoid reaction associated with histamine release [Tachon et al. 1983; Watkins 1986]). These untoward effects were frequent enough to warrant the removal of the human IV product from the market in the mid-1980s. It now appears, however, that the surfactant, not the solubilized steroid, was primarily responsible for the adverse effects (Clarke 1981). In addition, the Cremophor solvent base is known to be locally irritating to skeletal muscles in a manner qualitatively similar to Tween 80® (see Figure 13.4). Thus, cyclodextrins were considered as safer solubilizing agents.

Several chemically modified cyclodextrins, most notably HPβCD, were found to increase the aqueous solubility of alfaxalone (Brewster et al. 1989a). Phase-solubility analysis (Figure 13.7) indicated a linear increase in drug solubility as a function of solubilizer concentration, such that a 50 percent w/v solution of HPβCD would solubilize 77 mg/mL alfaxalone. This

Figure 13.7. Phase-solubility diagram for HPβCD and alfaxalone.

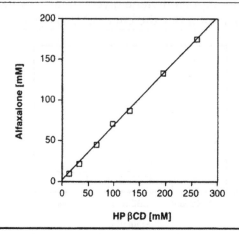

Chemical structure of various drug guests.

Alfaxalone

Prednisolone

Flurbiprofen

Nimodipine

Tiamulin

Chlorpromazine

Prochlorperazine

was almost 10-times greater than the solubility achievable using Cremophor (Brewster et al. 1989a). In rats, the two formulations (i.e., HPβCD and the Cremophor-based vehicle) were equipotent (Estes et al. 1991). In dogs, which are very sensitive to the allergic potential of Cremophor, the HPβCD formulation was significantly safer than the Cremophor-based system (Estes et al. 1991). The latter induced high blood histamine and low blood pressure, and the animals had to be manually ventilated. These positive findings have lead to the evaluation of alfaxalone as an IM agent in dogs (Clarke et al. 1991). Alfaxalone (at a dose of 4 mg/kg in HPβCD) was administered to dogs concurrently with medetomidine and xylazine. Following drug administration, anesthesia was induced within 15 min and lasted for at least 30 min. Dogs were sufficiently affected such that endotracheal intubation could be performed without response, and relaxation appeared to be excellent. The anesthesia lightened within 60 min. No allergic responses occurred, and the quality of anesthesia appeared to be good. No other side effects were noted.

The ability of SBEβCD to replace irritating cosolvents was examined using two formulations for IM prednisolone (Stella et al. 1994, 1995). The formulations included a 10 mg/mL prednisolone preparation solubilizer in either 15 percent w/v SBEβCD or in PEG 400:ethanol:water (40:10:50). As illustrated in Figure 13.8, SBEβCD linearly increases the solubility of prednisolone. Using CK as a marker for muscle damage, the cosolvent preparation was significantly more corrosive than that associated with the SBEβCD system (Table 13.1) (Stella et al. 1995). The two formulations were, however, bioequivalent in terms of drug delivery producing similar area under the curve (AUC), elimination constants, and T_{max} values. The

Figure 13.8. Phase-solubility profile of prednisolone and SBEβCD.

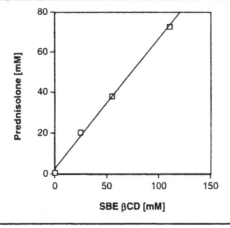

cyclodextrin-based system did significantly increase the C_{max} of prednisolone, consistent with higher initial rates of absorption and the increased water solubility afforded the steroid.

Use of Cyclodextrins to Reduce Intrinsic Drug-Related Toxicity

Pain on injection and muscle damage may also be related to intrinsic properties of the drug molecule, most notably its surface activity. The hemolytic potency of many drugs is correlated with their surface activity and muscle damage potential (Svendsen et al. 1985). On the other hand, alternative mechanisms may also be operating. In the case of the natural cyclodextrins, α- and β-cyclodextrin are thought to express their hemolytic action, at least in part, by their ability to complex fatty acids and cholesterol and extract them from red blood cell membranes (Irie et al. 1982). In any case, the large physiochemical change associated with complexation may well act to mask unwanted drug properties.

IM administration of nonsteroidal anti-inflammatory agents is widely used in pain management (Martens 1994). Such administration can, however, be complicated by the effect of these acidic drugs in the muscular matrix. Flurbiprofen is irritating to muscle and mucous membranes when administered in simple buffer formulations (Masuda et al. 1984). Irritation scores in rabbits are similar to those produced by organic solvents, and the drug is associated with pain on instillation to the eye. A β-cyclodextrin complex of flurbiprofen was found to be less hemolytic than the uncomplexed drug in human, rabbit, and dog blood. In the rabbit model of muscle irritation, the complex was significantly less toxic than flurbiprofen in a phosphate buffer compared to the vehicle alone (Masuda et al. 1984). When applied to rabbit eyes, the nonsteroidal anti-inflammatory agent induced severe discomfort as measured by blinking and other signs and symptoms. The β-cyclodextrin complex significantly reduced these untoward actions. An evaluation of the drug in 10 human volunteers also suggested that the β-cyclodextrin complex was more comfortable than the uncomplexed drug in the eye. While the complex was less irritating, the effectiveness of the flurbiprofen was not diminished, as shown by its ability to inhibit protein production in rabbit eyes induced by paracentesis. Decreased muscle damage for tiamulin was also observed when the drug was administered as a γ-cyclodextrin complex (Sato et al. 1982).

Nimodipine is a calcium channel blocker with selectivity for cerebral rather than peripheral blood vessels (Kazdu et al. 1982; Towart and Perzborn 1981). The utility of the drug is reduced by its poor oral bioavailability, suggesting the preparation of parenteral dosage forms. Unfortunately, IM administration of nimodipine to test animals is associated with significant muscle damage. HPβCD was therefore considered as an excipient in the configuration of an IM formulation for nimodipine (Yoshida et al. 1990).

A complex of nimodipine consisting of a 1:3 molar ratio of drug to HPβCD was administered as a suspension in saline into the vastus lateralis muscle of rabbits, and the pharmacokinetics and muscle irritation were compared to a nimodipine suspension similarly administered. Peak blood levels of nimodipine were more than doubled after complex administration and $AUC_{24\,h}s$ were increased by about 2.5-fold (Table 13.2).

Furthermore, nimodipine was found to produce less irritation (Shintani score: 0.85) than a simple suspension of the drug (Shintani score: 1.88) (Yoshida et al. 1990). Thus, IM administration of the nimodipine complex provided a significantly higher bioavailability for the complexed drug, and the dosage form was significantly less irritating to muscle than was the uncomplexed drug.

The neuroleptic chlorpromazine is widely used as a major tranquilizer, although IM administration has long been known to induce pain on injection and muscle damage (Hodges 1959; Swett 1974). Complexation of chlorpromazine with β-cyclodextrin was accomplished in an attempt to improve IM dosing (Irie et al. 1983a; Irie et al. 1984). IM administration of chlorpromazine (2.2 mg/mL saline), a β-cyclodextrin preparation (2.2 mg chlorpromazine + 16 mg β-cyclodextrin/mL saline), β-cyclodextrin (16 mg/mL saline), or saline (1 mL), to the vastus lateralis muscles of rabbits resulted in similar pharmacokinetic profiles (although the C_{max} values for the complex were higher than those of the unmodified drug, Table 13.3) but dramatically different histological presentation (Irie et al. 1984).

The chlorpromazine-treated muscle showed signs of hemorrhage, damage, and discoloration, giving a Shintani score of 3.5 at 5 days after treatment, and 2.8 at 10 days postinjection. Microscopic evaluation of chlorpromazine-treated muscle indicated loss of cross striations, collapse of the sarcoplasms, and general necrosis (Irie et al. 1983b). Stromal edema was also prominent. In cross-section, the muscle cells demonstrated vacuolization of the sarcoplasms, and atrophic sarcoplasms were observed to detach from the sarcolemmas. The presence of cells indicative of inflammation (polymorphs and phagocytes) were observed infiltrating into the stroma surrounding the lesions. In contrast, all other treatment yielded

Table 13.2. Pharmacokinetic Parameters for Nimodipine When Administered Intramuscularly Either as a Suspension of a HPβCD Complex (*$p < 0.05$)

Parameter	Suspension	HPβCD Complex
C_{max} (ng/mL)	9.13 ± 1.78	23.18 ± 2.94
T_{max} (h)	0.78 ± 0.21	0.35 ± 0.06*
AUC (ng·h/mL)	31.90 ± 8.78	82.55 ± 8.92*

Table 13.3. Physicochemical and Biological Properties (Muscle Irritation and Pharmacokinetic Parameters) of Chlorpromazine (CPZ) and a CPZ·β-Cyclodextrin Complex (β-CD) (*$p < 0.05$)

Property	Saline	βCD	CPZ	CPZ·βCD
Surface Tension (mN/m)	70.9	71.6	48.2	68.7
Muscle Irritation (Shintani score)				
Day 2	0	0.3	3.0	0.5
Day 5	0	0	3.5	0
Day 10	0	0	2.8	0
CPZ AUC (ng·min/mL)	—	—	114 ± 13	127 ± 10
CPZ MRT	—	—	2.8 ± 0.14	2.4 ± 0.15
CPZ C_{max} (min)	—	—	46 ± 7	96 ± 10*

similar results with the chlorpromazine·β-cyclodextrin complex being indistinguishable from normal saline at days 5 and 10 (Shintani score: 0).

Histologically, there were no abnormalities or notable findings. Other studies have also found that β-cyclodextrin significantly reduces the degree of CK depletion from rabbit muscle associated with chlorpromazine injection (Figure 13.9) (Svendsen 1988). These data are in keeping with the protective effects of β-cyclodextrin on the hemolytic potential of chlorpromazine. The ability of β-cyclodextrin to reduce chlorpromazine-induced

Figure 13.9. Effect of various IM formulations containing different molar ratios of chlorpromazine (CPZ) and β-cyclodextrin (β-CD) on creatine kinase (CK) depletion per gram muscle tissue in the rabbit.

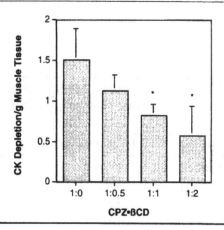

hemolysis as well as muscle damage may well be related to decreased availability of the drug for the target sites (Otagiri et al. 1981; Garay et al. 1994; Uekama et al. 1981; Irie et al. 1983a). This is a consequence of competition of chlorpromazine between the complex (which has a stability constant ($K_{1:1}$) of 12,000 M^{-1}) and the biological membranes (Irie et al. 1983b). In addition, β-cyclodextrin was shown to reduce the surface activity of chlorpromazine solutions (Table 13.3). Similarly, a β-cyclodextrin complex of prochlorperazine decreased the tendency for this neuroleptic to induce contact dermatitis in a guinea pig animal model (Uekama et al. 1982).

CONCLUSIONS AND FUTURE DIRECTIONS

The improvement of dosage forms intended for IM or other parenteral administration routes is possible through the use of cyclodextrins. These nontoxic pharmaceutical complexing agents can significantly increase the water solubility of drugs, allowing their substitution in otherwise irritating formulations. In addition, through microencapsulation of the drug molecule, cyclodextrins can decrease local toxicity by temporarily decreasing tissue availability, as well as mitigating drug effects on surface activity. Depending on the system examined, these effects may or may not affect systemic bioavailability.

In Europe and Japan, oral β-cyclodextrin complexes have already been introduced into the market; in the United States, a monograph for their use has been incorporated into the U.S. Pharmacopeia/National Formulary (USP/NF). In addition, the process of adding β-cyclodextrin to the Food and Drug Administration's (FDA) GRAS (generally recognized as safe) list has been initiated (Szejtli 1996). Chemically modified cyclodextrins, in particular HPβCD, are also receiving attention. A monograph has been prepared for the USP/NF and has already appeared in such compendial sources as the *Handbook of Pharmaceutical Excipients* (Nash 1994). HPβCD has been used as a excipient in IV dosage forms in several clinical trials in which well over 1,000 volunteers and patients have been treated (Estes et al. 1994; Brewster et al. 1996; Mesens et al. 1991).* In addition, HPβCD has entered clinical trials as a component of ocular and buccal formulation where its local irritation potentials has been proven to be very low (Salehian et al. 1995; Stuenkel et al. 1991; Loftsson et al. 1994a, b) Given a suitable formulation candidate, similar progress in the area of IM dosage forms is highly likely. In addition, new and promising derivatives such as SBEβCD are constantly being developed and tested.

---

*The first oral HPβCD product, Sporanox® Oral Solution, was approved in the United States in late 1997.

Acknowledgments

The authors would like to thank Dr. T. Murakami (Hiroshima University) and Dr. T. Irie (Kumamoto University) for their assistance in preparing this chapter.

References

Alper, P. R. 1978. Legitimate indications for intramuscular injections. *Arch. Intern. Med.* 138:1705–1710.

Brazeau, G. A., and H-L. Fung. 1989a. An in vitro model to evaluate muscle damage following intramuscular injections. *Pharm. Res.* 6:167–170.

Brazeau, G. A., and H-L. Fung. 1989b. Use of an in vitro model for the assessment of muscle damage from intramuscular injections: In vitro-in vivo correlations and predictability with mixed solvent systems. *Pharm. Res.* 6:766–771.

Brewster, M. E. 1991. Parenteral safety and applications of 2-hydroxypropyl-β-cyclodextrin. In *New trends in cyclodextrins*, edited by D. Duchene. Paris: Editions de Santé, pp. 313–350.

Brewster, M., and N. Bodor. 1990. Parenteral safety and use of 2-hydroxypropyl-β-cyclodextrin. In *Minutes, fifth international symposium on cyclodextrins*, edited by D. Duchene. Paris: Editions de Santé, pp. 525–534.

Brewster, M., K. Estes, and N. Bodor. 1989a. Development of a non-surfactant formulation for alfaxalone through the use of chemically modified cyclodextrins. *J. Parent. Sci. Technol.* 43:262–265.

Brewster, M. E., J. W. Simpkins, M. S. Hora, W. C. Stern, and N. Bodor. 1989b. The potential use of cyclodextrins in parenteral formulations. *J. Parent. Sci. Technol.* 43:231–240.

Brewster, M., K. Estes, and N. Bodor. 1990. An intravenous toxicity study of 2-hydroxypropyl-β-cyclodextrin, a useful drug solubilizer, in rats and monkeys. *Int. J. Pharm.* 59:231–243.

Brewster, M., J. Howes, W. Griffith, N. Garty, N. Bodor, W. Anderson, and E. Pop. 1996. Intravenous and buccal 2-hydroxypropyl-β-cyclodextrin formulations of E2-CDS—phase I clinical trials. In *Proceedings of the eighth international symposium on cyclodextrins*, edited by J. Szejtli and L. Szente. Dordrecht, The Netherlands: Kluwer Academic Publishers, pp. 0000.

Brewster, M. E., T. Loftsson, S. Amselem, D. Friedman, A. Yogev, W. R. Anderson, D. O. Helton, A. Dinculescu, N. Bodor, and E. Pop. 1995. Formulation development for a zidovudine chemical delivery system. 1. Parenteral dosage forms. *Int. J. Pharm.* 125:17–30.

Campbell, D., A. Forrester, D. Miller, I. Hutton, J. Kennedy, T. Lawrie, A. Lorimer, and D. McCall. 1971. A preliminary clinical study of CT1341, a steroid anesthetic agent. *Brit. J. Anaesth.* 43:14–24.

Chellman, G. J., G. F. Faurot, L. O. Lollini, and T. E. McCullough. 1990. Rat paw-lick/muscle irritation model for evaluating parenteral formulations for pain-on-injection and muscle damage. *Fund. Applied Toxicol.* 15:697–709.

Clarke, K. W., R. N. White, G. C. W. England, and C. E. Bryant. 1991. Alfaxalone/ cyclodextrin anaethesia in the dog. *Abstracts, Fourth international congress of veterinary anaesthesia.* Utrecht, The Netherlands, p. 59.

Clarke, R. 1981. Adverse effects of intravenously administered drugs used in anesthetic practice. *Drugs* 22:26–41.

Comereski, C. R., P. D. Williams, C. L. Bregman, and G. H. Hottendorf. 1986. Pain in injection and muscle irritation: A comparison of animal models for assessing parenteral antibiotics. *Fund. Applied Toxicol.* 6:335–338.

Coussement, W., H. Van Cauteren, J. Vandenberghe, P. Vanparys, G. Teuns, A. Lampo, and R. Marsboom. 1990. Toxicological profile of hydroxypropyl-β-cyclodextrin (HPβCD) in laboratory animals. In *Minutes, fifth international symposium on cyclodextrins,* edited by D. Duchene. Paris: Editions de Santé, pp. 522–524.

Duchene, D., ed. 1987. *Cyclodextrins and their industrial uses.* Paris: Editions de Santé.

Duchene, D. 1988. New trends in pharmaceutical applications of cyclodextrin inclusion complexes. In *Advances in inclusion science: Proceedings of the fourth international symposium on cyclodextrins,* edited by O. Huber and J. Szejtli. Dordrecht, The Netherlands: Kluwer Academic Publishers, pp. 389–398.

Estes, K., M. Brewster, and N. Bodor. 1994. Evaluation of an estradiol chemical delivery system (CDS) designed to provide enhanced and sustained hormone levels in the brain. *Adv. Drug Deliv. Rev.* 14:167–175.

Estes, K., M. Brewster, A. Webb, and N. Bodor. 1991. A non-surfactant formulation for alfaxalone based on an amorphous cyclodextrin: Activity studies in rats and dogs. *Int. J. Pharm.* 65:101–107.

Frank, D., J. Gray, and R. Weaver. 1976. Cyclodextrin nephrosis in the rat. *Am. J. Pathol.* 83:367–382.

Fromming, K-H., and J. Szejtli. 1994. *Cyclodextrins in pharmacy.* Dorcdrecht, The Netherlands: Kluwer Academic Publishers.

Garay, R. P., J. C. Feray, K. Fanous, C. Nazaret, M. J. Villegas, and J. F. Letavernier. 1994. A new approach for the in vitro evaluation of cyclodextrin effects on cellular membranes of human cells. In *Proceedings, seventh international cyclodextrin symposium.* Tokyo: Business Center for Academic Societies, pp. 373–376.

Gray, J. E. 1981. Appraisal of the intramuscular irritation test in the rabbit. *Fund. Applied Toxicol.* 1:290–292.

Greenblatt, D. J., and M. D. Allen. 1978. Intramuscular injection-site complications. *JAMA* 240:542–544.

Hashimoto, H. 1991. Preparation, structure, property and application of branched cyclodextrins, In *New trends in cyclodextrins,* edited by D. Duchene. Paris: Editions de Santé, pp. 99–156.

Hiasa, Y., M. Ohshima, Y. Kitahori, T. Yuasa, T. Fujita, C. Iwata, A. Miyashiro, and M. Konishi. 1981. Histochemical studies of β-cyclodextrin nephrosis in rats. *J. Nara Med. Assoc.* 31:316–326.

Higuchi, T., and K. Connors. 1965. Phase-solubility techniques. *Adv. Anal. Chem. Instrum.* 4:117–212.

Hirayama, F., and K. Uekama. 1987. Methods of investigating and preparing inclusion compounds. In *Cyclodextrins and their industrial uses,* edited by D. Duchene. Paris: Editions de Santé, pp. 131–172.

Hodges, R. J. 1959. Gangrene of the forearm after intramuscular chlorpromazine. *Brit. Med. J.* 2:918–919.

Irie, T., and K. Uekama. 1997. Pharmaceutical applications of cyclodextrins. III. Toxicological issues and safety evaluation. *J. Pharm. Sci.* 86:147–162.

Irie, T., M. Otagiri, M. Sunada, K. Uekama, Y. Ohtani, Y. Yamada, and Y. Sugiyama. 1982. Cyclodextrin-induced hemolysis and shape changes of human erythrocytes in vitro. *J. Pharm. Dyn.* 5:741–744.

Irie, T., M. Sunada, M. Otagiri, and K. Uekama. 1983a. Protective mechanism of β-cyclodextrin for the hemolysis induced with phenothiazine neuroleptics in vitro. *J. Pharm. Dyn.* 6:408–414.

Irie, T., S. Kuwahara, M. Otagiri, K. Uekama, and T. Iwamasa. 1983b. Reduction in the local tissue toxicity of chlorpromazine by β-cyclodextrin complexation. *J. Pharm. Dyn.* 6:790–792.

Irie, T., M. Otagiri, K. Uekama, Y. Okano, and T. Miyata. 1984. Alleviation of the chlorpromazine-induced muscular tissue damage by β-cyclodextrin complexation. *J. Incl. Phenom.* 2:637–644.

Irie, T., K. Fukunaga, A. Yoshida, K. Uekama, H. Fales, and J. Pitha. 1988. Amorphous water-soluble cyclodextrin derivatives. *Pharm. Res.* 5:713–717.

Kazda, S., B. Garthoff, H. P. Krause, and K. Schlossman. 1982. Cerebrovascular effects of the calcium antagonist dihydropyridine derivative nimodipine in animal experiments. *Arzneim.-Forsch.* 32:331–338.

Koizumi, K., Y. Okada, Y. Kubota, and T. Utamura. 1987. Inclusion complexes of poorly water soluble drugs with glucosyl-cyclodextrins. *Chem. Pharm. Bull.* 35:3413–3418.

Leroy-Lechat, F., M. Skiba, D. Wouessidjewe, and D. Duchene. 1992. Cytotoxicity of cyclodextrin and derivatives. In *Minutes, sixth international symposium on cyclodextrins,* edited by A. Hedges. Paris: Editions de Santé, pp. 292–297.

Loftsson, T. 1995. Effects of cyclodextrins on the chemical stability of drugs in aqueous solutions. *Drug Stability* 1:22–33.

Loftsson, T., and M. E. Brewster. 1996. Pharmaceutical applications of cyclodextrins. 1. Drug solubilization and stabilization. *J. Pharm. Sci.* 85:1017–1025.

Loftsson, T., E. Stefansson, H. Fridriksdottir, S. Thorisdottir, J. K. Kristinsson, and G. Gudmundsdottir. 1994a. Topical acetazolamide-HPβCD eye drop solution. In *Proceedings, seventh international cyclodextrin symposium.* Tokyo: Business Center for Academic Societies, pp. 447–450.

Loftsson, T., E. Stefansson, S. Thorisdottir, H. Fridriksdottir, and J. K. Kristinsson. 1994b. Dexamethasone-HPβCD-polymer co-complex in eye drops. In *Proceedings, seventh international cyclodextrin symposium.* Tokyo: Business Center for Academic Societies, pp. 451–454.

Martens, M. 1994. Oral beta-cyclodextrin-piroxicam versus intramuscular piroxicam for postoperative pain after orthopedic surgery. *Curr. Therap. Res.* 55:396–400.

Martin, A. 1993. *Physical pharmacy*, 4th ed. Philadelphia: Lea and Febiger.

Martin, A., P. Wu, A. Adjei, R. Lindstom, and P. Elworthy. 1982. Extended hilde-brand solubility approaches and the log linear solubility equation. *J. Pharm. Sci.* 71:849–856.

Masuda, K., A. Ito, T. Ikari, A. Terashima, and T. Matsuyama. 1984. Protective effects of cyclodextrin for the local irritation induced by aqueous preparations of flur-biprofen. *Yakugaku Zasshi* 104:1075–1082.

Menard, F. A., M. G. Dedhiya, and C. T. Rhodes. 1990. Physico-chemical aspects of the complexation of some drugs with cyclodextrins. *Drug Dev. Ind. Pharm.* 16:91–113.

Mesens, J. L., P. Putterman, and P. Verheyen. 1991. Pharmaceutical applications of 2-hydroxypropyl-β-cyclodextrin: Preclinical and current clinical development. In *New trends in cyclodextrins*, edited by D. Duchene. Paris: Editions de Santé, pp. 369–407.

Morgan, M., and J. Whitwar. 1985. Althesin. *Anaesthesia* 41:121–123.

Muller, B., and U. Brauns. 1985. Solubilization of drugs by modified β-cyclodextrins. *Int. J. Pharm.* 26:77–88.

Nash, R. A. 1994. Cyclodextrins. In *Handbook of pharmaceutical excipients*, edited by A. Wade and P. J. Weller. Washington, D.C.: American Pharmaceutical As-sociation, and London: Pharmaceutical Press, pp. 145–148.

Otagiri, M., K. Uekama, T. Irie, M. Sunada, T. Miyata, and Y. Kase. 1981. Effects of cyclodextrins on the hemolysis induced with phenothiazine neuroleptics. In *Ad-vances in inclusion science: Proceedings of the first international symposium on cyclodextrins*, edited by J. Szejtli. Budapest: Akademiai Kiado, pp. 389–398.

Pagington, J. 1987. β-cyclodextrin, the success of molecular inclusion. *Chem. Brit.*, pp. 455–458.

Perrin, J., P. Field, D. Hansen, R. Mufson, and G. Torosian. 1978. β-cyclodextrin as an aid to peritoneal dialysis: Renal toxicity of β-cyclodextrin in the rat. *Res. Commun. Chem. Pathol. Pharmacol.* 19:373–376.

Pitha, J., and T. Hoshino. 1992. Effect of ethanol on formation of inclusion com-plexes of hydroxypropylcyclodextrins with testosterone and methyl orange. *Int. J. Pharm.* 80:243–251.

Pitha, J., and J. Pitha. 1985. Amorphous water-soluble derivatives of cyclodextrins, non-toxic dissociation enhancing excipients. *J. Pharm. Sci.* 74:987–990.

Pitha, J., M. Harman, and M. Michel. 1986a. Hydrophilic cyclodextrin derivatives enable effective oral administration of steroid hormones. *J. Pharm. Sci.* 75:165–167.

Pitha, J., J. Milecki, H. Fales, L. Pannell, and K. Uekama. 1986b. Hydroxypropyl-β-cyclodextrin, preparation and characterization: Effects on solubility of drugs. *Int. J. Pharm.* 29:73–82.

Pitha, J., T. Irie, P. Sklar, and J. Nye. 1988. Drug solubilizers to aid pharmacologists: Amorphous cyclodextrin derivatives. *Life Sci.* 43:493–502.

Pitha, J., Y. Hoshino, J. Torres-Labandeira, and T. Irie. 1992. Preparation of drug:hy-droxypropylcyclodextrin complexes using ethanol or ammonia as co-solubiliz-ers. *Int. J. Pharm.* 80:253–258.

Rajewski, R. A., and V. J. Stella. 1996. Pharmaceutical applications of cyclodextrins. 2. In vivo drug delivery. *J. Pharm. Sci.* 85:1142–1169.

Rajewski, R., G. Traiger, J. Bresnahan, P. Jaberaboansari, V. J. Stella, and D. O. Thompson. 1995. Preliminary safety evaluation of parenterally administered sulfoalkyl ether β-cyclodextrin derivatives. *J. Pharm. Sci.* 84:927–932.

Rao, C., H. Fales, and J. Pitha. 1990. Pharmaceutical usefulness of hydroxypropyl cyclodextrins, "E Pluribus Unum" is an essential feature. *Pharm. Res.* 7:612–615.

Rekharsky, M. V., F. P. Schwarz, Y. B. Tewari, and R. N. Goldberg. 1994. A thermo-dynamic study of the reactions of cyclodextrins with primary and secondary aliphatic alcohols, with D- and L-phenylalanine, and with L-phenylala-nineamide. *J. Phys. Chem.* 98:10282–10288.

Rekharsky, M. V., R. N. Goldberg, F. P. Schwarz, Y. B. Tewari, P. D. Ross, Y. Ya-mashoji, and Y. Inoue. 1995. Thermodynamic and nuclear magnetic resonance study of the interactions of α- and β-cyclodextrin with model substances: Phenethylamine, ephedrines and related substances. *J. Am. Chem. Soc.* 117:8830–8840.

Saenger, W. 1980. Cyclodextrin inclusion compounds in research and industry. *Angew. Chem., Int. Ed. Engl.* 19:344–362.

Salehian, B., C. Wang, G. Alexander, T. Davidson, V. McDonald, N. Berman, R. E. Dudley, F. Ziel, and R. S. Swerdloff. 1995. Pharmacokinetics, bioefficacy, and safety of a sublingual testosterone cyclodextrin in hypogonadal men: Compar-ison to testosterone enanthate—a clinical research center study. *J. Clin. En-docrinol. Metab.* 80:3576–3575.

Sato, Y., H. Matsumaru, T. Irie, M. Otagiri, and K. Uekama. 1982. Improvement of local irritation induced with intramuscular injection of tiamulin by cyclodextrin complexation. *Yakugaku Zasshi* 102:874–880.

Shintani, S., M. Yamazaki, M. Nakamura, and I. Nakayama. 1967. A new method to determine the irritation of drugs after intramuscular injection in rabbits. *Toxi-col. Applied Pharmacol.* 11:293–301.

Shiotani, K., K. Uehata, K. Ninomiya, T. Irie, K. Uekama, D. O. Thompson, and V. J. Stella. 1994. Different mode of interaction of chlorpromazine with sulfated and sulfoalkylated cyclodextrins and effects on erythrocyte membranes. In *Pro-ceedings, seventh international cyclodextrin symposium.* Tokyo: Business Center for Academic Societies, pp. 492–495.

Steiness, E., F. Rasmussen, O. Svendsen, and P. Nielsen. 1978. A comparative study of serum creatine phosphokinase (CPK) activity in rabbits, pigs and humans af-ter intramuscular injection of local damaging drugs. *Acta Pharmacol. et Toxicol.* 42:357–364.

Stella, V. J., H. Y. Lee, and D. O. Thompson. 1994. The effect of a parenterally safe, anionic β-cyclodextrin derivative, SBE4-β-CD, on I.M. tissue damage and pred-nisolone pharmacokinetics in rabbits. In *Proceedings, seventh international cy-clodextrin symposium.* Tokyo: Business Center for Academic Societies, pp. 369–372.

Stella, V. J., H. K. Lee, and D. O. Thompson. 1995. The effect of SBE4-β-CD on I.M. prednisolone pharmacokinetics and tissue damage in rabbits: Comparison to a co-solvent solution and a water-soluble prodrug. *Int. J. Pharm.* 120:197–204.

Stuenkel, C. A., R. E. Dudley, and S. S. C. Yen. 1991. Sublingual administration of testosterone-hydroxypropyl-β-cyclodextrin inclusion complex stimulates episodic androgen release in hypogonadal men. *J. Clin. Endocrinol. Metab.* 72:1054–1059.

Svendsen, O. 1988. β-cyclodextrin and local muscle toxicity of intramuscular drug formulations. *Arch. Toxicol. (Suppl.)* 12:391–393.

Svendsen, O., F. Højelse, and R. E. Bagdon. 1985. Test for local toxicity of intramuscular drug preparations: Comparison of in vivo and in vitro methods. *Acta Pharmacol. et Toxicol.* 56:183–190.

Swett, C. 1974. Adverse reactions to chlorpromazine in psychiatric patients. *Dis. Nerv. Syst.* 35:509–511.

Szejtli, J. 1982. *Cyclodextrins and their inclusion complexes.* Budapest: Akademiai Kiado.

Szejtli, J. 1994. Medical applications of cyclodextrins. *Med. Res. Rev.* 14:353–386.

Szejtli, J. 1996. Good news from the FDA, cyclodextrin news 10:1 (see *Fed. Reg.* Vol. 61; No. 164, Sept. 20, 1996, Docket No. 96G-0324).

Tachon, P., J. Descotes, A. Laschi-Loqueric, J. Guillot, and J. Evreux. 1983. Assessment of the allergenic potential of althesin and its constituents. *Brit. J. Anaesth.* 55:715–717.

Tait, R. J., D. J. Skanchy, D. O. Thompson, N. C. Chetwyn, D. A. Dunshee, R. A. Rajewski, V. J. Stella, and J. F. Stobaugh. 1992. Characterization of sulphoalkyl ether derivatives of β-cyclodextrin by capillary electrophoresis with indirect UV detection. *J. Pharm. Biomed. Anal.* 10:615–622.

Towart, R., and E. Perzborn. 1981. Nimodipine inhibits carbocyclic thromboxane-induced contractions of cerebral arteries. *Eur. J. Pharmcol.* 69:213–215.

Uekama, K. 1981. Pharmaceutical application of cyclodextrin complexation. *Yakugaku Zasshi* 101:857–873.

Uekama, K., and M. Otagiri. 1987. Cyclodextrins as drug carrier system. *CRC Crit. Rev. Therap. Drug Carrier Systems* 3:1–40.

Uekama, K., F. Hirayama, and T. Irie. 1991. Modification of drug release by cyclodextrin derivatives. In *New trends in cyclodextrins*, edited by D. Duchene. Paris: Editions de Santé, pp. 411–446.

Uekama, K., M. Yamamoto, T. Irie, and F. Hirayama. 1992. Pharmaceutical evaluation of branched β-cyclodextrins as drug carriers in parenteral formulation. In *Minutes, sixth international symposium on cyclodextrins*, edited by A. Hedges. Paris: Editions de Santé, pp. 491–496.

Uekama, K., T. Irie, M. Sunada, M. Otagiri, Y. Arimatsu, and S. Nomura. 1982. Alleviation of prochlorperazine-induced primary irritation of skin by cyclodextrin complexation. *Chem. Pharm. Bull.* 30:3860–3862.

Uekama, K., T. Irie, M. Sunada, M. Otagiri, K. Iwasaki, Y. Okano, T. Miyata, and Y. Kase. 1981. Effects of cyclodextrin on chlorpromazine-induced haemolysis and central nervous system responses. *J. Pharm. Pharmacol.* 33:707–710.

Vikmon, M., A. Stadler-Szoke, and J. Szejtli. 1985. Solubilization of amphotericin B with g-cyclodextrin. *J. Antibiot.* 38:1822–1824.

Watkins, J. 1986. The allergic reaction to intravenous induction agents. *Brit. J. Hosp. Med.* 36:45–48.

Williams, P. D., B. G. Masters, L. D. Evans, D. A. Laska, and G. H. Hottendorf. 1987. An in vitro model for assessing muscle irritation due to parenteral antibiotics. *Fund. Applied Toxicol.* 9:10–17.

Wright, P., and J. Dundee. 1982. Forum: Attitudes to intravenous anesthesia. *Anaesthesia* 37:1209–1213.

Yalkowsky, S. H., and J. T. Rubino. 1985. Solubilization by cosolvents I: Organic solutes in propylene glycol–water mixtures. *J. Pharm. Sci.* 74:416–421.

Yamamoto, M., M. Yoshida, F. Hirayama, and K. Uekama. 1989. Some physicochemical properties of branched-β-cyclodextrins and their inclusion characteristics. *Int. J. Pharm.* 49:163–171.

Yamamoto, M., H. Aritomi, T. Irie, F. Hirayama, and K. Uekama. 1990. Pharmaceutical evaluation of branched β-cyclodextrins as parenteral drug carriers. In *Minutes, fifth international symposium on cyclodextrins,* edited by D. Duchene. Paris: Editions de Santé, pp. 541–544.

Yamamoto, M., H. Aritomi, T. Irie, K. Hirayama, and K. Uekama. 1991. Biopharmaceutical evalution of maltosyl-β-cyclodextin as a parenteral drug carrier. *S. T. P. Pharma Sci.* 1:397–402.

Yoshida, A., H. Arima, K. Uekama, and J. Pitha. 1988. Pharmaceutical evaluation of hydroxyalkyl ethers of β-cyclodextrin. *Int. J. Pharm.* 46:217–222.

Yoshida, A., M. Yamamoto, T. Irie, F. Hirayama, and K. Uekama. 1989. Some pharmaceutical properties of 3-hydroxypropyl- and 2,3-dihydroxypropyl-β-cyclodextrin and their solubilizing and stabilizing abilities. *Chem. Pharm. Bull.* 37:1059–1063.

Yoshida, A., M. Yamamoto, T. Itoh, T. Irie, F. Hirayama, and K. Uekama. 1990. Utility of 2-hydroxypropyl-β-cyclodextrin in an intramuscular injectable preparation of nimodipine. *Chem. Pharm. Bull.* 38:176–179.

14

Liposomal Formulations to Reduce Irritation of Intramuscularly and Subcutaneously Administered Drugs

Farida Kadir
Christien Oussoren
Daan J. A. Crommelin

Dept. of Pharmaceutics, Utrecht Institute for Pharmaceutical Sciences
Utrecht University
Utrecht, The Netherlands

Intramuscular (IM) and subcutaneous (SC) injections are well established and frequently used routes of drug administration. These injections cause disruption of the tissue. This almost unavoidably causes adverse reactions such as pain and discomfort which may be aggravated by the injected material. Several constituents of the injected product, including the drug, can be held responsible for the additional pain (Avis and Morris 1984; Kadir et al. 1992; Rasmussen 1978).

Local irritation, pain and muscle damage following injection may be assessed by several methods, including macroscopical examination, histological examination, and biochemical assays. These items are addressed extensively in Chapters 4 through 10.

If present, tissue damage can be treated in a number of ways, such as excision of necrotized tissue allowing proper healing to occur, application of local cooling or the use of antidotic agents (e.g., co-administration of local corticosteroids, anesthetics, antioxidants, antihistaminic agents, nonsteroidal anti-inflammatory drugs (NSAIDs) or hyaluronidase (Forssen and Tökes 1983; Geervliet et al. 1989; Reilly et al. 1980). In some cases, it is recommended to regularly change the site of injection, but this is not always possible or convenient.

The use of delivery systems to minimise tissue damage is an interesting alternative approach. In this chapter, the main focus will be on liposomes utilised to avoid local adverse drug effects.

LIPOSOMES: A SHORT INTRODUCTION

Liposomes have been studied for about three decades. The number of publications on liposomes demonstrates their importance as drug delivery systems. Pharmaceutical aspects of liposomes, including their behaviour in-vivo, and technological aspects have been reviewed extensively. The reader is referred to the many literature reviews available. In the following introduction, the liposome as a drug carrier system is briefly discussed with emphasis on the characteristics that are relevant to the reviewed issue.

Liposomes are vesicular structures composed of at least one bilayer surrounding water-filled compartments (Figure 14.1). They are highly versatile in terms of their physicochemical properties. The backbone of the bilayer consists of phospholipids of which phosphatidylcholine (PC), a neutral lipid, is most commonly used. Phosphatidylcholines are the major constituents of regular liposomes designed as drug delivery systems and they are essential constituents of cell membranes as well. They are biodegradable and have a relatively low toxicity.

Figure 14.1. (a) Morphology of different liposome structures: SUV—small unilamellar vesicle; LUV—large unilamellar vesicle; MLV—multilamellar vesicle; MVV multivesicular vesicle. (b) The gel to liquid-crystalline phase transition; T_c: transition temperature.

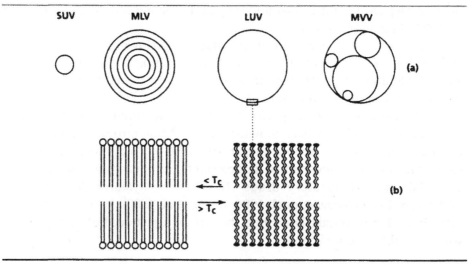

Charged phospholipids, e.g., phosphatidylglycerol (PG) or phosphatidylserine (PS), may be included into the phospholipid bilayer. The presence of these charge-inducing agents in the bilayer tends to improve the physical stability of the liposomes as a result of electrostatic repulsion.

Bilayer rigidity strongly depends on the bilayer components. In general, acyl chains in phosphatidylcholine bilayers make gel-like structures at temperatures below the phospholipid transition temperature (T_c). The transition temperature of a lipid is the temperature at which the fluidity of the lipid changes: at temperatures above T_c the mobility of the fatty acyl chains is increased compared to the gel state bilayers. As a result the fluidity of the membrane also increases and a lower rigidity of the bilayer is found. These liposomes are called fluid state liposomes. At temperatures below T_c, these gel state bilayers tend to be less permeable than fluid state bilayers. A bilayer with low rigidity may be "rigidified" by inclusion of cholesterol. At constant temperature addition of cholesterol reduces the mobility of the acyl chains in the liquid state resulting in a decreased fluidity and bilayer permeability. It has been shown that incorporation of cholesterol and cholesterol derivatives alters the in-vivo stability of the vesicle as well. If specific targeting is desired, other agents such as anchor molecules to connect homing devices can be included in the bilayer structure (Heeremans et al. 1992; Nässander et al. 1995; Vingerhoeds et al. 1994).

Traditionally, drugs can be incorporated into liposomal carriers in different ways. Water soluble drugs can be entrapped in the internal aqueous compartment(s) of the liposomes. Lipophilic and amphiphatic drugs can intercalate into or adsorb to the liposome membranes.

Liposomes are prepared by shaking dried films of phospholipids, or a mixture of phospholipids and other lipid soluble compounds, with aqueous solutions above their transition temperature. The liposomes prepared by these methods are multilamellar and heterogeneous with respect to size. By ultrasonication of such liposome dispersions, most of the multilamellar vesicles (MLVs) (with a size range up to a few micrometers), can be transformed into small unilamellar vesicles (SUVs) with a lower size range (tens of nanometers) (Crommelin and Schreier 1994; Barenholz and Crommelin 1994; Talsma 1991). Over the years, alternative preparation techniques for drug loaded liposomes were developed, including techniques to control their size, maximise drug loading capacity and ensure a long shelf life. A large number of publications and reviews on liposome chemistry and formulation strategies have been published (Gregoriadis 1992; Gregoriadis 1988; Jackson 1981; Nässander et al. 1995; Ostro and Cullis 1989; Ostro 1987; Szoka and Papahadjopoulos 1978; van Winden et al. 1997; Zierenberg et al. 1979). For further details about liposome formulation, the reader is referred to these references.

Liposomes have been studied as drug delivery systems. The therapeutic objectives for the use of liposomes can be summarised as follows. Upon parenteral administration, liposomes can act as a reservoir of the drug, inducing a sustained or delayed release effect. Alternatively, liposomes can be used for site-specific delivery of drugs through passive (mainly macrophages in liver and spleen) or active (homing device attached) targeting strategies (Nässander et al. 1990; Vingerhoeds et al. 1994).

The objective of this chapter is to review the potential use of liposomes to reduce irritation of drugs upon SC or IM injection. To do so properly, it is necessary to discuss first the fate of liposomes and liposome-associated drugs upon IM or SC injection. These sections will be followed by a critical review of actual studies on the topic of reduction of local irritation. A discussion section on the value of liposomes as protective agents concludes this chapter.

Liposomes as Intramuscular and Subcutaneous Drug Delivery Systems

Many drugs are routinely administered intramuscularly and subcutaneously. After IM or subcutaneous injection, therapeutically effective drug levels can be reached fairly rapidly if the drugs are administered in an aqueous solution. In cases of drugs that are rapidly eliminated, blood drug levels may decline quickly and the therapeutic response may be of short duration. For a number of drugs it is desirable to maintain the concentration of the drug in blood within the therapeutic range for a long time and to avoid toxic levels. In these cases, the use of drug delivery systems that provide slow release patterns of the drug over an extended period of time might be useful. Liposomes are among the many candidate formulations for depot systems (e.g., nanoparticles or microspheres, such as polylactid acids, polyglycolic acids, polyacrylamides, polyalkyl(cyano)acrylates, oil solutions, oil suspensions and emulsions). Liposomal encapsulation may avoid high, toxic peak levels in the blood and may limit dosing frequencies. The potential usefulness of liposomes as prolonged release carriers of therapeutic agents has been discussed extensively (Crommelin and Schreier 1994; Gregoriadis 1988; Kadir et al. 1992; Kadir et al. 1993; Ostro and Cullis 1989; Schäfer et al. 1987; Titulaer et al. 1990; Zierenberg and Betzing 1979).

Apart from a prolonged release capacity, another interesting potential application for local administration of liposomes involves targeting to regional lymph nodes for diagnostic and therapeutic purposes. When administered locally, liposomes may leave the injection site and enter draining lymphatic capillaries. Once in the lymphatic capillaries, liposomes will be transported to the blood circulation. On their way to the general circulation, a small fraction of the lymphatically absorbed liposomes may be retained in regional lymph nodes. Recent work in rats (Oussoren et al. 1997) shows that only small (smaller than about 100 nm) liposomes will be taken up by lymphatic capillaries after local injection. Larger liposomes will remain at the injection site.

The mechanism of drug release from liposomes after local administration has not yet been completely clarified. Several mechanisms have been suggested (Kadir et al. 1993; Oshawa et al. 1985; Schäfer et al. 1987; Zierenberg and Betzing 1979). Based on their findings, Ohsawa et al. (1985) presented a schematic illustration of drug absorption following IM injection of liposome encapsulated drugs. Similar mechanisms might hold for the subcutaneous administration route. Free drug and liposome-associated drug may reach the blood compartment either via absorption through the capillary wall of blood vessels or via lymphatic absorption. Liposomes remaining at the site of injection might gradually erode and eventually completely disintegrate (e.g., as a result of attack by enzymes or destruction by neutrophils). During this process the entrapped drug is released. Also, a considerable fraction of the drug can diffuse through the intact liposomal bilayer and move directly to the blood capillaries. A schematic representation is shown in Figure 14.2.

STUDIES ON REDUCTION OF LOCAL IRRITATION

As discussed before, IM and SC administration of liposomal formulations of drugs may be favourable compared to free drug adminstration as they release the incorporated drug gradually and may provide sustained release kinetics. Additionally, liposomes may act as drug carrier systems to

Figure 14.2. Schematic representation of the drug transfer following intramuscular or subcutaneous injection of liposomes. A: transfer of free drug; B: transfer of small liposomes; C: transfer of larger liposomes; D: erosion of liposomes (adapted from Ohsawa et al. 1985).

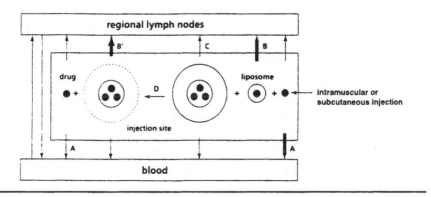

regional lymph nodes after IM and SC administration. A different advantageous effect of the use of liposomes is their tissue protective effect if irritating drugs are being injected (Al-Suwayeh et al. 1996; Axelsson 1989; Balazsovits 1989; Dorr et al. 1980; Forssen and Tökes 1983; Kadir et al. 1992; Litterst 1982; Storm et al. 1992). Upon IM or SC injection, liposomes may protect the muscular and subcutaneous tissue from direct exposition to the drug. To avoid local irritation these drugs are often injected intravenously. However, a serious problem associated with the intravenous (IV) delivery of these irritating drugs concerns accidental extravasation at the site of infusion. Extravasation then results in severe local tissue damage and necrosis of surrounding tissue.

Only a limited number of studies have focused on IM and SC administration of liposomal drugs and even fewer have focused on the protective effects of liposomal formulations. We will now summarise and discuss studies on the protective properties of liposomal encapsulation of irritating drugs. Two administration routes, the IM and the SC, will be discussed separately. The studies will be discussed in chronological order.

Studies on the Protective Effect After Intramuscular Administration

Novaminsulfone (NS) injected intramuscularly in "free" form is a strongly irritating drug, causing haemorrhage, cell necrosis, inflammatory reactions and eventually fibrosis. The ability of liposome encapsulation to diminish the irritating effects of intramuscularly applied NS (as a model) drug was studied by macroscopic (swelling, redness) and histopathological analysis over a period of 14 days in mice (Kadir et al. 1992). Although in the literature mention is made of the protective effect of liposome encapsulation this study, was—to our knowledge—the first published attempt to histologically analyze the irritating effects of intramuscularly injected liposomal formulations. Parameters for histological evaluation included cell necrosis, haemorrhage, fibrosis, infiltration by granulocytes and infiltration by macrophages upon a Masson-Trichrome (Goldner) staining. Liposomes were prepared according to the reverse evaporation method (Szoka and Papahadjopoulos). A detailed description of the preparation, characterisation and stability of this type of "gel state" liposomes is given by Peeters et al. (1989). In case of the preparation of empty liposomes, the internal aqueous phase of the liposomes, consisted of sterile saline without drug. Free NS was prepared from a commercially available injection solution of NS (500 mg/mL) by dilution with sterile, pyrogen-free, isotonic saline.

The liposomal NS (lip-NS) preparations contained 3.4 percent of free (i.e., not encapsulated) NS. The fraction of non-encapsulated NS increased from 3.4 percent to a maximum of 5 percent during incubation (2 weeks) at 37°C in saline or in normal mouse serum. In the same study, as a part of a larger study on the sustained release properties of liposomal chloroquine (antimalarial agent), this liposomal formulation was evaluated as well. Chloroquine liposomes (lip-CQ) were prepared according to the same procedure. The free CQ solution was prepared from a commercially available injection solution. The final concentration of CQ in this solution corresponded to the fraction of non-encapsulated CQ in the liposomal formulation. Some characteristics of the formulations tested in this study are summarised in Table 14.1.

The IM injection as such causes disruption of the tissue by "mechanical" damage. Occasionally, a small haemorrhage without any additional reaction and enlargement of the interstitial space between the muscle cells was observed independent of the substance injected. Injections of saline had no detectable irritating effect, which confirms previous observations (Svendsen et al. 1979). As expected (Axelsson [1984] and Surber and Sucker [1987]), intramuscularly injected free NS had a strongly irritating effect causing severe tissue damage, whereas the same dose of NS entrapped in liposomes did not. Macrophage accumulation caused by lip-NS was comparable to that observed after treatment with empty liposomes. No relationship between in-vivo and in-vitro release characteristics of intramuscularly injected liposome preparations could be established until today. But, if it is assumed that the in-vitro observed slow release pattern in serum or saline is indicative of the in-vivo situation, the absence of a peak concentration of the liposome encapsulated drug upon injection at the injection site may be held responsible for the observed local reactions.

Upon injection of liposome-encapsulated CQ, a small number of polymorphs was observed. The solution of free CQ with a CQ concentration

Table 14.1. Characteristics of the Formulations Tested

Formulation	Conc. Drug mg/mL	Lipid Content (μmol/mL*)	Particle Size[†] (μm)
saline	—	—	—
empty liposomes	—	231	0.29 ± 0.01
aqueous solution of NS	100	—	—
NS liposomes	105	260	0.29 ± 0.01
aqueous solution of CQ	0.87[‡]	—	—
CQ liposomes	28.3[‡]	239	0.30 ± 0.01

*μmol phospholipid per mL liposome dispersion

[†]mean ± s.d.

NS: novaminsulfone

[‡]calculated as CQ base

corresponding to the concentration of non-encapsulated CQ in the liposome dispersion, showed a comparable histological pattern. In summary, liposomes of the "gel-state" type described in this study were well tolerated in IM depots and may form protective drug carrier systems. A fraction (still to be quantified) of the liposomes is probably phagocytosed by macrophages infiltrating the injection site. This process might contribute to the in-vivo drug release process from liposomes that thus deviates with respect to rate and extent from in-vitro release pattern of the encapsulated drug.

More recently, Al-Suwayeh et al. (1996) obtained similar results with regard to myotoxicity of IM liposomal formulations. The objective of the study was to study in-vitro myotoxicity of empty liposomes, and to examine whether liposome size, charge and fluidity affect liposome myotoxicity. The second objective was to investigate the effect of liposomal encapsulation on the in-vitro and in-vivo myotoxicity of loxapine compared to the commercially available loxapine preparation.

The in-vitro myotoxicity of different types of empty liposomes and loxapine liposomes was evaluated by monitoring the cumulative efflux of the cytosolic enzyme creatine kinase (CK) from the isolated rat extensor digitorum longus (EDL) muscle over a 2 h period. In the in-vivo studies the area under plasma CK curve over 12 hours was used to evaluate muscle damage. The in-vitro myotoxicity for all empty liposomal formulations was not statistically different from negative controls (untreated control muscles and normal saline injected muscles). Moreover, these empty liposomal formulations were significantly less myotoxic than the positive controls: muscles injected with phenytoin solution and muscle sliced in half. In-vitro and in-vivo studies showed that the liposomal encapsulation of loxapine resulted in a significant ($p < 0.05$) reduction in myotoxicity (80 percent reduction in vitro and 60 percent in vivo) compared to an equal dose of the commercially available formulation which contains propylene glycol (70 percent) and polysorbate 80 (5 percent). These results again indicate that empty liposomes do not induce myotoxicity. Furthermore, under the chosen experimental conditions, liposomal size, charge and fluidity did not affect myotoxicity.

Several antitumor drugs are known to cause severe tissue damage when administered locally. In line with studies described above, findings by Oussoren et al. (1998) demonstrate the ability of liposomes to protect surrounding tissue against the damaging effect of an antitumor drug after IM administration. The study was performed with the antitumor drug mitoxantrone, which is an antitumor drug that causes severe inflammation and necrosis when injected intramuscularly at a dose of 0.2 mg in mice. When an equal dose of mitoxantrone encapsulated in liposomes was administered virtually no inflammatory response was observed 1 and 7 days after injection.

Studies on the Protective Effect After Intradermal and Subcutaneous Administration

Irritation of subcutaneous tissue has been frequently reported after inadvertent extravasation of vesicant antitumor drugs, such as doxorubicin. Extravasation of these highly toxic and irritating drugs results in large wounds which are often difficult to treat. Observations in the early eighties, suggesting that encapsulation of doxorubicin may lead to significant protection of surrounding tissue after extravasation, have led to the initiation of several studies on the effect of liposome encapsulation of tissue irritating antitumor drugs on local tissue irritation after subcutaneous administration. Most studies focused on the protective effect of liposomes on the damage induced by the antitumor drug doxorubicin. An overview of studies on the protective effect of liposomes against the damaging effect of antitumor drugs after subcutaneous and intradermal (ID) administration is given in Table 14.2.

Forssen and Tökes (1983) were the first to study the ability of liposomes to reduce vesicant properties of doxorubicin. Doxorubicin was encapsulated into liposomes by incorporation of a complex of PC with doxorubicin into the bilayers of negatively charged liposomes. Liposomes were injected intradermally into mice. The entrapment of doxorubicin in liposomes appeared to provide significant protection against the vesicant activity normally associated with extravasation one week after injection. Later, Balzasovits et al. (1989) studied the vesicant properties of doxorubicin encapsulated in liposomes using pH-gradient–driven encapsulation to provide improved trapping efficiency and stability. They demonstrated that liposomal encapsulation dramatically prevented doxorubicin from inducing necrosis at the site of infiltration. Mice receiving subcutaneous injections of liposomal doxorubicin experienced a slight inflammatory response and some discomfort, but at no time did the site of injection ulcerate. Hair regrowth occurred and the area of insult appeared normal by day 10. In contrast, mice receiving free doxorubicin experienced a pronounced inflammatory response that progressed to severe necrosis. Preclinical studies with doxorubicin encapsulated in polyethyleneglycol (PEG)–coated liposomes were performed by Gabizon et al. (1993). To study the protective effect of liposomes against the local toxic effects of doxorubicin, mice were intradermally injected with free doxorubicin or liposomal doxorubicin. In line with the findings of earlier investigators, they found that encapsulation in PEG–liposomes prevents vesicant damage of doxorubicin.

The influence of liposomal bilayer rigidity and PEG-coating on the protective effect of subcutaneously administered liposomes was studied by Oussoren et al. (1998). It was confirmed that liposomes can protect surrounding tissue at the subcutaneous injection site against the damaging effects of doxorubicin. The protective effect was stronger when gel-state

Table 14.2. Studies on the Protective Effect of Liposomes after Intradermal and Subcutaneous Administration of Vesicant Antitumor Drugs

Antitumor Drug	Animal	Route*	Formulation	Liposome Composition†	Antitumor Drug Dose (mg)	Results	Reference
Doxorubicin	mouse	ID	free drug		0.05	skin damage ranging from minimal changes to moderate induration with erythema in 4 of 5 mice	Forssen and Tökes (1983)
			liposomes	PC:PS:Chol (6:2:3)	0.10	skin damage ranging from moderate and severe skin damage to ulcerated lesions in all mice	
					0.05	mild induration in 1 of 5 mice	
					0.10	mild induration in 6 of 8 mice	
Doxorubicin	mouse	SC	free drug		0.40	progressing inflammatory reaction, necrotic lesions at day 4	Balazsovits et al. (1989)
			liposomes	EPC:Chol (55:45)	0.40	slight inflammatory reaction, no necrosis and ulceration within 30 days	
Doxorubicin	mouse	ID	free drug		0.10	erythema, ulceration and necrosis	Gabizon et al. (1993)
			liposomes	HPC:Chol:PEG: α-tocoferol (93:70:7.5:1)	0.10	minimal erythema	
Doxorubicin	mouse	SC	free drug		0.01	modest inflammation	Oussoren et al. (1998)

Antitumor Drug	Animal	Route*	Formulation	Liposome Composition†	Antitumor Drug Dose (mg)	Results	Reference
			liposomes		0.10	severe tissue damage and necrosis	
				EPC:EPG (2:1)	0.10	slight inflammation after 1 day, necrosis after 7 days	
				EPC:Chol:PEG (1.85:1:0.15)	0.10	slight inflammation after 1 day, necrosis after 7 days	
				DPPC:Chol (2:1)	0.10	modest inflammation, no tissue damage	
				DPPC:Chol: PEG (1.85:1:0.15)	0.10	modest inflammation, no tissue damage	Madhavan and Northfelt (1996)
Doxorubicin	human	inadvertent extravasation	liposomes	HPC:Chol:PEG: α-tocoferol (3:1:1:0.01)	0.25–1 (estimated extravasated amount)	mild edema and/or erythema, no clinically apparent tissue damage or necrosis	
Vincristine	mouse	SC	free drug		0.01	gross ulceration in all animals within 11 days after injection	Boman et al. (1996)
			liposomes	DSPC:Chol (55:45)	0.01	mild, prolonged inflammatory response	
Mitoxantrone	mouse	SC	free drug		0.02	mild tissue damage	
					0.20	severe inflammation and necrosis after 1 day	Oussoren et al. (1998)
			liposomes	EPC:EPG:Chol (10:4:4)	0.20	slight inflammation after 1 day, severe tissue damage and necrosis after 7 days	

*SC: subcutaneous; ID: intradermal

†PC: phosphatidylcholine; PS: phosphatidylserine; Chol: cholesterol; EPC: egg phosphatidylcholine; HPC: hydrogenated soybean phosphatidylcholine; EPG: egg phosphatidylglycerol; PEG: polyethylene glycol; DPPC: dipalmitoyl-phosphatidylcholine; DSPC: distearoyl-phosphatidylcholine

liposomes with more rigid bilayers (composed of dipalmitoyl-phosphatidylcholine:cholesterol [DPPC:Chol], molar ratio 2:1) were administered. Fluid-state liposomes (composed of egg phosphatidylcholine:cholesterol [EPC:Chol], molar ratio 2:1), which are less stable with regard to leakage of the liposomal content, initially protected the tissue. However, seven days post-injection necrosis at the subcutaneous injection site was observed. In contrast, seven days after administration of "gel-state" liposomes only modest inflammation was observed. The presence of a hydrophilic PEG– coating did not influence the protective effect of liposomes.

Recently, several clinical trials of intravenously administered long-circulating liposome encapsulated doxorubicin in patients with acquired immunodeficiency syndrome (AIDS)–related Kaposi's sarcoma were performed (Madhaven and Northfelt 1996). In eight cases, inadvertent extravasation of the liposomal formulation occurred. Extravasation of liposomal doxorubicin (estimated amount, 0.25–1.0 mg) resulted in a dramatically different course of events in these patients compared to historical experience with extravasation of conventional doxorubicin. In most cases, little more than mild edema and/or erythema were observed, whereas extravasation of free doxorubicin during infusion generally induced severe local inflammation and ulceration.

Since it has been shown that liposomal encapsulation of doxorubicin can dramatically reduce the vesicant properties of the drug after ID and SC administration, several studies have appeared on the protective effects of liposomes on the local toxicity of other antitumor drugs. The effect of liposomal encapsulation on the vesicant properties of the cytostatic vincristine was studied by Boman et al. (1996). Liposomal encapsulation of vincristine dramatically reduced soft-tissue damage by the drug. There was virtually no evidence of inflammatory response when liposomal vincristine was administered subcutaneously. In contrast, free drug produced gross ulceration in all treated animals. Histological analysis of the injection site suggested that liposomal vincristine induced a mild, but prolongnd inflammatory response that was distinct from the intense, short-lived inflammation response observed after free drug administration. Findings by Oussoren et al. (1998) indicate that liposomes can delay tissue damage after subcutaneous administration. Mitoxantrone, encapsulated in liposomes injected subcutaneously in mice, resulted in minimal tissue damage one day post-injection. However, seven days after administration, inflammation and necrosis were observed and tissue damage was as severe as after administration of free mitoxantrone.

The literature sources discussed above draw a mixed picture. Sometimes complete or considerable tissue protection is achieved, sometimes tissue damage is only delayed. Presumably, local tissue damage is caused by a cytotoxic effect of the drug. Slow release of the drug from the liposomal carrier may result in delayed tissue damage. The prolonged inflammatory response observed following subcutaneous injection of liposomal vincristine may be due to prolonged vincristine levels within the injection site. The drug leaks slowly from the liposomal interior, resulting in the tissue being exposed to a long-term low concentration of free drug. In comparison, when free drug is administered, there is a brief exposure of the tissue to the full drug dose before it disappears from the injection site. This peak level of exposure to free drug may be the cause for the occurrence of soft-tissue necrosis. This hypothesis is supported by the finding that fluid-state liposomes are less protective against local tissue damage than more stable, gel-state liposomes. Fluid-state liposomes release their contents faster than more stable liposomes. Therefore, surrounding tissue will be exposed to higher levels of the released drug and consequently, tissue irritation may be more severe.

DISCUSSION

The question should be raised as to what extent the findings reported in this chapter have general applicability and can guide the reader in making a rational choice regarding selection of liposomes. The studies discussed in this chapter differ in several ways. Different compounds were investigated, different lipid doses were used, different parameters for evaluation of drug toxicity were chosen, different study designs were followed, different parenteral formulations, including liposome compositions (size, charge, etc.), were administered and different experimental animals and sites of injections were studied. Also, injection techniques, pressure applied at the site of injection, injection site, volume of injection and frequency of dosing, play an important role in reducing the risk of local side effects.

Local irritation is not necessarily caused only by the drug compound itself. The role of solvent constituents used or present in the liposomal preparation should be considered carefully and study designs should not exclude evaluations of (co)solvent and other constituents. Therefore, study designs should be chosen carefully. Not only should "empty" liposomes be investigated but study of the behaviour of mixtures of empty liposomes plus free agents may provide useful information as well.

Another item to consider is that the drug under investigation might interfere with the results to be evaluated. For instance, NS, just like other NSAIDs, is able to reduce inflammation at the site of injection. These aspects should be considered carefully when evaluating the outcome of studies on local irritation.

Local tissue damage appeared to be strongly dependent on the route of administration. As reported by Oussoren et al. (1998), initially, surrounding tissue was protected efficiently against the toxic effects of the encapsulated mitoxantrone after injection, via the IM and subcutaneous route of administration. However, seven days post-injection remarkable differences were observed in the protective effect of liposomes. At this time-point, encapsulation of liposomes dramatically reduced toxic effects after IM administration but not after SC administration. The differences between the protective effect after SC and IM administration may be ascribed by the more complete and faster clearance of injected material after IM injection as compared to SC administration. Differences in the rate of clearance from the IM and SC injection site are attributed to a richer supply of blood and the presence of abundant lymphatic capillaries in muscle tissue and increased blood and lymph flow through muscles during body movement of the animal (Casley-Smith 1964). Released drugs may be cleared rapidly from the IM injection site. As surrounding tissue will only be exposed to very low concentrations of the free drug, tissue damage will be negligible. In contrast, the prolonged inflammatory response observed following subcutaneous administration of mitoxantrone- and doxorubicin-containing liposomes may be the result of a large proportion of the injected liposomal dose remaining at the injection site for a long period of time (Oussoren et al. 1997). Lack of clearance from the injection site may result in accumulation of the released drug and thus in prolonged exposure of surrounding tissue to high concentrations of the cytotoxic drug.

With regard to the methods to evaluate local irritation, Dorr et al. (1980) concluded that visual examination actually provided better correlations than did histological review, biochemical change or sulfan blue dye extravasation. Repetitive blood sampling itself may lead to increased levels of CK, thus CK monitoring may not be advisable in study designs with frequent blood sampling schemes.

In the studies discussed in this chapter, different experimental animals have been used. It is known that interspecies differences might complicate the extrapolation of study results. The predictive value for clinical use in humans, often under pathological conditions, is particularly the subject of such discussions. For instance, it is known that uptake of liposomes and other particulate agents by the regional lymph nodes is reduced when the injected tissue is inflamed, either chemically or as a result of the chronic disease itself (Tümer et al. 1983).

CONCLUSIONS

Liposomes are successful drug carrier systems and they can be used to reduce drug toxicity effectively. A number of liposomal formulations for IV administration (amphotericin B, doxorubicine, daunorubicin) are already commercially available, indicating that pharmaceutically acceptable production technologies for drug liposome combinations are now available (van Winden et al. 1998).

Only a few liposomal formulations intended for IM and SC administration have been marketed until now (Senior 1998). To our knowledge, these formulations do not contain tissue-irritating compounds. Before marketing liposomal formulations containing tissue-irritating drugs, a number of aspects should be further investigated. Since tissue damage is related to the injection frequency, dose, and site concentration of the drug and lipid, and to the chemical properties of the drug or components of the vehicle, each particular combination of drug and liposome should be tested carefully.

Liposomes consisting of regularly used (phospho)lipids such as PC, PG and cholesterol seem to be relatively nontoxic when administered as single injections. However, more information is needed concerning their safety when repeatedly administering them subcutaneously or intramuscularly at short intervals over several weeks or months.

REFERENCES

Al-Suwayeh, A. A., I. R. Tebbett, D. Wielbo, and G. A. Brazeau. 1996. In vitro-in vivo myotoxicity of intramuscular liposomal formulations. *Pharm. Res.* 13 (9): 1384–1388.

Avis, K. E., and B. G. Morris. 1984. The dosage form and its historical development. In *Pharmaceutical dosage forms: Parenteral medications*, edited by K. E. Avis and B. G. Morris. New York: Marcel Dekker, Inc.

Axelsson, B. 1989. Liposomes as carriers for anti-inflammatory agents. *Adv. Drug Deliv.* 3:391–404.

Balazsovits, J. A. E., L. D. Mayer, M. B. Bally, P. R. Cullis, M. Donell, R. S. Ginsberg, and R. E. Falk. 1989. Analysis of the effect of liposome encapsulation on the vesicant properties, acute and cardiac toxicities, and antitumor efficacy of doxorubicin. *Cancer Chemother. Pharmacol.* 23:81–86.

Barenholz, Y., and D. J. A. Crommelin. 1994. Liposomes as pharmaceutical dosage forms. In *Encyclopedia of Pharmaceutical Technology*, edited by J. Swarbrick and J. C. Boylan. New York: Marcel Dekker, Inc., pp. 1–39.

Boman, N. L., V. A. Tron, M. B. Bally, and P. R. Cullis. 1996. Vincristine-induced dermal toxicity is signifcantly reduced when the drug is given in liposomes. *Cancer Chemother. Pharmacol.* 37:351–355.

Casley-Smith, J. R. 1964. An electron microscopic study of injured and abnormally permeable lymphatics. *Ann. N.Y. Acad. Sci.* 116:803–830.

Crommelin, D. J. A., and H. Schreier. 1994. Liposomes. In *Colloidal drug delivery systems*, edited by Kreutzer J. New York: Marcel Dekker, Inc., pp. 73–90.

Dorr, R. T., D. S. Alberts, and G. C. Hsiao-Sheng. 1980. Experimental model of doxorubicin extravasation in the mouse. *J. Pharmacol. Methods* 4:237–250.

Forssen, E. A., and Z. A. Tökes. 1983. Attenuation of dermal toxicity of doxorubicin by liposome encapsulation. *Cancer Treatment Reports* 67 (5):481–484.

Gabizon, A. A., O. Pappo, D. Goren, M. Chemla, D. Tzemach, and A. Horowitz. 1993. Preclinical studies with doxorubicin encapsulated in polyethyleneglycol-coated liposomes. *J. Liposome Res.* 3:517–528.

Geervliet, E., J. H. Beijnen, S. L. Verweij, F. T. M. Peters, A. C. Dubbelman, G. P. C. Simonetti, and W. J. M. Underberg. 1989. Extravasatie van oncolytica, *Pharmaceutisch Weekblad* 124:843–852.

Gregoriadis, G. 1988. *Liposomes as drug carriers: Recent trends and progress.* Chichester, UK: John Wiley & Sons.

Gregoriadis, G. 1992. *Liposome technology,* vols. 1–3, 2nd ed. Boca Raton, Fla., USA: CRC Press Inc.

Heeremans, J. L. M., J. J. Kraaijenga, P. Los, C. Kluft, and D. J. A. Crommelin. 1992. Development of a procedure for coupling the homing device glu-plasminogen to liposomes. *Biochim. Biophys. Acta* 1117:258–264.

Jackson, A. J. 1981. Intramuscular absorption and regional lymphatic uptake of liposome-entrapped insulin. *Drug Met. Dispos.* 9 (6):535–540.

Kadir, F., W. M. C. Eling, D. Abrahams, J. Zuidema, and D. J. A. Crommelin. 1992. Tissue reaction after intramuscular injection of liposomes in mice. *Inter. J. Clin. Pharm. Ther. Tox.* 30 (10):374–382.

Kadir, F., W. M. C. Eling, J. Zuidema, and D. J. A. Crommelin. 1992. Kinetics and efficacy of increasing dosages of liposome-encapsulated chloroquine after intramuscular injection into mice. *J. Controlled Release* 20:47–54.

Kadir, F., J. Zuidema, and D. J. A. Crommelin. 1993. Liposomes as drug delivery systems for intramuscular and subcutaneous injections. In *Pharmaceutical particulate carriers in medical applications,* edited by A. Rolland. New York: Marcel Dekker, Inc., pp. 165–198.

Lichtenberg, D., and Y. Barenholz. 1988. Liposomes: preparation, characterization and preservation. In *Methods of biological analysis,* edited by D. Glick. New York: John Wiley & Sons, pp. 337–461.

Litterst, C. L., S. M. Sieber, M. Copley, and R. J. Parker. 1982. Toxicity of free and liposome-encapsulated adriamycin following large volume, short-term intraperitoneal exposure in the rat. *Toxicol. Appl. Pharmacol.* 64:517–528.

Madhavan, S., and D. W. Northfelt. 1996. Lack of vesicant injury following extravasation of liposomal doxorubicin. *J.N.C.I.* 87:1556–1557.

Nässander, U. K., G. Storm, P. A. M. Peeters, and D. J. A. Crommelin. 1990. Liposomes. In *Biodegradable polymers as drug delivery systems,* edited by M. Chasin and R. Langer. New York: Marcel Dekker, pp. 261–338.

Nässander, U. K., P. A. Steerenberg, W. H. De Jong, W. O. W. M. van Overveld, C. M. E. te Boekhorst, L. G. Poels, P. H. K. Jap, and G. Storm. 1995. Design of immunoliposomes directed against human ovarian carcinoma. *Biochim. Biophys. Acta* 1235:126–139.

Ohsawa, T., Y. Matsukawa, Y. Takakura, M. Hashida, and H. Sezaki. 1985. Fate of lipid and encapsulated drug after intramuscular administration of liposomes prepared by the freeze-thawing method in rats. *Chem. Pharm. Bull.* 33 (11): 5013–5022.

Ostro, M. 1987. *Liposomes: From biophysics to therapeutics.* New York: Marcel Dekker.

Ostro, M. J., and P. R. Cullis. 1989. Use of liposomes as injectable-drug delivery systems. *Am. J. Hosp. Pharm.* 46:1576–1587.

Oussoren, C., W. M. C. Eling, D. J. A. Crommelin, G. Storm, and J. Zuidema. 1998. The influence of the route of administration and liposome composition on the potential of liposomes to protect tissue against local toxicity of two antitumor drugs. *Biochim. Biophys. Acta* 1369:159–172.

Oussoren, C., J. Zuidema, D. J. A. Crommelin, and G. Storm. 1997. Lymphatic uptake and biodistribution of liposomes after s.c. injection. II. Influence of liposomal size, lipid composition and lipid dose. *Biochim. Biophys. Acta* 1328:261–272.

Peeters, P. A. M., C. W. E. M. Huiskamp, W. M. C. Eling, and D. J. A. Crommelin. 1989. Chloroquine containing liposomes in the chemotherapy of murine malaria. *Parasitology* 98:381–386.

Rasmussen, F. 1978. Tissue damage at the injection site after intramuscular injection of drugs. *Vet. Sci. Commun.* 2:173–182.

Reilly, J. J., J. P. Neifield, and S. A. Rosenberg. 1980. Clinical course and management of accidental adriamycin extravasation. *Cancer* 40:1543–1544.

Schäfer, H., W. Schmidt, H. Berger, and J. Bergfeld. 1987. Pharmacokinetics of gonadotropin-releasing hormone and stimulation of luteinizing hormone secretion after single dose administration of GnRH incorporated into liposomes. *Pharmazie* 42:689–693.

Senior, J. H. 1998. Medical applications of multivesicular lipid-based particles. In *Medical applications of liposomes,* edited by D. D. Lasic and D. Papahadjopoulos. Amsterdam: Elsevier, pp. 733–750.

Storm, G., C. Oussoren, P. A. M. Peeters, and Y. Barenholz. 1992. Tolerability of liposomes in vivo. In *Liposome technology,* 2nd ed., edited by G. Gregoriadis. Boca Raton, Fla., USA: CRC Pess Inc.

Surber, C., and H. Sucker. 1987. Tissue tolerance of intramuscular injectables and plasma enzyme activities in rats. *Pharm. Res.* 4:490–494.

Svendsen, O. F., F. Rasmussen, P. Nielsen, and E. Steiness. 1979. The loss of creatine phosphokinase (CK) from intramuscular injection sites in rabbits. A predictive tool for local toxicity. *Acta Pharmacol. Toxicol.* 44:324–328.

Szoka, F., and D. Papahadjopoulos. 1978. Procedure for preparation of liposomes with large internal aqueous space and high capture by reverse-phase evaporation. *Proc. Natl. Acad. Sci. USA* 75:4194–4198.

Talsma, H. 1991. Preparation, characterization and stabilization of liposomes. PhD thesis, Utrecht University.

Titulaer, H. A. C., W. M. C. Eling, D. J. A. Crommelin, P. A. M. Peeters, and J. Zuidema. 1990. The parenteral controlled release of liposome encapsulated chloroquine in mice. *J. Pharm. Pharmacol.* 42:529–532.

Tümer, A., C. Kirby, J. Senior, and G. Gregoriadis. 1983. Fate of cholesterol-rich liposomes after subcutaneous injection into rats. *Biochem. Biophys. Acta* 760:119–125.

Van Winden, E. C. A., K. J. Zuidam, and D. J. A. Crommelin. 1998. Strategies for large scale production and optimised stability of pharmaceutical liposomes for parenteral use. In *Medical applications of liposomes,* edited by D. D. Lasic and D. Papahadjopolous. Amsterdam: Elsevier, pp. 567–624.

Vingerhoeds, M. H., G. Storm, and D. J. A. Crommelin. 1994. Immunoliposomes in vivo (review). *ImmunoMethods* 4:259–272.

Zierenberg, O., and H. Betzing. 1979. Pharmacokinetics and metabolism of intramuscular injected polyenylphosphatidylcholine liposomes. *Arzneim.-Forsch./ Drug Res.* 29 (I):4949–498.

15

Biodegradable Microparticles for the Development of Less-Painful and Less-Irritating Parenterals

Elias Fattal

University of Paris-Sud
Châtenay-Malabry, France

Fabiana Quaglia

University of Paris-Sud and University of Naples
Châtenay-Malabry, France, and Napoli, Italy

Pramod Gupta

TAP Holdings, Inc.
Deerfield, Illinois, USA

Gayle Brazeau

University of Florida
Gainesville, Florida

Microparticles are polymeric particles whose diameter can vary from 1 to 1,000 μm. They can be made of natural or synthetic polymers, biodegradable or not degradable. It is possible to distinguish two types of forms: microcapsules, which are micrometric reservoir systems, or microspheres, which are micrometric matrix systems.

There are several advantages of using microparticles for intramuscular (IM) or subcutaneous delivery, including protection of fragile drugs against degradation and controlled release from the site of administration, thus reducing the number of injections.

These systems have been studied extensively during the past two decades first as long-term controlled-release systems for active drugs, including contraceptive steroids, local anesthetics, antibiotics, cytostatics, anti-inflammatories, and neuroleptics. Microparticles were also proposed for the delivery of peptides and proteins (hormones, cytokines, monoclonal antibodies, and growth factors). These drugs have became a very important class of therapeutic agents as a result of a greater understanding of their role in physiology and pathology, as well as the rapid advances in the field of biotechnology/genetic engineering. In addition, the efforts of synthetic chemists have in many cases given rise to analogues of endogenous compounds with greater potency than the parent compound. More recently, nucleic acids, such as antisense oligonucleotides and deoxyribonucleic acid (DNA) were also encapsulated in microparticles (Jones et al. 1997; Cleek et al. 1997).

Biodegradable microparticles have thus been investigated extensively to see which molecules achieve satisfactory efficiency and increase patient compliance. However, few papers have addressed the question of whether microparticles can reduce pain and irritation of intramuscularly or subcutaneously administered drugs. In this review, we discuss the advantages of biodegradable microparticles in this particular application.

RATIONALE FOR USING MICROPARTICLES IN THE DEVELOPMENT OF LESS-PAINFUL AND LESS-IRRITATING PARENTERALS

The main advantages of using microparticles are threefold: 1) to protect the active molecule against degradation, 2) to reduce the number of injections, and 3) to allow the controlled release of the active drugs. In addition, due to several factors, the encapsulation of drugs into microparticles potentially favors the reduction of pain/irritation of drugs (Table 15.1).

In most cases, association of drugs with microparticles occurs through an encapsulation process. Thus, the drug that is encapsulated is

Table 15.1. Reduction of Pain and Irritation of Intramuscularly Administered Drugs by Microencapsulation

Drawbacks of Free Drug Administration	Advantages of Microencapsulation
Direct contact with the tissue	Contact is avoided by the presence of microparticles
All of the drug is released at once	Slow delivery
Presence of irritating solvent	Solvent is water
Irritation by degradation products produced locally	Microencapsulation protects against degradation
Frequent injections	Reduction of the number of administrations

contained within a polymeric matrix, thus avoiding direct contact with the tissue. Hence, local cytotoxicity is reduced. The drug is then liberated in a controlled-release fashion, which means that there is always a small amount of free drug available to the tissue, minimizing fast drug release and its associated pain/irritation. In some cases, for solubility reasons, the solvent but not the drug can induce pain and irritation upon administration. The choice of biodegradable, biocompatible polymers can eliminate the presence of some solvents and the associated toxicity. If some local degradation leading to strongly toxic degradation products occurs, this can be avoided by encapsulation into microparticles that allows protection against degradation. Finally, reducing the frequency of administration is obviously an advantage in order to decrease the occurrence of pain and irritation upon IM administration.

POLY(LACTIDE-CO-GLYCOLIDE) MICROPARTICLES AS DELIVERY SYSTEMS IN THE DEVELOPMENT OF LESS-PAINFUL AND LESS-IRRITATING PARENTERALS

Polymer Selection

Biodegradable polymers are clearly the materials of choice for sustained parenterals drug delivery. The polymeric drug carrier needs to be treated as a drug itself in terms of safety, biocompatibility, and lack of toxicity of the polymer and its degradation products. Polymers where degradation is hydrolytically rather than enzymatically controlled are preferred because of less patient-to-patient variation. A range of biodegradable polymers has been considered for the sustained release of drugs, e.g., poly(alkyl-cyanoacrylates), poly(orthoesters), poly(amino acids), poly(dihydropyrans), poly(anhydrides) and the group of aliphatic polyesters: poly(lactic acid) (PLA), poly(glycolic acid) (PGA), poly(ε-caprolactone), and poly(hydroxy-butyrate).

However, because PLA and PGA and copolymers of both (PLGA) have a long and safe history of use as bioerodible suture materials, this system occupies a preeminent place among bioerodible drug delivery devices. Indeed, they are the most investigated and advanced polymers in regard to available toxicological and clinical data. PLA and PGA are nontoxic, biocompatible, and biodegradable polymers (Bos et al. 1991) approved by the Food and Drug Administration (FDA) for human use.

Production of Poly(Lactide-co-Glycolide) Polymers

Low molecular weight polymers (< 20, 000 Daltons) are produced by the direct condensation of lactic and/or glycolic acids. High molecular weight products are formed by the ring opening method using catalysts such as dialkyl zinc, trialkyl aluminum, and tetraalkyl tin, in which the lactide and/or glycolide rings form a cyclic dimer (Kulkarni et al. 1971). Polymers with a particular molecular weight can be manufactured by the choice of adequate polymerization conditions, (e.g., amount of catalyst, time of reaction, etc.) (Marcotte and Goosen 1989). Lactic acid contains an asymmetric carbon atom and has two optical isomers poly(D-lactic-acid) and poly(L-lactic-acid): the L-, or D-polymers have a crystalline form, and the D,L-polymers are amorphous and more rapidly degradable (Li and Vert 1994). Copolymers of lactic and glycolic acids (PLGA) form structures with lower crystallinity that have, among other factors, a hydrolysis rate controllable by their composition and hydrophobicity. Concerning hydrophobic properties, the lactic acid polymer is more hydrophobic than the glycolic acid polymer due to the presence of the methyl group (Yan et al. 1994), and this disfavors dissolution and degradation and slows drug release kinetics. The degradation products of PLA and PLGA polymers consist of the natural metabolites glycolic and lactic acid, which are naturally eliminated from the body (Figure 15.1) (Heller 1984; Lewis 1990). The degradation rate is controlled by factors including polymer molecular weight, polymer crystallinity and, for PLGA, the lactide/glycolide ratio (Cutright et al. 1974). Because the rate of hydrolysis of the polymer chain is dependent only on significant changes in temperature or pH, or on the presence of catalyst, very little difference is observed in the rate of degradation at different body sites. This is obviously an advantage in regard to drug delivery formulations (Lewis 1990).

Safety and Biocompatibility of Microparticles Products

Polymers used as drug delivery systems for pharmaceuticals need to exhibit biocompatible characteristics in terms of both the polymer effects on the organism receiving the drug delivery systems and, the polymer effects on the drug to be delivered. Several aspects of polymeric delivery systems ultimately contribute to its overall biocompatibility or lack thereof. The polymer itself, which consists of a repeating monomer species, may be antigenic (De Lustro et al. 1986, 1990), carcinogenic (Weiss et al. 1991, Nakamura et al. 1994) or toxic (Yoshida et al. 1993, Busch 1994). The shape of the implanted material has been implicated in its biocompatibility as well, smooth surfaces being less irritating and more biocompatible than rough surfaces (Matlaga et al. 1976). A key factor that influences the biocompatibility of an implanted polymer is the presence of low molecular weight extractables or unreacted residual monomers and polymerization initiators (King and Noss 1989). These residual materials are usually extracted by organic solvent prior to manufacture or preparation of a drug delivery system. However, residual solvents may also have adverse biological effects and must be removed prior to administration of a degradable drug delivery system. In some cases,

Figure 15.1. Structure, synthesis, and metabolism of poly(lactide-co-glycolide) polymer. The copolymer is synthesized by opening of the cyclic dimers in the presence of a catalyst.

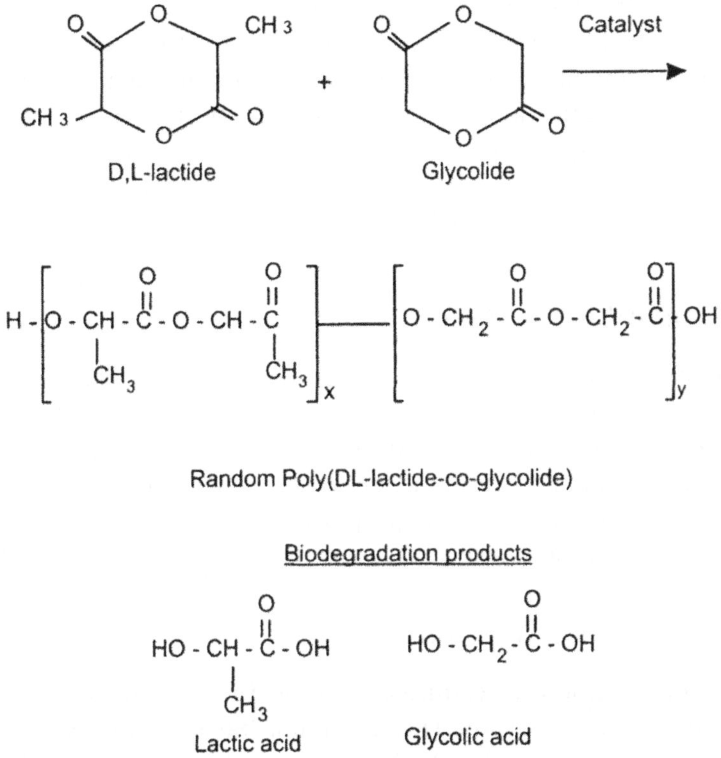

soluble polymers or breakdown products are sequestrated within organs, resulting in long-term adverse effects. The accumulation of high molecular weight polyvinyl pyrrolidone in the liver following prolonged exposure is one such example (Roske-Nielsen et al. 1976).

Generally, polymers described for use in drug delivery systems have had long histories as implants or excipients used in the pharmaceutical industry (e.g., PLGA copolymers). The use of PLA and PLGA in sutures has originally shown their biocompatibility (Cutright et al. 1971). In general, these biomaterials have demonstrated satisfactory biocompatibility and an absence of significant toxicity in vitro and in vivo. Concerning in vitro studies, cell proliferation of fibroblasts, osteosarcoma, and epithelial cells in the presence of PLA were determined under culture condition. The biocompatibility was judged satisfactory, although some cell inhibition was noted (Van Sliedgert et al. 1990, 1992). However, after degradation, PLA and PLGA produced acidic derivatives that were shown in only one experiment in vitro to be toxic (Taylor et al. 1994). It is worth noting that these experimental conditions do not emulate the in vivo situation, and that these tests cannot be considered extensive. In fact, numerous other studies have demonstrated successful in vivo biocompatibility characteristics of these biomaterials when utilized for different fracture fixations (Christel et al. 1983; Matsusue et al. 1992). PLA and PLGA have also been considered to be immunologically inert and well tolerated (Santavirta et al. 1990). The results of all these studies appear to support the in vivo use of PLA–PLGA biomaterials inducing no adverse biological responses. These observations have surely opened the door to the use of these polymers in other clinical applications such as microparticles fabrication for sustained delivery.

Microencapsulation Technique

During microparticle preparation, a number of process parameters have to be optimized, namely the mean size and size distribution, the drug loading and drug release rates, and the degradation rate of the matrix. Other aspects, such as sterility and residual solvent content need to be considered.

The methods widely used for preparing PLGA microparticles are the solvent evaporation, the phase separation methods and the spray drying.

Solvent Evaporation Methods

The solvent evaporation procedure can be useful for entrapping both water insoluble and soluble drugs. This method is based on the evaporation of the internal phase of a simple oil-in-water (o/w) or a multiple water-in-oil-in-water (w/o/w) emulsion and allows the formation of microspheric matrix systems whose diameter can vary from one to hundreds of micrometers.

In the single emulsion technique, the polymer is dissolved in a volatile organic solvent (usually methylene chloride), and the drug is added to the same organic phase. This phase is emulsified with an aqueous solution containing a suitable emulsifier, and the solvent is removed to form discrete, hardened, monolithic types of microparticles. The o/w solvent evaporation method is very useful for the entrapment of lipophilic drugs. This technique was proposed for the encapsulation of steroidal hormones (Beck et al. 1980; Beck and Pope 1984; Beck et al. 1985), local anesthetics (Wakiyama et al. 1981, 1982), antibiotics (Gupta et al. 1993), cytostatics (Spenlehauer et al. 1986, 1988; Deyme et al. 1992; Mestiri et al. 1993), anti-inflammatories (Cavalier et al. 1986; Bodmeier and Chen 1989; Chandrashekar and Udupa 1996) and neuroleptics (Fong et al. 1986). Because of their partition coefficient in favor of the external aqueous phase, the encapsulation of water-soluble compounds by this technique is rather difficult. Reducing the solubility of drugs in the external phase was achieved by modifying the pH of this phase (Bodmeier and McGinity 1987a), saturating it with drugs, or adding electrolytes (Wakiyama et al. 1981; Bodmeier and McGinity 1987a).

In order to increase the amount of hydrophilic molecules entrapped in microparticles, the w/o/w multiple emulsion solvent evaporation method (also called the in-water drying method) was developed (Ogawa et al. 1988a; Jeffery et al. 1993; Blanco-Prieto et al. 1994; Cohen et al. 1991). This method consists of dissolving the drug in distilled water or in a buffer solution (inner water phase) and dissolving the polymer in a volatile organic solvent that is not miscible to water (organic phase). The inner water phase in the absence or presence of a surfactant is then poured into the organic phase. This mixture is generally emulsified forming the first inner emulsion or the primary emulsion w/o. This w/o emulsion is then poured, under vigorous mixing using a mechanical stirrer (Blanco-Prieto et al. 1994), into an aqueous phase (outer water phase) that contains an emulsifier forming the w/o/w multiple emulsion. The resulting multiple emulsion is continuously stirred, and the solvent is allowed to evaporate, inducing polymer precipitation and, thereby, the formation of solid drug-loaded microparticles. This technique was mostly proposed for peptides and proteins (Cohen et al. 1991; Cleland 1997; Couvreur 1997) and more recently for nucleic acids (Cleek et al. 1997; Jones et al. 1997).

In both methods, the presence of an emulsifying agent in the outer water phase is critical for the successful formation of individual spherical microparticles (Parikh et al. 1993). The role of the emulsifier is to prevent the coagulation of microparticles during solvent removal. Different types of emulsifiers have been used, such as gelatin, alginates, methylcellulose, polyvinhilic alcohol, cetyltrimethylammonium bromide, sodium dodecyl sulfate, sodium lauryl sulfate, and sodium oleate (Fong et al. 1986; Arshady 1991; Jeffery et al. 1991).

Solvent evaporation can take place at atmospheric or reduced pressure, and under various temperatures. The complete evaporation of the solvent can be obtained in three different ways:

1. Interrupted process: the evaporation, performed at room temperature, is stopped when the solvent is not completely eliminated. The partially solid microparticles are transferred into a low concentrated emulsifier solution or an emulsifier-free medium where the evaporation is continued (Cohen et al. 1991).

2. Continuous process: the preparation is continuously stirred at room temperature until solvent evaporation is completed (Blanco-Prieto et al. 1994).

3. The multiple emulsion is placed into a rotatory evaporator and warmed to approximately 30°C (Ogawa et al. 1988a).

The solid microparticles are then isolated by filtration or centrifugation, washed several times in order to eliminate the emulsifier agent, and then dried under vacuum or freeze-dried.

According to several mechanical and physical-chemical parameters, particle diameter can vary from a few micrometers to hundreds of micrometers. For both single and multiple emulsion solvent evaporation methods, the amount and the nature of the surfactant used in the continuous external phase may influence the final diameter of the particles. When increasing the amount of surfactant, the diameter decreases (Jeffery et al. 1991; Sansdrap and Moes 1993; Blanco-Prieto et al. 1994). At high surfactant concentration, the rate at which the emulsion stabilizing molecules diffuse at the emulsion droplets/aqueous phase interface may increase, resulting in a greater presence of stabilizer at the surface of the emulsion droplets. This would provide an improvement in the protection of droplets against coalescence, resulting in the formation of smaller emulsion droplets at higher surfactant concentrations. As the solvent evaporates from the system, these droplets harden to form the microparticles. Therefore, the size of the finally obtained microparticles is dependent on the size and stability of the emulsion droplets formed during the agitation process. At low surfactant concentration, small emulsion droplets are not stable, and the resulting microparticles are larger in size than those prepared with higher surfactant concentrations. Increasing the concentration of the dissolved polymer increased the viscosity of the organic phase, which resulted in the reduction of the stirring efficiency (Blanco-Prieto et al. 1994). The higher the viscosity of polymer solution the more difficult the formation of small emulsion droplets (Blanco-Prieto et al. 1994).

In the multiple emulsion solvent evaporation technique, when adding a hydrosoluble stabilizing agent (gelatin or ovalbumin) to the inner water phase, particle size increases due to the rise in the diameter of the internal globules. Also, the particle size increases when the polymer concentration in the organic phase increases (Yan et al. 1994). Particle mean diameter also depends on the mixing methods used to prepare the first inner emulsion and the second emulsion (Bodmeier et al. 1989). When both emulsions are prepared by vortex mixing, the microparticles obtained are large. However, when the inner emulsion is prepared by sonication and the second emulsion by vortex mixing, a microfine inner emulsion is formed (Bodmeier et al. 1989). The resulting microparticles become smaller and very homogenous (Bodmeier et al. 1989). Finally, when the inner emulsion is formed with a homogenizer and the second emulsion with a vortex mixer, the particle diameter is intermediate between sizes of the microparticles obtained by both methods (Bodmeier et al. 1989).

Concerning the encapsulation rate of low water-soluble molecules in microparticles prepared by the solvent evaporation technique, this method of preparation has allowed the encapsulation of molecules with an aqueous solubility of 0.02 mg/mL or less (Okada and Toguchi 1995). The loading efficiency is generally very high, varying from 10 to 80 percent. However, this loading efficiency depends on several parameters (Table 15.2): Drug loading increased with the initial amount of drug dissolved in the organic solvent (Parikh et al. 1993). However, at high concentrations, drugs start to

Table 15.2. Factors Influencing Drug Encapsulation Efficiency in Microparticles Prepared by the Single Emulsion Solvent Evaporation Method

Parameters		Effect	Reference
Inner organic phase	increasing the volume	+	Bodmeier and McGinity (1988b)
	increasing the viscosity	+	Spenlehauer et al. (1988)
Outer water phase	increasing the volume	+	Bodmeier and McGinity (19887)
	adjustment of the pH	+	Bodmeier and McGinity (1987a)
Drug	increasing the amount	+	Parikh et al. (1993)

crystallize outside the polymeric matrix, modifying morphologically the surface aspect of the microparticles (Bodmeier et al. 1989; Spenlehauer et al. 1988). Moreover, it was also shown that the percent of drug incorporated decreased inversely in proportion to the octanol-water partition coefficient (Cha 1989). The amount of drug incorporated increased with increases in the mean particle size (Spenlehauer et al. 1986; Parikh et al. 1993). The role of the viscosity and polymer concentration was clearly demonstrated. Increasing polymer concentration resulted in a higher viscosity of the organic phase and a better distribution of the drug in the matrix (Spenlehauer et al. 1986). On the contrary, lowering the viscosity of the organic phase allows drugs to come close to the surface during microparticle formation and to dissolve in the surrounding aqueous medium, resulting in a lower drug content (Spenlehauer et al. 1988).

Water-soluble molecules are generally entrapped in microparticles prepared by the multiple emulsion solvent evaporation method. Parameters involved in loading efficiency are more numerous than those influencing the formation of microparticles prepared by the single emulsion evaporation method. Stability of the primary emulsion is a prerequisite for the successful stabilization of a multiple emulsion and the loading of a large amount of drug within the solid microparticles (Nihant et al. 1994; Blanco-Prieto et al. 1996a). In addition, key parameters for the successful encapsulation of drugs are the small droplet size of the internal aqueous phase and the insolubility of the drug in the organic polymer solution. The organic polymer solution acts as a barrier between the internal drug-containing aqueous phase and the continuous aqueous phase.

When large proteins are encapsulated, they generally stabilize the primary emulsion, (e.g., ovalbumin) (Nihant et al. 1994; Blanco-Prieto et al. 1997). On the other hand, when small water-soluble molecules (e.g., small peptides) are entrapped, the addition of a surfactant is often necessary to obtain high loading efficiency (Blanco-Prieto et al. 1996a).

Among the factors controlling the entrapment of a drug into microparticles prepared by the w/o/w multiple emulsion method are the concentration of the polymer in the organic phase, the viscosity of the internal aqueous phase, and the volume of the inner and outer aqueous phases (Table 15.3). Increasing the amount of polymer in the organic phase augmented the encapsulation efficiency because raising the amount of polymer increased the viscosity of the w/o primary emulsion. This high viscosity stabilized the internal aqueous phase against coalescence and thus reduced drug loss to the external aqueous phase (Herrmann and Bodmeier 1995; Blanco-Prieto et al. 1996a).

Increasing the volume fraction of the internal aqueous phase in the primary emulsion resulted in lower encapsulation efficiencies (Herrmann and Bodmeier 1995). It is assumed that increasing the proportion of the internal aqueous phase will promote contact and subsequently exchange (drug loss) between the internal and the external aqueous phase across the surface of microparticles droplets. In addition, the thickness of the layer of the organic phase decreases with a larger volume of the internal aqueous phase. This could also lead to less stable w/o primary emulsions with larger droplets of the internal aqueous phase being formed. The viscosity of the internal aqueous phase also influences the encapsulation efficiency. Ogawa et al. (1988a) reported an increase in the entrapment efficiency of the hydrophilic peptide leuprolide acetate following the addition of gelatin (and lowering the temperature) to the peptide solution prior to the emulsification. In agreement with this, Heya et al. (1991) also observed an increase in the encapsulation efficiency of thyroid releasing hormone (TRH) into PLGA microparticles when the viscosity of the first emulsion was augmented. Finally, a raise in the volume of the external aqueous phase resulted in an increase of both OVA entrapment and particle size (Jeffery et al. 1993). As a result of

Table 15.3. Factors Influencing Drug Encapsulation Efficiency in Microparticles Prepared by the Multiple Emulsion Solvent Evaporation Method

Parameters		Effect	Reference
Inner organic phase	increasing the volume	–	Herrmann and Bodmeier (1995
	increasing the viscosity	+	Ogawa et al. (1988a)
Outer water phase	increasing the volume	+	Jeffery et al. (1993)
	adjustment of the pH	+	Blanco-Prieto et al. (1997)
Organic phase	increasing the viscosity	+	Herrman and Bodmeier (1995)
Drug	increasing the amount	+	Blanco-Prieto et al. (1996a)

increasing particle size, there is an associated increase in particle volume, which enables more OVA to be incorporated into microparticles. Linear relationships were shown to exist between the volume of the external aqueous phase and the amount of OVA entrapped (Jeffery et al. 1993).

As mentioned before, the formation of a very stable w/o/w multiple emulsion is of the utmost importance for an effective encapsulation efficiency (Blanco-Prieto et al. 1996a). However, in general, high water-soluble substances, especially those with low molecular weights are easily released to the outer aqueous phase during solvent evaporation, even after the formation of a stable w/o/w multiple emulsion. In this case, the adjustment of the pH in the outer water phase to the minimal solubility of the entrapped drug, can significantly augment the encapsulation efficiency. For example, the trapping efficiency of a water-soluble seven amino acid peptide (pBC 264, which is a cholecystokinin derivative) was improved by the creation of a pH gradient between the inner and outer aqueous phase (Blanco-Prieto et al. 1997). The pH of the outer water phase was adjusted to the minimal solubility of the peptide in order to reduce its leakage. This pH gradient between the inner and the outer aqueous phase of the multiple emulsion led to a significant increase in the retention of the peptide within microparticles. This phenomena was also observed for β-lactoglobulin, but in this case strong adsorption of the protein on the microparticles surface occurred (Leo et al. 1998).

Phase Separation Methods

Phase separation microencapsulation procedures, also referred as coacervation, are suitable for entrapping water-soluble agents in PLGA excipients. Generally, the phase separation process involves coacervation of the polymer from an organic solvent by addition of a nonsolvent such as silicone oil (Ruiz 1989). This technique leads to the production of microcapsules and, under certain circumstances, of microparticles. It has proven useful for microencapsulation of water-soluble peptides and macromolecules (Ruiz et al. 1989).

Spray Drying

The principle of spray drying consists of the atomization of a solution, suspension, or emulsion. According to the nature of the molecule to encapsulate-polymer mixture, microparticles or microcapsules can be obtained (Bodmeier and Chen 1988). Spray drying allows a one-step processing, with quite good production yields, but it might be a little difficult to carry out all processing during aseptic conditions. As a modified spray drying technique involving milder drying conditions, the aerosol solvent extraction system utilizing the extraction properties of supercritical gases has been developed. PLA solution in methylene chloride, containing drug, was sprayed into the supercritical gas of carbon dioxide and the organic solvent was extracted, leading to the formation of solid microparticles (Bleich et al. 1993).

Drug Release

Release from biodegradable microparticles is dependent on both diffusion of the entrapped material through the polymer matrix, and on polymer degradation. The general properties of drug release are described in Figure 15.2. It occurs as follows: initial release from the microparticle surface due to the molecule absorbed on or embedded in the surface. Then, drug release from PLA or PLGA matrix can occur by two main routes: diffusion or matrix degradation (Figure 15.2). The latter occurs when drug release from the matrix follows erosion of the polymer surface and/or bulk matrix. One of these two mechanisms plays a role in the release process depending on properties of the polymer, the morphology of microparticles, the solubility and the diffusion properties of the entrapped material. The kinetics of drug release from microparticles of PLGA is generally biphasic (Sanders et al. 1985), (a negligible or slow rate of drug release followed by a more rapid rate). The induction period prior to rapid release has prompted the development of delivery systems that either incorporate this temporal feature to advantage (e.g., for vaccine delivery), or seek to minimize it by varying the polymer composition to achieve zero-order delivery. Without going

Figure 15.2. Schematic diagram of two possible mechanisms for drug release from PLA or PLG matrices: (A) Initial release from microparticle surface, the drug is then released through the pores depending on the morphology, or upon degradation. (B) Initial release from microparticle surface, the drug contained in the matrix is then able to diffuse out from the microparticles before microparticles degrade.

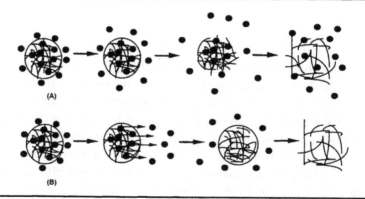

(A)

(B)

into the details of release mechanisms, it should be noted that it is very difficult to model drug release from microparticles. Many mathematical models have been tried, but it is rarely possible to draw conclusions about the release profiles and to generalize release kinetics.

Parameters involved in drug release from PLA and PLGA microparticles have been investigated in both in vitro and in vivo studies. These studies have shown that release kinetics are predominantly dependent on the polymer erosion rate. The more stable polymers yield the slowest rates, while microparticles prepared with quickly degradable polymers gradually release the encapsulated material. An increase in glycolide content induces an increase in the release rate from microparticles (Beck et al. 1983; Tabata and Ikada 1988). Also, polymer molecular weight is able to affect drug release such that higher molecular weight induces slower release (Wakiyama et al. 1982; Jalil and Nixon 1990; Cohen et al. 1991; Heya et al; 1991; O'Hagan et al. 1994). However, in some cases (e.g., proteins) diffusion is impossible so the drug is only released when the polymer degrades.

The effect of drug loading on drug release rates has also been studied (Parikh et al. 1993; O'Hagan et al. 1994; Sah et al. 1994; Leo et al. 1998). These studies found that increasing drug loading over a certain value causes an elevation of the initial release due to a higher absorption of the molecule on a microparticle surface and an increase in aqueous channels by connecting the drug cores. Microparticle size is also a very important factor influencing the drug release profile. The release rate will increase with a reduction in particle size as a result of the increase in surface area (Aisina et al. 1994). In fact, the particle system often departs from a polysized distribution that implies a range of release rates, with the smaller particles exhibiting rapid release and the larger ones a slower liberation.

In some studies, in vitro release was similar to in vivo (Maulding et al. 1986; Blanco-Prieto et al. 1996b), and some authors found that release is faster in vivo in vitro (Wakiyama et al. 1982). This difference might be due to faster degradation occurring in vivo. Plasma concentration of drug release from microparticles after IM or subcutaneous administration indicates that microspheres can, in vivo, induce a total release of their content according to their properties and in a time span ranging from few days to months. For instance, Lupron Depot®, which is a commercial biodegradable PLGA microsphere delivery system for luteinizing hormone releasing hormone (LHRH) analog releases the drug over one month (Ogawa et al. 1988b, 1989; Okada et al. 1991). In addition, a second formulation product allowing drug release for three months was also described (Okada et al. 1994). For Maulding (1987), the route of administration between IM and subcutaneous played an important role in the duration of a LHRH when given encapsulated in PLGA microparticles. This observation is, however, in contradiction with the findings of Ogawa and coworkers (1989), showing that there are insignificant differences in the pharmacokinetics from either subcutaneous or IM injection of microcapsules containing a LHRH agonist.

Sterilization

Sterilization techniques used for PLGA biomaterials were reviewed by Athanasiou et al. (1996). PLGA polymers, in addition to being susceptible to damage by moisture and radiation, are heat sensitive because of their thermoplastic nature. Therefore, the selection of the correct sterilization technique for PLGA microparticles is crucial to their physical and mechanical properties, and, thus, to their performance in vivo (Athanasiou et al. 1996). Steam sterilization techniques commonly use high moisture and temperatures in excess of 100°C. Such temperatures can approach or exceed the thermal transition temperatures of PLGA polymers and potentially alter their physical and mechanical properties (Rozema et al. 1991). Gamma radiation sterilization is known to cause chain scission in PLGA polymers. At doses of 2.5 Mrad, ^{60}Co gamma radiation causes deterioration of the polymer in sutures. In addition, there is a rapid decrease in the molecular weight of PLGA sutures with increasing doses of gamma radiation (Gilding and Reed 1979).

The effect of gamma radiation on drug release from PLGA microparticles has also been studied. It was found that radiation does not affect drug release in the initial few days (Spenlehauer et al. 1989). There is, however, massive drug release upon collapse of the matrix. Gamma radiation causes the matrix collapse to occur at 10 to 15 days rather than at the 60 to 70 days as observed for nonradiated materials (Spenlehauer et al. 1989). Finally, chemical sterilization by gases such as ethylene oxide is often used for polymers that are sensitive to heat and moisture, such as PLGA. However, it is noteworthy that chemical sterilization can leave residues in toxic quantities on the surface of and within the polymer. The amount of gases adsorbed into the polymer depends on the equilibrium absorption and diffusion coefficient (Vink and Pleijser 1986). Taking into account these parameters, it is clear that sterilization techniques can affect microparticle characteristics, and, in some cases, can leave harmful residues in vivo. The choice of a sterilization technique should, therefore, be carefully considered.

Residual Solvents

The volatile organic solvent used in the preparation of the microparticles by both single and multiple emulsion solvent evaporation techniques needs to possess a low boiling point to overcome the problems associated with residual solvent. Many solvents can be used for the preparation of microparticles: acetonitrile, ethyl acetate, chloroform, benzene, and methylene chloride. This last solvent is considered the most suitable for the preparation of microparticles by the solvent evaporation method (Bodmeier and McGinity 1988). Methylene chloride has a high volatility that facilitates easy removal by evaporation, and it also shows a good solubility towards a range of encapsulating polymers. The limit proposed by the U.S. Pharmacopeia (USP) is 500 ppm. Bitz and Doelker (1996) showed that methylene chloride residue was only well below the 500 ppm limit in batches prepared by spraydrying at an inlet temperature of 60°C. However, using the solvent evaporation technique, Yamamoto et al. (1985) succeeded to reduce the methylene chloride residue to below 100 ppm by well programmed heating during the freeze-drying process. It is particularly noteworthy that chlorinated solvents are generally undesirable for manufacturing processes, and they may be banned in the future for environmental and health reasons. However, recent studies have shown that there is no link between exposure to methylene chloride and cancer in humans (Jones 1996). In addition, methylene chloride does not deplete the stratospheric ozone layer, and it has a proven low potential to create low-level ozone (Jones 1996). Finally, a number of nonchlorinated solvents are potentially suitable for microparticle preparation (e.g., ethyl acetate or acetonitrile) (Bodmeier and Chen 1988; Arshady 1990).

Stability of the Encapsulated Drug and Microparticle Products

Stability issues are also critical when dealing with drugs that are sensitive to degradation. In the process of preparing microparticles, drugs may be exposed to extreme stresses. Manufacturing steps should not include excessive exposure to heat, shear forces, pH extremes, organic solvents, freezing, and drying. During storage, the incorporated drugs may become hydrated and, in this type of environment, may become more susceptible to degradation (Liu et al. 1991). Also, when a polymer begins to degrade following administration, a highly concentrated microenvironment is created in and around the microparticles due to polymer breakdown by-products (acidic monomers). The active drug may be susceptible to hydrolytic degradation and/or chemical modification in such an environment (Park et al. 1995). Finally, some drugs may undergo reversible or irreversible adsorption to the polymers, which can affect drug delivery rate (Crotts and Park 1997).

Special attention should also be paid to microparticle products. Drug-polymer interactions can lead to an accelerated hydrolytic process, particularly in the case of basic drugs (Maulding et al. 1986). Microparticles can also aggregate if suspended in a medium that does not contain any stabilizing agent (Arshady 1991). Long-term storage might be accompanied by polymer degradation, and freeze-drying should be considered for microparticles. However, this process should be applied in conditions in which it does not modify morphology and release of microparticles.

PROTECTION AGAINST MYOTOXICITY BY INTRAMUSCULARLY/SUBCUTANEOUSLY ADMINISTERED MICROPARTICLES

Microparticles have been used for IM/subcutaneous delivery of many drugs. In a few cases, the purpose of the formulation was to study at the reduction of toxicity of the drug upon injection. In this section, we will discuss in detail the different studies achieved for this application.

Visscher et al. (1985, 1986) reported in detail the tissue response after IM injection of PLGA and PLA microparticles (30 μm) and morphological changes in the microparticles based on histological observations. In the case of a device with a one-month lifespan, a minimal inflammatory reaction characterized by infiltration of lymphocytes, plasma cells, and histocytes, and acute myositis was observed soon after injection. This inflammatory response remained until complete erosion and breakdown of the polymer occurred. At that point, the tissue response disappeared completely.

Acute myotoxicity of unloaded microparticles was studied using the isolated rodent skeletal muscle model (Brazeau et al. 1996). Briefly, measuring the cumulative release of creatine kinase (CK) from an isolated rat extensor digitorum longus muscle assessed myotoxicity. This in vitro system has been previously validated for its potential to discriminate between the myotoxicity of various parenterals formulations (Brazeau and Fung 1989; Brazeau et al. 1992). Using a high molecular weight poly(D,L-lactide-co-glycolide) copolymer, the myotoxicity of two different size microparticles formulations (3.6 μm and 19 μm) in normal saline or distilled water was quantified using the previously validated isolated rat muscle system (Brazeau et al. 1996). Overall, microparticles were found to be relatively nontoxic compared to known myotoxic agents (e.g., phenytoin) and control muscles. The smaller microparticles were found to be significantly more myotoxic than larger microparticles (Brazeau et al. 1996). Furthermore, the myotoxicity was lower in large microparticles reconstituted with normal saline or normal saline with 0.5 percent (w/v) carboxymethylcellulose (to prevent aggregation) compared to those reconstituted with distilled water (Brazeau et al. 1996).

Reducing pain and irritation of drugs using microparticles was investigated with a number of drugs such as clarithromycin, progesterone, and naltrexone. It was found that the naltrexone-loaded microparticles induced a larger inflammation response than the unloaded microparticles. According to the authors (Yamaguchi and Anderson 1992), this was due to the release of the drug from the microparticles. However, in that study, myotoxicity was not compared to that of the free drug.

Clarithromycin is an antibiotic from the macrolide group with a methoxy group attached to the C6 position of erythromycin, which makes it more acid stable than erythromycin. Clarithromycin is recommended for the treatment of upper respiratory tract infections. However, it is a very painful drug during intravenous administration (IV) and it is irritating following IM administration. An IM formulation of clarithromycin was developed by encapsulation in biodegradable PLA microparticles ranging from 5 to 40 μm in diameter (Gupta et al. 1993). In vitro drug release revealed that 40 to 60 percent drug was released from the microparticles during the first 24 h, as opposed to complete dissolution of bulk during the same time period. A total of 80 to 90 percent drug was released from the microparticles in 120 to 160 h, suggesting the potential possibility of sustained drug release.

Bulk or PLA microsphere-encapsulated drug was administered to dogs. Blood samples were collected over time to monitor CPK concentrations. CPK concentrations in both groups were low, and compared well with those observed following the administration of placebo microspheres. The animals receiving drug/PLA microspheres demonstrated minor swelling at the site of injection that lasted for 12 to 24 h. However, the bulk drug treatment group exhibited much greater swelling, lasting for 2 to 3 days.

In a separate study, progesterone, an endogenous hormone playing a major role in the regulation of the reproductive cycle and fertility, was investigated in mares. The current regimen involves IM administration of drug dissolved in an alcoholic-oil solution, either daily (200 mg) or twice a week (1 g) for 6 to 8 months. This has resulted in several occurrences of abscesses, inflammation, infection, and even permanent scars in mares. The drug causes pain at the site of injection and hence is very distressing to the animal. To avoid these problems progesterone was encapsulated in PLA microparticles with the aim of maintaining progesterone levels of 2 to 6 ng/mL for 10 to 14 days after IM administration in mares (Gupta et al. 1992). Results suggest that microparticles might reduce muscle damage and local inflammation due to progesterone at the site of injection.

CONCLUSIONS

Obviously, biodegradable polyester microparticles offer interesting perspectives for clinical applications. They have been shown to extensively improve the delivery of drugs that are administered intramuscularly or subcutaneously. The main advantage of these systems is the absence of toxicity, the possibility of entrapping hydrophilic and lipophilic molecules, and their ability to control in vivo and in vitro release. Recent studies have shown that microspheres can also reduce the acute toxicity of drugs that are painful and tissue irritating upon IM and/or subcutaneous administration. This appears to be an additional advantage for polyester microparticles.

REFERENCES

Aisina, R. B., N. B. Diomina, T. N. Ovchinnikova, and S. D. Varfolomeyev. 1994. Microencapsulation of somatropic growth hormone. *S. T. P. Pharma Sciences.* 4:437–441.

Arshady, R. 1990. Microspheres and microcapsules: A survey of manufacturing techniques, Part 2. Coacervation. *Polym. Eng. Sci.* 30:905–914.

Arshady, R. 1991. Preparation of biodegradable microspheres and microcapsules: 2. Polylactides and related polyesters. *J. Control. Rel.* 17:1–22.

Athanasiou, K. A., G. C. Niederauer, and C. M. Agrawal. 1996. Sterilization, toxicity, biocompatibility and clinical applications of polylactic acid.polyglycolic acid copolymers. *Biomaterials* 17:93–102.

Beck, L. R., and V. Z. Pope. 1984. Controlled-release delivery systems for hormones. A review of their properties and current therapeutic use. *Drugs* 27:528–547.

Beck, L. R., V. Z. Pope, D. R. Cowsar, D. H. Lewis. and Tice T. R. 1980. Evaluation of three-month contraceptive microspheres system in primates. *J. Contracept. Deliv. System.* 1:79–82.

Beck, L. R., V. Z. Pope, C. E. Flowers, D. R. Cowsar, T. R. Tice, D. H. Lewis, R. L. Dunn, A. B. Moore, and R. M. Gilley. 1983. Poly(DL-lactide-co-glycolide)/ norethisterone microcapsules: An injectable biodegradable contraceptive. *Biol. Reprod.* 28:186–195.

Beck, L. R., V. Z. Pope, T. R. Tice, and R. M. Gilley. 1985. Long-acting injectable microsphere formulation for the parenteral administration of levonorgestrel. *Adv. Contracept.* 1:119–29.

Bitz, C., and E. Doelker. 1996. Influence of the preparation method on residual solvents in biodegradable microspheres. *Int. J. Pharm.* 131:171–181.

Blanco-Prieto, M. J., F. Delie, E. Fattal, A. Tartar, F. Puisieux, A. Gulik, and P. Couvreur. 1994. Characterization of V3 BRU peptide-loaded small PLGA microspheres prepare by a (W1/O)W2 emulsion solvent evaporation method. *Int. J. Pharm.* 111:137–145.

Blanco-Prieto, M. J., Leo E., F. Delie, A. Gulik, P. Couvreur, and E. Fattal. 1996a. Study of the influence of several stabilizing agents on the entrapment and in vitro release of pBC 264 from poly(lactide-co-glycolide) microspheres prepared by a W/O/W solvent evaporation method. *Pharm. Res.* 13:1127–1129.

Blanco-Prieto, M. J., C. Durieux, V. Dauge, E. Fattal, P. Couvreur, and B. P. Roques. 1996b. Slow delivery of the selective cholecystokinin agonist pBC264 into the rat nucleus accumbens using microspheres. *J. Neurochem.* 67:2417–2424.

Blanco-Prieto, M. J., E. Fattal, A. Gulik, J. C. Dedieu, B. P. Roques, and P. Couvreur. 1997. Characterization and morphological analysis of a cholecystokinin derivative peptide-loaded poly(lactide-co-glycolide) microspheres prepared by a water-in-oil-in-water emulsion solvent evaporation method. *J. Control. Rel.* 43:81–87.

Bleich, J., B. W. Müller, and W. Wassmus. 1993. Aerosol solvent extraction system, a new microparticle production technique. *Int. J. Pharm.* 97:111–117.

Bodmeier, R., and J. W. McGinity. 1987a. Polylactic acid microspheres containing quinidine base and quinidine sulfate prepared by the solvent evaporation technique. I-Methods and morphology. *J. Microencapsulation* 4:279–288.

Bodmeier, R., and J. W. McGinity. 1987b. Polylactic acid microspheres containing quinidine base and quinidine sulfate prepared by the solvent evaporation technique. II. Some process parameters influencing the preparation and properties of microspheres. *J. Microencapsulation* 4:289–297.

Bodmeier, R., and J. W. McGinity. 1988. Solvent selection in the preparation of poly(D,L-lactide) microspheres prepared by the solvent evaporation method. *Int. J. Pharm.* 43:179–186.

Bodmeier, R., and H. Chen. 1988. Preparation of biodegradable polylactide microparticles using a spray-drying technique. *J. Pharm. Pharmacol.* 40:754–757.

Bodmeier, R., and H. Chen. 1989. Preparation and characterization of microspheres containing the anti-inflammatory agents indomethacin, ibuprofen and ketoprofen. *J. Control. Rel.* 10:167–175.

Bodmeier, R., K. H. Oh, and H. Chen. 1989. The effect of the addition of low molecular weight poly(DL-lactide) on drug release from biodegradable poly(DL-lactide) drug delivery systems. *Int. J. Pharm.* 51:1–8.

Bos, R. R. M., F. R. Rozema, G. Boering, A. J. Nijhenius, A. B. Verwey, P. Nieuwenhius, and H. W. B. Jansen. 1991. Degradation and tissue reaction to biodegradable poly(L-lactide) for the use as internal fixation of fractures: A study in rats. *Biomaterials* 12:32–36.

Brazeau, G. A., and H. L. Fung. 1989. An in vitro model to evaluate muscle damage following intramuscular injection. *Pharm. Res.* 6:167–179.

Brazeau, G., S. Arthus, and J. Mott. 1992. No correlation between pain an in vitro myotoxicity after intramuscular injection of three cephalosporins. *Curr. Therap. Res.* 51:839–842.

Brazeau, G. A., M. Sciame, S. A. Al-Suwayeh, and E. Fattal. 1996. Evaluation of PLGA microsphere size effect on myotoxicity using the isolated rodent skeletal muscle model. *Pharm. Dev. Technol.* 1:279–283.

Busch, H. 1994. Silicone toxicology. *Semin. Arthritis. Rheum.* 24:11–17.

Cavalier, M., J. P. Benoit, and C. Thies. 1986. The formation and characterization of hydrocortisone-loaded poly(lactide) microspheres. *J. Pharm. Pharmacol.* 38:249–253.

Cha, Y., and C. G. Pitt. 1989. The acceleration of degradation-controlled drug delivery from polyester microspheres. *J. Control. Rel.* 8:259–265.

Chandrashekar, G., and N. Udupa. 1996. Biodegradable injectable implant systems for long-term drug delivery using poly (lactic-co-glycolic) acid copolymers. *J Pharm Pharmacol.* 48:669–674.

Christel, P. S., M. Vert, F. Chabot, Y. Abols, and J. L. Leary. 1983. Polylactic acid for intramedullary plugging. In *Biomaterials and biomechanics,* vol. 5, edited by P. Ducheyne. Amsterdam: Elsevier Science Publishers, pp. 1–6.

Cleek, R. L., A. A. Rege, L. A. Denner, S. G. Eskin, and A. G. Mikos. 1997. Inhibition of smooth muscle cell growth in vitro by an antisense oligodeoxynucleotide released from poly(DL-lactic-co-glycolic acid) microparticles. *J. Biomed. Mater. Res.* 35:525–530.

Cleland, J. L. 1997. Protein delivery from biodegradable microspheres. *Pharm Biotechnol.* 10:1–43.

Cohen, S., T. Yoshioka, M. Lucarelli, L. H. Hwang, and R. Langer. 1991. Controlled delivery system for protein based on poly(lactic/glycolic acid) microspheres. *Pharm. Res.* 8:713–720.

Couvreur, P., M. J. Blanco-Prieto, F. Puisieux, B. Roques, and E. Fattal. 1997. Multiple emulsion technology for the design of microspheres containing peptides and oligopeptides. *Adv. Drug Deliv. Rev.* 28:85–96.

Crotts, G., and T. P. Park. 1997. Stability and release of bovine serum albumin encapsulated within poly(D,L lactide-co-glycolide) microparticles. *J. Control. Rel.* 44:123–134.

Cutright, D. E., J. D. Beasley, and B. Perez. 1971. Histologic comparison of polylactic and polyglycolic acid sutures. *J. Oral Surg.* 32:165–173.

Cutright, D. E., E. Perez, J. D. Beasley, W. J. Larson, and W. R. Posey. 1974. Degradation of poly (lactic acid) polymer and co-polymers of poly (glycolic acid). *J. Oral. Surg.* 37:142–152.

De Lustro, F., R. A. Condell, M. A. Nguyen, and J. M. McPherson. 1986. A comparative study of the biologic and immunologic response to medical devices derived from dermal collagen. *J. Biomed. Mat. Res.* 20:109–120.

De Lustro, F., J. Dasch, J. Keefe, and L. Ellingsworth. 1990. Immune response to allogenic and xenogenic implants of collagen and collagen derivatives. *Clin. Orthop.* 260:263–279.

Deyme, M., G. Spenlehauer, and J. P. Benoit. 1992. Percolation and release of cisplatin-loaded in poly(lactide-co-glycolide) microspheres for chemoembolization. *J. Bioact. Com. Polym.* 7:150–160.

Fong, J. W., J. P. Nazareno, J. E. Pearson, and H. V. Maulding. 1986. Evaluation of biodegradable microspheres prepared by a solvent evaporation process using sodium oleate as emulsifier. *J. Control. Rel.* 3:119–130.

Gilding, D., and A. M. Reed. 1979. Biodegradable polymers for use in surgery-polyglycolic/poly(lactic acid) homo- and copolymers. *Polymers* 20:1459–1464.

Gupta, P. K., H. Johnson, and C. Allexon. 1993. In vitro and in vivo evaluation of clarithromycin/poly(lactic acid) microspheres for intramuscular drug delivery. *J. Control. Rel.* 26:229–238.

Gupta, P. K., R. C. Mehta, R. H. Douglas, and P. P. De Luca. 1992. In vivo evaluation of biodegradable progesterone microspheres in Mares. *Pharm. Res.* 9:1502-1506.

Heller, J. 1984. Biodegradable polymers in controlled drug delivery. *CRC Crit. Rev. Ther. Drug Carrier Syst.* 1:30–90.

Herrmann, J., and R. Bodmeier. 1995. Somatostatin containing biodegradable microspheres prepared by a modified solvent evaporation method based on W/O/W-multiple emulsions. *Int. J. Pharm.* 126:129–138.

Heya, T., H. Okada, Y. Tanigawara, Y. Ogawa, and H. Toguchi. 1991. Effects of counteranion of TRH and loading amount on control of TRH release from copoly(dl-lactic/glycolic acid) microspheres prepared by an in-water drying method. *Int. J. Pharm.* 69:69–75.

Jalil, R., and J. R. Nixon. 1990. Microencapsulation using poly(DL-lactic acid) III: Effect of polymer molecular weight on the release kinetics. *J. Microencapsulation* 7:357–374.

Jeffery, H., S. S. Davis, and D. T. O'Hagan. 1991. The preparation and characterization of poly(lactide-co-glycolide) microparticles. I. Oil-in-water emulsion solvent evaporation. *Int. J. Pharm.* 77:169–175.

Jeffery, H., S. S. Davis, and O'Hagan D. T. 1993. The preparation and characterization of poly(lactide-co-glycolide) microparticles. II. The entrapment of a model protein using a (water-in-oil-in-water) emulsion solvent evaporation technique. *Pharm. Res.* 10:362–368.

Jones, D. H., S. Corris, S. McDonald, J. C. Clegg, and G. H. Farrar. 1997. Poly(DL-lactide-co-glycolide)-encapsulated plasmid DNA elicits systemic and mucosal antibody responses to encoded protein after oral administration. *Vaccine* 15:814–817.

Jones, E. 1996. Methylene chloride—an overview of human and environmental effects. *Pharmaceutical Technology Europe* 8:30–32.

King, D. J., and R. R. Noss. 1989. Toxicity of polyacrylamide and acrylamide monomer. *Rev. Environ. Health* 8:3–16.

Kulkarni, R. K., E. G. Moore, A. F. Hegyeli, and F. Leonard. 1971. Biodegradable poly(lactic acid) polymers. Biodegradable poly(lactic acid) polymers. *J. Biomed. Mat. Res.* 5:169–181.

Leo, E., S. Pecquet, J. Rojas, P. Couvreur, and E. Fattal. 1998. Changing the pH of the external aqueous phase may modulate protein entrapment and delivery from poly(lactide-co-glycolide) microspheres prepared by a w/o/w solvent evaporation method. *J. Microencapsulation* 15:421–430.

Lewis, D. H. 1990. Controlled release of bioactive agents from lactide/glycolide polymers. In *Biodegradable polymers as drug delivery systems: Drugs and the pharmaceutical sciences,* edited by M. Chasin and R. Langer. New York: Marcel Dekker, pp. 1–41.

Li, S. M., and M. Vert. 1994. Morphological changes resulting from the hydrolytic degradation pf stereocopolymers derived from L- and DL-lactides. *Macromolecules* 27:1307–1310.

Liu, W. R., R. Langer, and A. M. Klibanov. 1991. Moisture-induced aggregation of lyophilized proteins in the solid state. *Biotech. Bioeng.* 37:177–184.

Marcotte, N.. and M. F. A. Goosen. 1989. Delayed release of water-soluble macromolecules from polylactide pellets. *J. Control. Rel.* 9:75–85.

Matlaga, B. F., L. P. Yasenchak, and T. N. Salhouse. 1976. Tissue response to implanted polymers: the significance of shape. *J. Biomed. Mater. Res.* 10:391–397.

Matsusue, Y., T. Yamamuro, M. Oka, Y. Shikinami, S. H. Hyon, and Y. Ikada. 1992. In vitro and in vivo studies on bioabsorbable ultra-high-strength poly(L-lactide) rods. *J. Biomed. Mat. Res.* 26:1553–1567.

Maulding, H. V., T. R. Tice, D. R. Cowsar, J. W. Fong, J. E. Pearson, and J. P. Nazareno. 1986. Biodegradable microcapsules: Acceleration of polymeric excipient hydrolytic rate by incorporation of a basic medicament. *J. Control. Rel.* 3:103–117.

Maulding, H. V. 1987. Prolonged delivery of peptides by microcapsules. In *Advances in drug delivery systems*, vol. 3, edited by J. M. Anderson and S. W. Kim. Amsterdam: Elsevier Science Publishers, pp. 167-176.

Mestiri, M., F. Puisieux, and J. P. Benoit. 1993. Preparation and characterization of cisplatin-loaded polymethyl methacrylate microspheres. *Int. J. Pharm.* 89:229–234.

Nakamura, T., Y. Shimizu, N. Okumura, Matsui T., S. H. Hyon, and T. Shimamoto. 1994. Tumorigenicity of poly-L-lactide (PLLA) plates compared with medical-grade polyethylene. *J. Biomed. Mater. Res.* 28:17–25.

Nihant, N., C. Schugens, C. Grandfils, R. Jêrome, and P. Teyssié. 1994. Polylactide microparticles prepared by double emulsion/evaporation technique. I. Effect of primary emulsion stability. *Pharm. Res.* 11:1479–1484.

Ogawa, Y., M. Yamamoto, H. Okada, T. Yashiki, and T. Shimamoto. 1988a. A new technique to efficiently entrap leuprolide acetate into microcapsules of polylactic acid or copoly(lactic/glycolic) acid. *Chem. Pharm. Bull.* 36:1095–1103.

Ogawa, Y., H. Okada, M. Yamamoto, and T. Shimamoto. 1988b. In vivo profiles of leuprolide acetate from microcapsules prepared with polylactic acids or copoly(lactic/glycolic) acids and in vivo degradation of these polymers. *Chem. Pharm. Bull.* 36:2576–2581.

Ogawa, Y., H. Okada, T. Heya, and T. Shimamoto. 1989. Controlled Release of LHRH agonist, leuprolide acetate from microspheres: Serum drug level profiles and pharmacological effects in animals. *J. Pharm. Pharmacol.* 41:439–444.

O'Hagan, D. T., H. Jeffery, and S. S. Davis. 1994. The preparation and characterization of poly(lactide-co-glycolide) microparticles: III. Microparticle/polymer degradation rates and the in vitro release of a model protein. *Int. J. Pharm.* 103:37–45.

Okada, H., Y. Inoue, T. Heya, H. Ueno, Y. Ogawa, and H. Toguchi. 1991. Pharmacokinetics for once-a-month injectable microspheres of leuprolide acetate. *Pharm. Res.* 8:787-791.

Okada, H., Y. Doken, Y. Ogawa, and H. Toguchi. 1994. Preparation of three-month depot injectable microspheres of leuprolin acetate using biodegradable polymers. *Pharm. Res.* 11:1143–1147.

Okada, H., and H. Toguchi. 1995. Biodegradable microspheres in drug delivery. *Crit. Rev. Ther. Drug Carrier Sys.* 12:1–99.

Parikh, B. V., S. M. Upadrashta, S. H. Neau, and N. O. Nuessle. 1993. Oestrone loaded poly(l-lactic acid) microspheres: Preparation, evaluation and in vitro release kinetics. *J. Microencapsulation* 10:141–153.

Park, T. G., W. Lu, and G. Crotts. 1995. Importance of in vitro experimental conditions on protein release kinetics, stability and polymer degradation in protein encapsulated poly(D,L-lactic acid-co-glycolic acid) microspheres. *J. Control. Rel.* 33:211–222.

Roske-Nielsen, E., M. Bojsen-Moller, M. Vetner, and J. C. Hansen. 1976. Polyvinylpyrrolidone-storage disease. *Acta Pathol. Microbiol. Scand., Sect. A.* 84:397–401.

Rozema, F. R., R. R. M. Bos, G. Boering, J. A. A. M. Van Asten, A. J. Nijenhuls, and A. J. Pennings. 1991. The effects of different steam-sterilization programs on material properties of poly(L-lactide). *J. Appl. Biomater.* 2:23–28.

Ruiz, J. M., B. Tissier, and J. P. Benoit. 1989. Microencapsulation of peptide: a study of the phase separation of poly(DL-lactic acid-co-glycolic acid) copolymers. *Int. J. Pharm.* 49:69–77.

Sah, H., R. Toddywala, and Y. W. Chien. 1994. The influence of biodegradable microcapsule formulations on the controlled release of a protein. *J. Control. Rel.* 30:201–211.

Sanders, L. M., G. I. Mc Rae, K. M. Vitale, and B. A. Kell. 1985. Controlled delivery of an LHRH analogue from biodegradable injectable microspheres. *J. Control. Rel.* 2:187–195.

Sansdrap, P., and A. J. Moes. 1993. Influence of manufacturing parameters on the size characteristics and the release profiles of nifedipine from poly(DL-lactide-co-glycolide) microspheres. *Int. J. Pharm.* 98:157–164.

Santavirta, S., Y. T. Konttinen, and T. Saito. 1990. Immune response to polyglycolic acid implants. *J. Bone Joint Surg.* 72B:597–600.

Spenlehauer, G., M. Veillard, and J. P. Benoit. 1986. Formation and characterization of cisplatin loaded poly(d,l lactide) microspheres for chemoembolization. *J. Pharm. Sci.* 75:750–755.

Spenlehauer, G., M. Vert, J. P. Benoit, F. Chabot, and M. Veillard. 1988. Biodegradable cisplatin microspheres prepared by the solvent evaporation method: Morphology and release characteristics. *J. Control. Rel.* 7:217–229.

Spenlehauer, G., M. Vert, J. P. Benoit, and A. Bodaert. 1989. In vitro and in vivo degradation of poly(D,L lactide/glycolide) type microspheres made by the solvent evaporation method. *Biomaterials* 10:557–563.

Tabata, Y., and Y. Ikada. 1988. Macrophage phagocytosis of biodegradable microspheres composed of L-lactic/glycolic acid homo- and copolymers. *J. Biomed. Mat. Res.* 22:837–858.

Taylor, M. S., A. U. Daniels, K. P. Andriano, and J. Heller. 1994. Six bioabsorbable polymers: In vitro acute toxicity of accumulated degradation products. *J. Appl. Biomater.* 5:151–157.

Van Sliedgert, A., C. A. Van Blitterswijk, S. C. Hesseling, J. J. Grotte, and K. De Groot. 1990. The effect of the molecular weight of polylactic acid on in vitro compatibility. *Adv. Biomater.* 9:207–212.

Van Sliedgert, A., M. Radder, K. De Groot, and C. A. Van Blitterswijk. 1992. In vitro biocompatibility testing of polylactides. Part I: Proliferation of different cell types. *J. Mater. Sci.: Mater. Med.* 3:365–370.

Vink, P., and K. Pleijser. 1986. Aeration of ethylene oxide-sterilized polymers. *J. Biomaterials* 7:225–230.

Visscher, G. E., R. L. Robinson, H. V. Maulding, J. W. Fong, J. E. Pearson, and G. J. Argentieri. 1985. Biodegradation of and tissue reaction to 50:50 poly(DL-lactide-co-glycolide) microcapsules. *J. Biomed. Mat. Res.* 19:349–365.

Visscher, G. E., R. L. Robinson, H. V. Maulding, J. W. Fong, J. E. Pearson, and G. J. Argentieri. 1986. Biodegradation of and tissue reaction to poly(DL-lactide) microcapsules. *J. Biomed. Mat. Res.* 20:667–676.

Wakiyama, N., K. Juni, and M. Nakano. 1981. Preparation and evaluation in vitro of polylactic acid microspheres containing local anaesthetics. *Chem. Pharm. Bull.* 29:3363–3368.

Wakiyama, N., K. Juni, and M. Nakano. 1982. Preparation and evaluation in vitro and in vivo of polylactic acid microspheres containing dibucaine. *Chem. Pharm. Bull.* 30:3710–3727.

Weiss, W. M., T. S. Riles, T. H. Gouge, and H. H. Mizrachi. 1991. Angiosarcoma at the site of a Dacron vascular prosthesis: A case report and literature review. *J. Vasc. Surg.* 14:87–91.

Yamaguchi, K., and J. M. Anderson. 1992. Biocompatibility studies of naltrexone sustained release formulations. *J. Control. Rel.* 19:299-314.

Yamamoto, M., S. Takada, and Y. Ogawa. 1985. Method for producing microcapsule. Japan Patent #22978 .

Yan, C., J. H. Resau, J. Hewetson, M. West, W. L. Rill, and M. Kende. 1994. Characterization and morphological analysis of protein-loaded poly(lactide-co-glycolide) microparticles prepared by water-in-oil-in-water emulsion technique. *J. Control. Rel.* 32:231–241.

Yoshida, S. H., C. C. Chang, S. S. Teuber, and M. E. Gershwin. 1993. Silicone and silicone: Theoretical and clinical implications of breast implants. *Regul. Toxicol. Pharmacol.* 17:3–18.

16

Emulsions

Pramod K. Gupta

TAP Holdings, Inc.
Deerfield, Illinois

John B. Cannon

Abbott Laboratories
North Chicago, Illinois

Emulsions are pharmaceutical dosage forms that can be used topically, orally, and/or parenterally. Control of the viscosity in emulsion formulations permits their development as free-flowing liquids to semisolid creams. Unlike solutions for oral or parenteral administrations, which are usually homogeneous one-phase systems or molecular dispersions, emulsions are colloidal dispersions of at least two immiscible phases stabilized with the aid of a third component, usually referred to as the emulsifying agent. This attribute of emulsions has offered unique scope for their application in pharmaceutical drug delivery. For example, emulsions offer an opportunity to deliver immiscible phases in a reliable and reproducible manner. Hence, if a medicament could be dissolved in a small (or dispersed) phase of formulation, and if this phase could be suspended in a larger (or continuous) phase in a physically stable manner, the resulting system would allow delivery of medicament without being adversely affected by the larger (or continuous) phase.

Emulsions, either oil-in-water (o/w) or water-in-oil (w/o), generally have droplet diameters of less than 200 nm, and thus are opaque or milky in appearance. Oil-in-water emulsions have been used for quite some time as intravenous (IV) nutritional mixtures. These are generally emulsions of soybean, sesame, or safflower oil (10–20 percent) emulsified with phospholipids, e.g., egg lecithin containing 60–70 percent phosphatidylcholine (PC). Lipsoyn® and Intralipid® are two examples of the most widely used total parenteral emulsions. Studies have shown that the soybean emulsion can be substituted for glucose to supply one- to two-thirds of the total calories, and they can be administered peripherally without significant vein irritation (Hansen et al. 1975). Multiple (e.g., w/o/w) emulsions can also be prepared, but these are less widely used in pharmaceutical applications. A general description of the methods of preparing emulsions, and their physical-chemical properties, has been recently reviewed (Gupta and Cannon 1998).

The use of emulsion formulations in parenteral drug delivery is usually based on one or more of the following fundamental facts:

- The drug has high a log *P* value, i.e., the drug prefers to partition into lipophilic versus aqueous media. For example, o-alky-N-aryl thiocarbamate has poor solubility in water or water-containing cosolvents; however, its solubility is two to three orders of magnitude higher in oils (Strickley and Anderson 1993).

- The drug is marginally soluble in lipophilic media; however, the solubilization can be improved with the aid of excipients. For example, the solubility of clarithromycin has been increased with the aid of counterions like hexanoic and oleic acid (Lovell et al. 1994).

- The drug partitioning into the lipophilic phase can be retained over time regardless of normal handling and storage conditions.

- The drug's solubilization and delivery using emulsions does not alter its stability, efficacy, and/or safety.

Conformance to one or more of the above criteria generally qualifies development of emulsion formulations for drugs that otherwise cannot be successfully administered orally or parenterally. However, this chapter mainly focuses on demonstrating the usefulness of emulsion systems for improved drug efficacy and patient compliance upon parenteral administration, i.e., reduced pain and/or irritation after parenteral delivery. Several supportive experimental and clinical examples are included. Finally, some of the challenges encountered in developing these formulations are also discussed.

RATIONALE OF USING EMULSIONS FOR REDUCING PAIN AND IRRITATION UPON INJECTION

When an emulsion formulation is administered parenterally, the body is first exposed to the larger external or continuous phase. Subsequent physical disruption of the emulsion releases the smaller internal or dispersed phase of the formulation. Only then is the medicament contained in the internal phase of the emulsion exposed to the body. This process, in turn, provides an opportunity to minimize any sudden unpleasant painful and/or irritating property of the drug to the body, which is generally encountered after drug administration as a solution. The success of this process depends, among others, on the following factors:

- The relative solubility of the drug in hydrophilic versus lipohilic phases: Generally, the higher the log *P* value, the higher the probability that an emulsion formulation would reduce pain/irritation upon injection. At times, it may be advantageous to enchance intrinsic log *P* by the aid of approved excipients (i.e., increase the drug's solubility in the oil phase).

- The ratio of lipophilic versus hydrophilic phases: The reduction in the lipophilic phase volume of the emulsion is known to improve its physical stability. Hence, if log *P* is relatively high, the reduction in the lipophilic phase reduces exposure of the body to the delivered painful/irritating drug.

- The droplet size: The importance of the droplet size of an emulsion on pain/irritation stems from the correlation between droplet size and surface area, and the correlation between surface area of droplets and exposure of the drug to the body. This complex issue should be carefully balanced, since droplet size may influence the process of product sterilization (i.e., filtration vs. heat application), physical stability, and also drug partitioning to the hydrophilic phase.

POTENTIAL MECHANISMS OF PAIN ON INJECTION

The rationale behind using emulsions to decrease the pain on injection of drugs can also be considered in relation to the causal mechanisms of pain on injection. These can be classified into osmotic or hemolytic effects, precipitation or crystallization effects, and inherent drug-receptor effects. Pain normally associated with certain drugs may be more a function of the formulation conventionally used with the drug (because of solubilization requirements); i.e., a given formulation may give pain on injection even for placebo formulation. Osmotic effects fall into this category; if a drug has sufficiently low aqueous solubility such that a conventional formulation requires high organic solvent content (e.g., ethanol and/or propylene glycol), the resulting hyperosmolarity will cause hemolysis and pain on injection. Emulsion droplets generally contribute little to the osmolarity of a mixture, and it is possible to design emulsions that are isotonic and yet can incorporate large amounts of a drug, unlike cosolvent-based systems. For example, conventional formulations of etomidate in propylene glycol are over

2,000 mosmol/L even after dilution for injection, whereas an etomidate lipid emulsion was 400 mosmol/L (Doenicke et al. 1992). Similarly, the conventional lorazepam formulation (Ativan®) in propylene glycol caused over 95 percent hemolysis in human blood, while a lorazepam emulsion resulted in only 9 percent hemolysis. The organic solvent and emulsion vehicles alone yielded 98 percent and 6 percent hemolysis, respectively (Yalin et al. 1997). Surfactant-based formulations can also be hemolytic, whereas emulsions can be generally relatively benign in this regard. In some cases, the drug itself is hemolytic, due to interactions of the drug with red blood cell membranes. Amphotericin B is such a drug, and it is occasionally observed to cause pain at the injection site (PDR 1996). Incorporation of a drug into the oil phase of an emulsion will decrease the concentration of that drug available to interact with red blood cell membranes.

Another possible cause of pain on injection for conventional formulations is precipitation of a drug in the blood after injection due to dilution of the cosolvent or surfactant in the formulation. It has been proposed that the resulting microcrystals may cause irritation and pain in the blood vessel walls (Yalkowsky et al. 1983). If, instead, the drug is solubilized into the internal phase of an emulsion, dilution will generally not cause its precipitation. If any repartitioning occurs between the emulsion droplet and the external aqueous media upon dilution, it will still be below the solubility limit in the aqueous media.

A final and probably much narrower mechanism for pain on injection would be specific interactions of the drug with pain receptors in the blood vessel walls. In this case, incorporation into the internal phase of an emulsion protects the offending moieties of the drug molecule from the receptors.

Examples of the rationales for decreasing pain on injection outlined above will be discussed in the sections that follow, although it must be remembered that it is frequently impossible to determine which mechanism for eliciting pain is most important for a given drug. A combination of effects may be operating.

CASE STUDIES

Propofol (Diprivan®)

One drug for which there is considerable data on pain on injection for emulsion formulations is propofol (2,6-diisopropylphenol). This rapidly acting anesthetic is lipophilic (log P = 3.8), has a molecular weight of 178.3 and a melting point of 19°C, and is very slightly soluble in water. Propofol was originally formulated in a Cremophor® EL vehicle, but anaphylactic reactions due to this solubilizer led to withdrawal of this product. Thus, propofol is now formulated as an emulsion (Diprivan® of Zeneca

Pharmaceuticals), containing 10 mg/mL of propofol along with 10 percent soybean oil, 1.2 percent egg lecithin as emulsifier, 2.25 percent glycerol to adjust tonicity, and 0.005 percent disodium edetate. The Diprivan® injectable emulsion is isotonic and has a pH of 7 to 8.5. Although anesthesia generally occurs within 40 sec from the start of injection, pain on injection is sometimes observed. An early report indicated that 8 out of 12 patients showed severe pain on injection into a hand vein (Hynynen et al. 1985). Pain is particularly evident in pediatric patients if small veins (e.g., of the hand) are used; there was a 45 percent incidence of pain in these cases (PDR 1996). However, the pain is minimized (to < 10 percent incidence) by using larger veins (e.g., in the forearm or antecubital fossa). Alternatively, pretreatment by IV injection of 1 mL of a 1 percent lidocaine (lignocaine) solution is also recommended to reduce the pain on injection to less than 10 percent incidence (PDR 1996). McCulloch and Lees (1985) performed a study examining the effects of site of injection and lignocaine pretreatment in 3 groups of adult patients (40 each) receiving 2.5 mg/kg Diprivan® intravenously. Of the group receiving the drug in the dorsum of the hand, 37.5 percent showed pain on injection, whereas only 2.5 percent of those receiving the drug in the forearm or antecubital fossa felt pain—a significant difference ($p < 0.001$). Pretreatment with 10 mg lidocaine before administration of propofol into the dorsum of the hand gave 17.5 percent of the group pain on injection, but this difference was not statistically different from those with no pretreatment. Thus, choice of the injection site (large veins vs. small veins) is the more important factor. Premixing the lidocaine into the propofol infusion is an alternative to pretreatment and somewhat reduces the pain on injection (Dundee and Clarke 1989). It has been shown that the addition of 0.05 percent lidocaine to the emulsion is optimal (Tham and Khoo 1995).

The mechanism by which propofol causes pain on injection appears to be a direct interaction between propofol molecules and pain receptors in the veins. This is suggested by the facts that Diprivan® is isotonic, and that propofol is a liquid at room temperature. This goes against osmotic and precipitation effects, respectively, for the occasional pain on injection observed with Diprivan®. There are no reports of propofol causing hemolysis; in fact, administration to cats resulted in no hemolysis (Andress et al. 1995). Results for pain on injection with the older Cremophor-based propofol formulation are similar to those detailed above for Diprivan®, in that 30–80 percent of patients complained of pain when the drug was injected into the hand vein, whereas this was reduced to 3–30 percent when larger veins were used (Rutter et al. 1980; Briggs et al. 1982). This is also consistent with a direct interaction of propofol with pain receptors.

More direct evidence for this mechanism is offered by the studies of Klement and Arndt (1991) and of Doenicke et al. (1996), who independently hypothesized that it is the free (aqueous) concentration of the drug that is responsible for the pain on injection. For the 1 percent propofol in the

Diprivan® formulation, this value is 19 µg/mL (Doenicke et al. 1996), and it can be decreased by increasing the lipid content of the vehicle because of repartitioning of the drug into the lipid phase. Klement and Arndt (1991) observed that dilution of Diprivan® in 10 percent Intralipid® fat emulsion was more effective in decreasing pain on injection than dilution in 5 percent glucose, and the pain on injection was directly related to the propofol concentration (Klement and Arndt 1991). Similarly, Doenicke et al. (1996) examined the role of lipid dilution by administering different propofol formulations into the hand veins of 3 groups of 12 patients each. Group A received 10 mL Diprivan® diluted with 10 mL of saline; Group B received 10 mL Diprivan® diluted with 5 mL of a long-chain triglyceride (LCT) fat emulsion and 5 mL of saline; and Group C received 10 mL Diprivan® diluted with 10 mL of LCT fat emulsion. The propofol emulsion was injected over a 30–60 sec period into a dorsal vein of the hand. In group A, 67 percent of the patients reported moderate or severe pain on injection, whereas only mild pain was reported in 50 percent of the patients in group C. This supports the conclusion that addition of more lipid to the formulation leads to a repartitioning of the drug into the lipid phase of the emulsion, which in turn decreases the amount of drug in the aqueous phase available for causing pain on injection. This also suggests that in patients for which pain on injection is a problem, dilution of Diprivan® in a parenteral lipid emulsion, such as Intralipid® or Liposyn®, may be a useful technique to decrease pain on injection.

Diazepam

The IV administration of diazepam has warranted the use of propylene glycol and ethanol to aid drug dissolution (see composition in Table 16.1). However, the use of such drug solutions has been known to cause high incidences of pain, thrombophlebitis, erythema, edema, necrosis, and/or inflammation of the surrounding tissue. To minimize these unpleasent side effects, o/w emulsion formulations of this drug have been explored (see representative composition in Table 16.1).

Among the first few studies to thoroughly evaluate the acceptability of a diazepam emulsion formulation is one in which 314 patients received this product intravenously. The results were compared with a group of 63 patients that received a cosolvent-based drug solution. Whereas 1 patient in the emulsion group (0.3 percent) reported pain on injection, 22 patients (34.9 percent) receiving drug solution reported similar pain (see Table 16.2) (Van Dardel et al. 1976). In another study, 247 patients randomly received IV injections of either diazepam solution or diazepam emulsion prior to routine upper gastrointestinal endoscopy. During the first week, both treatments resulted in comparable local symptoms. However, in the 3 to 7 weeks after dosing, 25 percent of patients receiving solution indicated objective thrombosis as opposed to only 3.6 percent patients in the emulsion group,

Table 16.1. Composition of Hydroalcoholic (Valium®) and Emulsion Formulation of Diazepam (Diazemuls®)

Valium®		Diazemuls®	
Diazepam	5 mg	Diazepam	5 mg
Propylene glycol	414.4 mg	Soyabean oil	150 mg
Ethanol	80.6 mg	Acetyl monoglycerides	50 mg
Sodium benzoate	48.8 mg	Phospholipids	12 mg
Benzoic acid	1.2 mg	Glycerol	22 mg
Benzyl alcohol	15.7 mg	Water for Injection to	1 mL
Water for Injection to	1 mL		

Adapted from Von Dardel et al. (1983).

Table 16.2. Patient Reaction upon Intravenous Injection of Diazepam in Hydroalcoholic Solution (Valium®) and Emulsion Formulation

Reaction	Percent of Patients with Reaction	
	Valium® ($n = 63$)*	Emulsion ($n = 314$)**
No reaction	22.2	94.6
Discomfort	42.9	5.1
Pain	34.9	0.3

*Dose = 7.67 mg (range: 5 to 20 mg)

**Dose = 8.82 mg (range: 2.5 to 20 mg)

Adapted from Von Dardel et al. (1976).

which indicated similar symptoms ($p = 0.0018$) (Glesson et al. 1983). Several other studies have reported similar findings, supporting the use of diazepam emulsion over its solution formulations. For example, in one study, the emulsion formulation was reported to be painful in 13.5 percent of patients ($n = 35$) as opposed to 67.7 percent of patients who experienced pain following the IV administration of a glycoferol-based aqueous drug solution ($n = 31$). In addition, 2.7 and 22.6 percent of patients in the respective groups reported occurrence of thrombophlebitis (Selander et al. 1981). In another study involving 20 patients, IV dosing of diazepam emulsion was found to be significantly less painful ($p < 0.01$) than drug solution in ethyl ether and glycofurolium (Kromann et al. 1982). In a study by Bullimore (1982), 11 out of 47 patients undergoing endoscopy who received Valium®

reported moderate to severe pain on injection. However, none of the 58 patients receiving a comparable drug dose as emulsion (15 mg) reported such pain.

From 1975 to 1980, diazepam emulsion was tested in 9,492 patients without incidence of serious side effects. In this study, 2,435 patients were specifically evaluated with respect to pain and clinical effect. Whereas the intended clinical effect was observed in 99 percent of patients, pain was experienced in only 0.4 percent of patients (Van Dardel et al. 1983). Following intramuscular (IM) administration in groups of 30 patients, 6.7 and 43.3 percent of patients reported pain following emulsion and solution administrations (see Table 16.3). The plasma concentration profiles were comparable after IV administration of the two formulations. However, after IM administration, the emulsion formulation yielded peak drug concentrations that were about half of those estimated with the solution formulation.

One recent study compared the venous sequelae (i.e., change in color and/or thickness of the injected vein along with erythema, edema, necrosis and/or inflammation of the surrounding tissue) following injection of 0.3 mg/kg diazepam through the ear vein of rabbits as a 5 mg/mL o/w emulsion or 5 mg/mL hydroalcoholic solution. The results of the induction of venous sequelae were compared using saline as a negative control. The emulsion was found to cause significant reduction in local tissue reactions as compared to the hydroalcoholic formulation of diazepam ($p = 0.05$; see Figure 16.1). No statistically significant difference was observed in local tissue reaction with saline and the emulsion formulation. The scoring results were confirmed pathologically. Overall, the results suggested that avoidance of irritating solubilizing agents in the formulation and minimization of drug precipitation in vivo may reduce local tissue reactions (Levy et al. 1989).

Table 16.3. Patient Reaction on Intramuscular Injection of 5 mg/mL Diazepam in Hydroalcoholic Solution (Valium®) and Emulsion Formulation (Diazemuls®)

Reaction	Percent of Patients with Reaction	
	Valium® (*n* = 30)*	Diazemuls® (*n* = 30)**
No reaction	30	70
Slight discomfort	26.6	23.3
Pain	43.3	6.7

Adapted from Von Dardel et al. (1983).

Figure 16.1. Mean venous sequelae scores after IV injection of saline emulsion containing diazepam and hydroalcoholic solution of diazepam to rabbits. The increase in score is indicative of increased severity of drug reaction. Bars refer to standard deviation; *indicates significant difference from control ($p < 0.05$). Adapted from Levy et al. (1989).

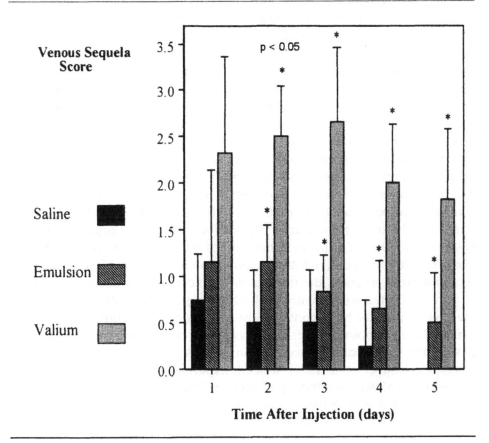

Generally, following IV administration, emulsion formulations demonstrate plasma profiles similar to those obtained with other solubilized formulations (e.g., micelles and cosolvent systems). However, some studies have reported controversial results. For example, one study reported significant differences in the pharmacokinetics of diazepam delivered as an emulsion (Diazemuls®) and in solubilized form (Valium®) (Fee et al. 1984). However, another study failed to find significant pharmacokinetic differences among these formulations in humans. In 8 healthy volunteers, the maximum drug concentrations (Cmax) as well as area under the plasma drug concentration versus time curve (AUC) over 60 min after dosing were found to be comparable for the two formulations (Naylor and Burlingham 1985).

Etomidate

Like diazepam, etomidate is insoluble in aqueous media and, hence, cosolvents have been used to enable its parenteral delivery. However, such formulations have been found to be painful on injection. In order to confirm this possibility, one study compared pain on injection and venous sequalae after IV injection of a propylene glycol–based drug solution and emulsion formulation in groups of 50 patients. Almost 36 percent of patients receiving the drug solution experienced pain on injection. On the first postoperative day, 19 percent of patients indicated phlebitis and 6 percent indicated thrombosis. Significant venous reaction was evident in 22 percent of patients, even up to 7 days after solution dosing. However in the group receiving the emulsion formulation, neither pain nor venous reaction was observed (Doenicke et al. 1990).

Pain on injection of propylene glycol–based etomidate solution has been hypothesized to be associated with the extremely high osmolality of this formulation. In order to gain better insight into this possibility, one study monitored serum haptoglobin in 12 healthy volunteers after administration of 0.3 mg/kg etomidate. Six subjects reveived propylene glycol–based drug solution with an osmolality of 4,965 mosmol/kg, and the remaining 6 subjects received drug in emulsion (400 mosmol/kg). In patients receiving drug solution, the haptoglobin concentrations decreased almost 40 percent from baseline within 2 h of dosing and were 27 percent lower than baseline at 24 h. In contrast, the emulsion formulation resulted in a maximal haptoglobin concentration reduction of 10.5 percent; at 24 h after dosing, the haptoglobin concentration was 4.4 percent above the baseline estimate (Nebayer et al. 1992). Indeed, hyperosmolar solutions have been suggested to affect the integrity of cells and may trigger the release of mediators. In vitro studies have indicated histamine release from human basophils exposed to hyperosmolar solutions (Findlay et al. 1981).

Pregnanolone (Eltanolone®)

Pregnanolone is a naturally occuring metabolite of progesterone with good anesthetic properties. However, the clinical utility of this and other steroidal drugs has been hampered due to their limited aqueous solubility and the unpleasant side effects of cosolvent-based formulations. An emulsion formulation of pregnanolone has indicated good promise for its application in therapeutics. One study compared the anesthetic properties of pregnanolone emulsion with existing IV anaesthetic agents (e.g., alphaxolone/alphadolone, propofol, thiopental, and midazolam) in a rat model. The therapeutic index of pregnanolone emulsion was found to be 6–8 times higher than those of propofol, thiopentone, and midazolam. No cumulative effects were observed on repeated administration of the emulsion, and no venous sequalae were observed. Hence, this study indicated that pregnanolone emulsion may provide a short-acting, less cumulative, and less toxic alternative to other anesthetic agents (Hogskilde et al. 1987). Similar results were reported in a study by Larsson-Backstrom et al. (1988), where pregnanolone emulsion was found to be significantly more effective and safer than thiopental.

In another study, pregnanolone emulsion was administered intravenously to 13 healthy volunteers to assess induction of anesthesia. Each subject received 0.5, 0.75 and 1.0 mg/kg of the drug on successive occasions at a constant rate. The injections were painless in all subjects at all doses. The emulsion formulation was found to produce smooth and dose-linear induction of general anesthesia (see Table 16.4), with cardiorespiratory effects comparable to those of other IV induction agents (Gray et al. 1992).

Methohexital and Thiopental

Methohexital (Brevital®) and thiopental (Pentothal®) are both anesthetics of the ultrashort-acting barbiturate class, administered as the sodium salts. Both are known to cause pain on injection in a manner similar to propofol. In a study involving 100 patients for each drug, the number of individuals experiencing pain on injection were 9 and 12 for thiopental and methohexital, respectively (Kawar and Dundee 1992). As with propofol, the incidence of pain was greater when smaller veins were used: 8-fold and 3-fold greater than large veins for thiopental and methohexital, respectively. A methohexital emulsion (1 percent drug in Intralipid®) has been investigated clinically for reduction of pain on injection. For 1 percent methohexital in saline, there was an 87 percent incidence of pain or discomfort on injection when using a small forearm vein, compared to 35 percent for drug in lipid

Table 16.4. Duration of Anesthesia (Time from Start of Induction to Eye Opening and to Head Lift on Command) Following IV Administration of Pregnanolone Emulsion to 11 Subjects

Dose (mg/kg)	Duration (min) (mean ± SD)	
	Eye Opening	Head Lift
0.5	4.68 (1.55)	7.30 (2.50)
0.75	10.95 (3.31)	13.38 (4.11)
1.0	17.69 (3.90)	20.24 (3.44)

Adapted from Gray et al. (1992).

emulsion. The "pain scores" were calculated to be 44.5 versus 0.5 for the saline and emulsion formulations, respectively; the anesthetic potency was not reduced by the emulsion formulation (Westrin et al. 1992). The same methohexital-Intralipid® formulation was found to be effective in children as well, with only 1 out of 75 patients indicating marked pain on injection (Westrin 1992). Thiopental is 2.5 times less potent than methohexital, but it is generally regarded as less likely to cause pain on injection than methohexital.

Amphotericin B

Amphotericin B is a polyene antibiotic well known to cause hemolysis arising from a direct interaction with the erythrocyte membrane and pore formation within the membrane. This is the mechanism of cytotoxicity to fungal cells, for which it shows selectivity relative to mammalian cell membranes. However, it still shows considerable toxicity to mammalian cells. In the conventional Fungizone® formulation with colloidal deoxycholate dispersion, the bile salts tend to exacerbate this hemolytic and cell damage tendency. While the primary side effects of amphotericin B are chills, fever, nephrotoxicity, and central nervous system (CNS) damage, pain on injection has also been reported (PDR 1996). Vein irritation with inflammation and thrombus formation has been documented in the rabbit ear vein model (Hoover et al. 1990). These side effects are probably related to its hemolytic tendencies and similar damage to other cell types.

Several liposomal formulations have recently been examined in clinical trials, one of which (AmBisome® of Nexstar) is marketed in Europe. These have been shown to exhibit a marked decrease in toxicity and side effects and cause less damage to mammalian cells relative to the conventional formulation (Ringden et al. 1991). Emulsions have also been examined as alternatives to decrease the toxicity of amphotericin B. Davis et al. (1987) prepared an emulsion from 20 percent soybean oil and egg lecithin. Fungizone® showed complete hemolysis at amphotericin B concentrations above 12 μg/mL, whereas the amphotericin B emulsion showed no hemolysis even at 16 μg/mL. For an emulsion containing 10 percent soybean oil and 200 μg/mL amphotericin B, there was only 10 percent hemolysis (Forster et al. 1988). Similar trends were observed for cultured canine kidney cell monolayers: Fungizone® led to a loss of monolayer integrity (as measured by electrical resistance) at concentrations as low as 10 μg/mL, while there was no measurable loss of integrity at 100 μg/mL for the amphotericin B emulsion. The formulations were equally efficacious in their antifungal activity to yeast cells (Lamb et al. 1991). Some clinicians have used an extemporaneous emulsion formulation wherein the lyophilized Fungizone® preparation is reconstituted into an Intralipid® or Liposyn® emulsion. There is apparently comparable efficacy but reduced toxicity relative to the conventional Fungizone® formulation reconstituted in dextrose (Chavanet et al. 1992; Moreau et al. 1992). However, there is evidence that such extemporaneous preparations can contain large amounts (up to 95 percent) of precipitated drug (Washington et al. 1993), thus partially negating the benefit of the emulsion formulation, especially with regard to pain reduction.

The mechanisms by which liposomal and emulsion formulations reduce the toxicity of amphotericin B are not completely understood. They are believed to be a combination of several effects: (1) the vehicle affords an increased selectivity toward fungal cells as opposed to mammalian cells, leading to decreased hemolysis and mammalian cell damage; (2) the lipid matrix provides a slow release of the drug, which alleviates the toxic effects; and (3) the liposomal or emulsion particles are taken up by the reticuloendothelial cells of the liver and spleen, which in turn can release the drug back into circulation over an extended period of time. How these mechanisms translate into decrease in pain on injection is not clear. The AmBisome® formulation is reported to cause a decrease in pain on injection relative to Fungizone® (Meunier et al. 1991), but there are no reports on injection pain of amphotericin B emulsions. The decreased hemolysis and cell damage (e.g., to cells of vein walls and nerves) would certainly be expected to lead to a decrease in pain on injection, but definitive data must await further experience in the clinic.

Clarithromycin

The feasibility of emulsion formulation for the delivery of a painful macrolide, clarithromycin, has been evaluated. The currently marketed IV formulation of clarithromycin is known to cause pain on injection. Hence, a 5 mg/mL emulsion formulation was developed. Drug dissolution in the oil phase was facilitated using oleic and hexanoic acids as lipophilic counterions (Lovell et al. 1994). The extent of pain reduction, compared to a lactobionate aqueous solution of drug, was assessed using various animal models, e.g., mouse scratch, rat paw lick, rabbit ear vein irritation, and rat tail vein irritation tests. In the mouse scratch test, the pain with 5 mg/mL emulsion formulation was found to be comparable to 1.6 to 2.7 mg/mL drug solution (see Figure 16.2). In the rat paw-lick test, only 70 percent of the animals receiving the emulsion were found to respond to pain, as opposed to 100 percent of the animals responding to pain after the injection of drug solution. The degree of paw lick (i.e., number of licks per rat and total licking time) was reduced by 50 percent. In vein irritation tests in rabbits and rats, the extent of reaction at the site of injection was significantly lower with emulsion than that with the drug solution. In addition, the emulsion formulation did not alter plasma drug distribution, toxicity, or efficacy of the drug (Lovell et al. 1994).

Figure 16.2. Results of mouse scratch test. Reprinted with permission of Lovell et al. (1994).

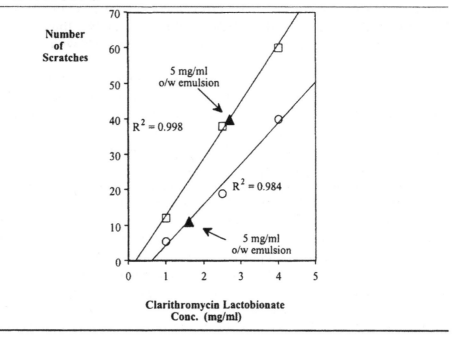

Investigation of the stability of this emulsion indicated a constant reduction in its pH over at least 9 months at 30°C. Nonetheless, it should be noted that emulsions have an intrinsic tendency to undergo hydrolysis resulting in liberation of free fatty acids, which in turn cause a drop in bulk pH over time (Herman and Groves 1992, 1993). This is particularly true for emulsions utilizing phosphatides as emulsifying agents. The extent of pH reduction of emulsions depends on the formulation and its storage condition. As can be anticipated, the higher the storage temperature, the higher the rate of hydrolysis, and the greater the reduction in pH. Thus, if the drug incorporated in emulsion is sensitive to pH changes, the hydrolysis of emulsion may result in poor product stability. In the case of clarithromycin emulsion, pH reduction following 30°C storage did not induce significant loss of drug. Real-time studies as well as accelerated stability study suggested that the shelf life of clarithromycin emulsion at 25°C was greater than or equal to 21 months (Lovell et al. 1995). These studies together suggest that use of emulsion techniques allows development of stable, less-painful formulations of otherwise painful compounds.

Challenges in the Use of Emulsions as Pharmaceutical Dosage Forms

Apart from challenges encountered with conventional formulations (e.g., drug solubility and chemical stability), the development of an emulsion formulation poses additional challenges such as relatively poor physical stability of the product, potential for altered efficacy, and patient compliance.

Physical Stability

The physical stability of emulsion products is perhaps one of the most important characteristics that governs its commercial success. Being a heterogeneous and thermodynamically unstable system, it has a significantly higher tendency to lose its physical stability than other dosage forms. Whereas an optimized emulsion formulation may undergo limited change in particle size upon destabilization, a poorly formulated emulsion has a large probability of particle coalescence and irreversible phase separation in a short time. This, in turn, can effect the efficacy of the delivered drug. The type and concentration of surfactant used to stabilize the emulsion, the phase volume ratio (i.e., ratio of oil vs. aqueous phase), droplet size, compatibility of drug and excipients with the emulsion, and storage condition of the emulsion are critical factors that affect the physical stability of emulsions.

Efficacy

Upon introduction of a drug-containing emulsion into the biological milieu, i.e., into plasma by IV administration, the drug release from emulsion droplets may occur by diffusion. To some extent, the kinetics of this process are governed by such properties as the distribution coefficient of drug between the emulsion oil phase, interface, and external aqueous phases. For treatments warranting immediate efficacy following administration, generally typical of IV dosing, success in the use of an emulsion dosage form requires that all drug in the dispersed phase be released relatively quickly in vivo after administration. In some cases, emulsion formulations have been found to be less efficacious than solution formulation of a drug (Wang et al. 1995). In fact, phospholipid oil-based emulsions resemble chylomicrons, which are rapidly cleared by the liver. Almost 65 percent of exogenously injected chylomicrons are recovered in the liver within 30 min after injection (Van Berkel et al. 1991). Triglycerides are removed and digested by lipoprotein lipases present in the capillary endothelium, and the remnant emulsion droplets are almost completely taken up by the liver within a few hours (Handa et al. 1994). Thus, if the diffusion of drug from the emulsion is slow, then a high uptake of drug by the reticuloendothelial system (RES) cells will be expected. This could have a significant impact on the pharmacokinetics and biodistribution of the emulsified drug, and therapeutic response profile may be altered. Nonetheless, this may be desirable in some cases where the liver and spleen are the therapeutic targets, and/or where subsequent slow release of drug from these sites is desirable, and/or where toxicity of drug to sites of low emulsion uptake would otherwise be a problem. On the other hand, if diffusion of drug from the emulsion is rapid compared to the metabolism and clearance of the emulsion droplets, then the pharmacokinetics and distribution of the drug will be little different from those of aqueous formulations. Under such circumstances, the efficacy of the drug administered as an emulsion is likely to be comparable to its solution form.

Dose Volume

As mentioned earlier, the use of emulsions as a dosage form stems from the fact that drugs can be solubilized in oils. However, depending on the dose of drug, the intrinsic solubility of the drug in oil, and physical and chemical stability, an emulsion with limited drug concentration may not be commercially viable. At times, drug concentrations in emulsion may be in the range that is practical for dosing (e.g., dosing volume = 5 mL for local parenteral administration). However, for large dose compounds, emulsion formulation may require administration of inconveniently large volumes. Hence, this issue should be kept in mind during development of this dosage form. It should be noted, however, that for drugs requiring IV dosing, the administration volume is generally a less critical issue.

Other Issues

Apart from the challenges outlined above, it should be appreciated that the use of emulsions as an injectable warrants an assurance of product sterility. Whereas the Food and Drug Administration (FDA) preferred heat sterilization process is acceptable for total parenteral nutritional (TPN) emulsions, it could affect the chemical as well as physical stability of emulsions containing therapeutic agents. Recently, data supporting the filter sterilization of emulsions have been published. On a separate note, maintenance of acceptable physical and chemical stability of emulsion formulations may warrant storage at 5°C. Upon approval and during marketing, this aspect limits the manufacturing volume, as well as product storage in distribution centers.

Conclusions

Despite several unique attributes of emulsion systems, their development for parenteral or oral use have been much slower. The historical reluctance of the pharmaceutical industry to use emulsions as a formulation tool in oral and parenteral drug delivery perhaps stems from parenteral safety concerns, difficulty in manufacturing, and perceived lack of patient acceptability. However, the scope of pharmaceutical emulsions is likely to grow in the future. Reasons for this observation include efforts in the synthesis of excipients that mimic the property of natural oils previously used in the manufacture of emulsions, design and development of high efficiency processing equipment that allow the formation of relatively stable emulsions with smaller amounts of stabilizers, and better understanding of the in vivo fate of medicaments parenterally administered as emulsions.

References

Andress, J. L., T. K. Day, and D. Day. 1995. The effects of consecutive day propofol anesthesia on feline red blood cells. *Vet. Surg.* 24:277–282.

Briggs, L. P., M. Bahar, H. T. Beers, R. S. J. Clarke, J. W. Dundee, P. J. Wright, D. M. McAuley, and M. P. O'Neill. 1982. The effect of preanesthetic medication on anesthesia with ICI35868. *Br. J. Anesth.* 54:303.

Bullimore, D. W. 1982. A comparison of the incidence of injection pain with two different diazepam formulations—Valium and Diazemuls. *Clin. Ther.* 4:367–368.

Chavanet, P. Y., I. Garry, N. Charlier, D. Caillot, J. P. Kisterman, M. D'Athis, and H. Portier. 1992. Trial of glucose versus fat emulsion in preparation of amphotericin for use in HIV infected patients with candidiasis. *Brit. Med. J.* 305:921–925.

Davis, S. S., C. Washington, P. West, L. Illum, G. Liversidge, L. Sternson, and R. Kirsh. 1987. Lipid emulsions as drug delivery systems. *Ann. NY Acad. Sci.* 507:75–88.

Doenicke, A., A. Kugler, and N. Vollmann. 1990. Venous tolerance to etomidate in lipid emulsion or propylene glycol (hypnomidate). *Can. J. Anaesth.* 37:823–824.

Doenicke, A, A. E. Nebauer, R. Hoernecke, M. Mayer, M. F. Roizen. 1992. Osmolalities of propylene glycol-containing drug formulations for parenteral use. Should propylene glycol be used as a solvent? *Anesth Analg.* 75:431–435.

Doenicke, A. W., M. F. Roizen, J. Rau, W. Kellermann, and J. Babl. 1996. Reducing pain during propofol injection: The role of the solvent. *Anesthesia & Analgesia* 82:472–474.

Dundee, J. W., and R. S. J. Clarke. 1989. Propofol. *Eur. J. Anaesthesiol.* 6:5–22.

Fee, J. P. H., J. W. Dundee, P. S. Collier, and E. McClean. 1984. Bioavailability of intravenous diazepam. *Lancet* 2:813.

Findlay, S. R., A. M. Dvorak, A. Kagey-Sobotka, and L. M. Lichtenstein. 1981. Hyperosmolar triggering of histamine release from human basophils. *J. Clin. Invest.* 67:1604–1613.

Forster, D., C. Washington, and S. S. Davis. 1988. Toxicity of solubilized and colloidal amphotericin B formulations to. human erythrocytes. *J. Pharm. Pharmacol.* 40:325–328.

Glesson, D., J. D. R. Rose, and P. M. Smith. 1983. A prospective randomised controlled trial of diazepam (Valium) vs. emulsified diazepam (Diazemuls) as a premedication for upper gastrointestinal endoscopy. *Br. J. Clin. Pharamcol.* 16:448–450.

Gray, H., B. L. Holt, D. K. Whitaker, and P. Eadsforth. 1992. Preliminary study of a pregnanolone emulsion (Kabi 2213) for i.v. induction of general anesthesia. *Br. J. Anaesth.* 68:272–276.

Gupta, P., and J. Cannon. 1998. Emulsions and microemulsions for drug solubilization. In *Water insoluble drug formulations,* edited by R. Liu. Buffalo Grove, Ill., USA: Interpharm Press, Inc.

Handa, T., Y. Eguchi, and K. Miyajima. 1994. Effects of cholesterol and cholesteryl oleate on lipolysis and liver uptake of triglycerides/phosphatiylcholine emulsions in rats. *Pharm. Res.* 11:1283–1287.

Hansen, L. M., W. Richard Hardie, and J. Hidalgo. 1975. Fat emulsion for intravenous administration: Clinical experience with Intralipid 10 percent. *Ann. Surg.* 184:80–88.

Herman, C. J., and M. J. Groves. 1992. Hydrolysis kinetics of phospholipids in thermally stressed intravenous lipid emulsion formulations. *J. Pharm. Pharmacol.* 44:539–542.

Herman, C. J., and M. J. Groves. 1993. The influence of free fatty acid formation on the pH of phospholipid-stabilized triglyceride emulsions. *Pharm. Res.* 10:774–776.

Hogskilde, S., J. Wagner, P. Carl, and M. Sorenson. 1987. Anesthetic properties of pregnanolone emulsion. *Anaesthesia* 42:1045–1050.

Hoover, D. M., J. B. Gardner, T. L. Timmerman, J. A. Klepfer, D. A. Laska, S. L. White, J. P. McGrath, M. K. Buening, and P. D. Williams. 1990. Comparison of in vitro and in vivo models to assess venous irritation of parenteral antibiotics. *Fundam. Appl. Toxicol.* 14:589–597.

Hynynen, M., K. Korttila, and T. Tammisto. 1985. Pain on i.v. injection of propofol (ICI 35868) in emulsion formulation. *Acta Anaesthesiol. Scand.* 29:651–652.

Kawar, P., and J. W. Dundee. 1982. Frequency of pain on injection and venous seqelae following the I.V. administration of certain anesthetics and sedatives. *Br. J. Anaesth.* 54:935–939.

Klement, W., and J. O. Arndt. 1991. Pain on injection of propofol: Effects of concentration and diluent. *Br. J. Anaesth.* 67:281–284.

Kromann, B., J. Jorgensen, and S. Larsen. 1982. Diazepam in an oil emulsion. *Anesth. Analges.* 61:544.

Lamb, K. A., C. Washington, S. S. Davis, and S. P. Denyer. 1991. Toxicity of amphotericin B emulsion to cultured canine kidney cell monolayers. *J. Pharm. Pharmacol.* 43:522–524.

Larsson-Backstrom, C., L. Lutteman Lustig, A. Eklund, and M. Thorstensson. 1988. Anaesthetic properties of pregnanolone in mice in an emulsion preparation for intravenous administration: A comparison with thiopentone. *Pharmacol. Toxicol.* 63:143–149.

Levy, M. Y., L. Langerman, S. Gottschalk-Sabag, and S. Benita. 1989. Side effect evaluation of a new diazepam formulation venous sequalae reduction following I.V. injection of diazepam emulsion in rabbits. *Pharm. Res.* 6:510–516.

Lovell, M. W., H. W. Johnson, and P. K. Gupta. 1995. Stability of a less-painful intravenous emulsion of clarithromycin. *Int. J. Pharm.* 118:47–54.

Lovell, M. W., H. W. Johnson, H.-W. Hui, J. B. Cannon, P. K. Gupta, and C. C. Hsu. 1994. Less-painful emulsion formulations for intravenous administration of clarithromycin. *Int. J. Pharm.* 109:45–57.

McCulloch, M. J., and N. W. Lees. 1985. Assessment and modification of pain on induction with propofol (Diprivan). *Anaesthesia* 40:1117–1120.

Meunier, F., H. G. Prentice, and O. Ringden. 1991. Liposomal amphotericin B (AmBisome): Safety data from a phase II/III clinical trial. *J. Antimicrob. Chemother.* 28 Suppl. B:83–91.

Moreau, P., N. Milpied, N. Fayette, J. F. Ramee, and J. L. Harousseau. 1992. Reduced Renal toxicity and improved clinical tolerance of amphotericin B mixed with Intralipid compared to conventional amphoterin B in neutropenic patients. *J. Antimicrob. Chemother.* 30:535–541.

Naylor, H. C. and A. N. Burlingham. 1985. Pharmacokinetics of diazepam emulsion. *Lancet* 1:518–519.

Nebayer, A. E., A. Doenicke, R. Hoernecke, R. Angster, and M. Mayer. 1992. Does etomidate cause haemolysis? *Brit. J. Anaesthes.* 69:58–60.

PDR. 1996. Diprivan® 1% Injection. In *Physicians desk reference,* 50th ed. Montvale, N.J., USA: Medical Economics Co., pp. 2833–2839.

PDR. 1996. Fungizone® Intravenous. In *Physicians desk reference,* 50th ed. Montvale, N.J., USA: Medical Economics Co., pp. 506–507.

Ringden, O., F. Meunier, J. Tollemar, P. Ricci, S. Tura, and E. Kuse. 1991. Efficacy of amphotericin B encapsulated into liposomes (AmBisome) in the treatment of invasive fungal infections in immunocompromised patients. *J. Antimicrob. Chemother.* 30:418.

Rutter, D. V., M. Morgan, J. Lumley, and R. Owen. 1980. ICI 35868 (Diprivan): A new intravenous induction agent: A comparison with methohexitone. *Anaesthesia* 35:1188–1192.

Selander, D., I. Curelaru, and T. Stefansson. 1981. Local discomfort and thromophlebitis following intravenous injection of diazepam. A comparison between a glycoferol-water solution and a lipid emulsion. *Acta Anaesth. Scand.* 25:516–518.

Strickley, R. G., and B. D. Anderson. 1993. Solubilization and stabilization of an anti-HIV thiocarbamate, NSC 629243, for parenteral delivery, using extemporaneous emulsions. *Pharm. Res.* 10:1076–1082.

Tham, C. S., and S. T. Khoo. 1995. Modulating effects of lignocaine on propofol. *Anaesth. Intensive Care* 23:154–157.

Van Berkel, T. J. C., J. Kar Kruijt, P. C. De Schmidt, and M. K. Bijsterbosch. 1991. Receptor-dependent targeting of lipoproteins to specific cell types of the liver. In *Lipoproteins as carriers of pharmacological agents,* edited by S. M. Shaw. New York: Marcel Dekker, pp. 225–249.

Von Dardel, O., C. Mebius, and T. Mossberg. 1976. Diazepam in emulsion form for intravenous use. *Acta Anaesth. Scand.* 20:221–224.

Von Dardel, O., C. Mebius, T. Mossberg, and B. Svensson. 1983. Fat emulsion as a vehicle for diazepam. A study of 9492 patients. *Br. J. Anesthes.* 55:41–47.

Wang, M. D., G. Wahlstrom, K. W. Gee, and T. Backstrom. 1995. Potency of lipid and protein formulation of 5α-pregnanolone at induction of anesthesia and the corresponding regional brain distribution. *Br. J. Anesthes.* 74:553–557.

Washington, C., M. Lance, and S. S. Davis. 1993. Toxicity of amphotericin B emulsion formulations. *J. Antimicrob. Chemother.* 31:806–808.

Westrin, P. 1992. Methohexital dissolved in lipid emulsion for intravenous induction of anesthesia in infants and children. *Anesthesiology* 76:917–921.

Westrin, P., C. Jonmarker, and O. Werner. 1992. Dissolving methohexital in a lipid emulsion reduces pain associated with intravenous injection. *Anesthesiology* 76:930–934.

Yalin, M., F. Oner, L. Oner, and A. A. Hincal. 1997. Preparation and properties of a stable intravenous lorazepam emulsion. *J. Clin. Pharm. Thera.* 22:39–44.

Yalkowsky, S. H., S. C. Valvani, and B. W. Johnson. 1983. In vitro method for detecting precipitation of parenteral formulations after injection. *J Pharm Sci.* 72:1014–1017.

Section D

FUTURE PERSPECTIVES IN THE DEVELOPMENT OF LESS-PAINFUL AND LESS-IRRITATING INJECTABLES

17

Formulation and Administration Techniques to Minimize Injection Pain and Tissue Damage Associated with Parenteral Products

Larry A. Gatlin

Biogen, Inc.
Cambridge, Massachusetts

Carol A. Brister Gatlin

Genzyme
Cambridge, Massachusetts

Parenteral products significantly contribute to global health by providing effective and immediate therapy through direct delivery of therapeutic compounds to the patient. However, as with most routes of delivery, parenteral drug administration has both real and perceived disadvantages. The two potential disadvantages that are typically associated with parenteral therapy are tissue damage and injection pain. Whether this pain is real or imagined makes little difference to the patient, and there exists a significant literature that both highlights the pain caused by injectable drug products and offers methods to reduce these effects.

The first section of this chapter provides a strategy that can be used to develop a parenteral product. Emphasis is placed on the two formulation parameters, pH and tonicity, that are usually associated with tissue damage and injection pain. It is through the adjustment of these parameters that the product formulator can minimize adverse effects. The second section of this chapter describes administration techniques used by healthcare professionals to reduce tissue damage or pain caused by commercial parenteral products. By recognizing the potential risks these alterations may confer to commercial formulations (such as decreased product stability or modified efficacy), the formulator will be better prepared to support the "real-world" use of the product.

FORMULATION DEVELOPMENT

The development strategy for parenteral products is similar for all products. The challenge is in the details of solving the physical/chemical difficulties encountered with a specific molecule within the timeline allowed for development. This section provides a parenteral product development outline with an emphasis on two formulation parameters, pH and tonicity, which may be modified to minimize tissue damage and pain caused by a parenteral product.

The activities necessary to develop a parenteral product can be placed into the following three broad areas: preformulation, formulation, and scale-up. While there are alternative development perspectives, all development ultimately needs to accomplish the same activities. Preformulation includes the characterization of the bulk drug plus initial screening for excipient compatibility with the drug. Formulation activities include the identification and selection of a suitable vehicle (aqueous, nonaqueous, or cosolvent system), necessary excipients with appropriate concentrations (buffers, antioxidants, antimicrobials, chelating agents, and tonicity contributors), and the container/closure system. Scale-up activities aid in moving the product to a manufacturing site (although not discussed here, references are available to provide guidance).

Preformulation

Preformulation studies provide fundamental data and the experience necessary to develop formulations for a specific compound. Activities are initiated and experiments performed for the purpose of characterizing specific and pharmaceutically significant physicochemical properties of the drug substance. These properties include interactions of the drug with excipients, solvents, packaging materials, and, specifically relating to the subject of this book, biological systems. These investigations also evaluate the drug under standard stress conditions of temperature, light, humidity, and oxygen. Many of these factors should be considered critically prior to animal testing, since these data will influence activities such as samples prepared for toxicology and animal testing, solubilization techniques, and design of subsequent studies.

Areas of specific interest during preformulation are provided in outline form below, along with an outline of additional characterization information needed to formulate a protein drug substance. Since analytical methods are usually developed concurrently with the preformulation data and then refined during formulation activities, the team must effectively communicate and collaborate to ensure appropriate assays are used to obtain data having sufficient accuracy and precision.

Preformulation Physicochemical Properties

1. Molecular weight

2. Color

3. Odor

4. Particle size, shape, and crystallinity

5. Thermal characteristics

    5.1. Melting profile

    5.2. Thermal profile

6. Hygroscopicity

7. Absorbance spectra

8. Solubility

    8.1. Selected solvents (water, ethanol, propylene glycol, polyethylene glycol 400, plus others as necessary)

    8.2. pH profile

    8.3. Temperature effects

    8.4. Partition coefficient

9. Stability

    9.1. Selected solvents

    9.2. pH profile

10. Ionization constant (pK or pI)

11. Optical activity

Additional Characterization for Protein Drugs

1. Physical stability

    1.1. Aggregation

2. Solubility

3. Chemical stability

    3.1. Beta-elimination

    3.2. Deamidation

    3.3. Isomerization/cyclization

    3.4. Oxidation

    3.5. Thiol disulfide exchange

4. Analytical methods

    4.1. Fluorescence spectroscopy

    4.2. Electrophoresis

    4.3. Calorimetry

    4.4. Size exclusion chromatography

    4.5. Reverse phase high performance liquid chromatography (HPLC)

    4.6. Circular dichroism

    4.7. Mass spectrometry

    4.8. Light scattering

Formulation

Formulation activities include the identification and selection of a suitable vehicle (aqueous, nonaqueous, or cosolvent system), necessary excipients with appropriate concentrations (buffers, antioxidants, antimicrobials, chelating agents, and tonicity contributors), and the container/closure system. The formulator is interested in the same list of activities given for preformulation; however, the activities are focused on specific excipients and characterization of the formulation. The principles of formulating a parenteral product have been outlined by several authors, although most do not specifically include the evaluation of tissue damage or pain caused by injection of the final product. This is likely due to the assumption that deviation of pH or tonicity from physiological conditions causes these effects. It is, however, important to consider that a product may cause tissue damage with little associated pain, pain with little tissue damage, or both pain and tissue damage. Therefore, the models utilized to assess either the pain or tissue damage associated with a product need to be selected carefully. Several complementary methods may be needed, and these models are provided throughout this book.

Significant formulation activities begin with initial preformulation data and knowledge of the specific route of administration. These data provide the formulator with the requirements and limitations for the final formulation. Due to the location of human pain receptors, formulation approaches to reduce pain are more critical for subcutaneous (SC) and intradermal injections and less critical for intramuscular (IM) and intravenous (IV) administration.

Injection volume is one of the most important considerations in the formulation development of a commercial product. This volume is selected based on the proposed injection route. Since veins have a relatively large volume and blood flow rate, a product administered by the IV route can have a volume greater than 10 mL; as the volume increases, the delivery rate may need to be controlled. This is in contrast to IM injections, which are normally limited to 3 mL, SC injections to 1 mL, and intradermal injections to 0.2 mL. Recommended maximum injection volumes are author dependent but not radically different.

Thus, the factors that need to be considered in evaluating the hemolysis caused by a product include both the quantity and proportions of the substances and how rapidly the blood dilutes the product. The data in Table 17.1 provide some perspective on the vascular system's capability of diluting an injected IV product, in terms of both volume and rate. The choice of solvent is dependent both on the route of administration, which

Table 17.1. Physical Characteristics of the Arteriovenous System

Anatomical Section	Volume (cm^3)	Velocity (cm/sec)
Aorta	100	40
Arteries	325	40–100
Arterioles	50	10–0.1
Capillaries	250	0.1
Venules	300	0.3
Veins	2,200	0.3–5
Vena cava	300	5–30

as noted above imparts volume limitations, and on drug solubility in the selected solvent. IV injections are typically restricted to dilute aqueous solutions to ensure compatibility with the blood; however, IM or SC injections allow for oily solutions, cosolvent systems, suspensions, or emulsions. Pain, soreness, and inflammation of tissues are frequently observed in the administration of parenteral suspensions, particularly with products having a high solid content.

A third important consideration in the development of a parenteral product is compatibility of the formulation with the tissue. An isotonic solution is less irritating, causes less toxicity and pain, and minimizes hemolysis. An isotonic product, however, is not always the goal since for SC or IM injections a hypertonic solution may facilitate drug absorption. Having an isotonic product is, however, very important for intraspinal injections, where the fluid circulation is slow and abrupt changes in osmotic pressure can contribute to unwanted and potentially severe side effects.

The choice of acceptable excipients in parenteral product development remains limited compared to other dosage forms, due to concerns of injection safety and feasibility of sterilization. In order to avoid uncertainty and reduce development time, most formulators select excipients successfully used in marketed products. A short list of commonly used additives, their functions, and typical concentrations is given in Tables 17.2 and 17.3. As the number of biotechnology products increases, excipients such as human serum albumin (HSA), amino acids, and sucrose are finding increasing utility. In Europe, the use of animal-derived excipients such as HSA and some polysorbate surfactants has become problematic due to the increasing concern with bovine spongiform encephalitis (BSE). This concern is expanding to the rest of the world and has impact on the selection of excipients.

An excipient selected for a parenteral product may serve one or more purposes. For example, benzyl alcohol is primarily a preservative; however, it has a transient local anesthetic property. Dual roles may help in the goal to minimize both the number of product ingredients and their quantity. The justification for each selection will become a part of the formulation development report.

Antimicrobials

Preservatives are always included in a product when multiple doses will be drawn from a single vial unless the drug itself is bacteriostatic. The addition of an antimicrobial is not a substitute for good manufacturing practices; however, many times they are added to single-use containers. They are specifically excluded from large-volume products intended for infusion. In some cases, as with benzyl alcohol, the excipient may have multiple functions. Therefore, the decision whether or not to include a preservative in a single-use product may be product specific. The rationale

Table 17.2. Additives Commonly Used in Parenteral Products

Substance	Concentration (percent)
Antimicrobial	
Benzalkonium chloride	0.01
Benzethonium chloride	0.01
Benzyl alcohol	1–2
Chlorobutanol	0.25–0.5
Chlorocresol	0.1–0.3
Metacresol	0.1–0.3
Phenol	0.5
Methyl p-hydroxybenzoate	0.18
Propyl p-hydroxybenzoate	0.02
Butyl p-hydroxybenzoate	0.015
Antioxidants	
Acetone sodium bisulfite	0.2
Ascorbic acid	0.1
Ascorbic acid esters	0.015
Butylhydroxyanisole (BHA)	0.02
Butylhydroxytoluene (BHT)	0.02
Cysteine	0.5
Monothioglycerol	0.5
Sodium bisulfite	0.15
Sodium metabisulfite	0.2
Tocopherols	0.5
Glutathione	0.1
Surfactants	
Polyoxethylene sorbitan monooleate	0.1–0.5
Sorbitan monooleate	0.05–0.5

for any preservative addition should be a part of the product development report.

Common antimicrobial agents are given in Table 17.2. These agents are grouped into five chemical classes: quaternary ammonium compounds, alcohols, esters, mercurials, and acids. The alcohols and esters are commonly used in parenteral products. The quaternary compounds, which are commonly used in ophthalmic products, are not compatible with negatively charged ions or molecules.

Table 17.3. Common Buffers Used in Parenteral Formulations

Buffer	pK_a	Usual Buffering Range
Acetic acid	4.8	3.5–5.7
Citric acid	3.14, 4.8, 5.2	2.1–6.2
Glutamic acid	2.2, 4.3, 9.7	8.2–10.2
Phosphoric acid	2.1, 7.2, 12.7	2–3.1, 6.2–8.2
Benzoic acid	4.2	3.2–5.2
Lactic acid	3.1	2.1–4.1
Ascorbic acid	4.2, 11.6	3.2–5.2
Tartaric acid	3.0, 4.3	2.0–5.3
Succinic acid	4.2, 5.6	3.2–6.6
Adipic acid	4.4, 5.28	3.4–6.3
Glycine	2.34, 9.6	1.5–3.5, 8.8–10.8
Malic acid	3.4, 5.1	2.4–6.1
Triethanolamine	8.0	7–9
Diethanolamine	9.0	8.0–10.0
Tromethamine	8.1	7.1–9.1

The literature reports interactions of the parabens with surfactants and formation of molecular complexes with gelatin, methylcellulose, polyvinyl pyrrolidone, and polyethylene glycol. These interactions may decrease preservative efficacy. Some antimicrobial compounds, such as benzyl alcohol, may be adsorbed by the container closure. Thus, microbial preservation must be demonstrated for the final formulated product.

Buffers

The buffer system establishes and maintains the product pH. A specific buffer system is selected such that the pK_a of the system is within one pH unit of the pH desired for the product. A list of common buffers is provided in Table 17.3. The selection of the product pH is based on the stability of the active drug. When alternative buffers are available, a comparison of their respective effects on stability will usually aid in the final choice. The acetate buffer system is not a good choice for a lyophilized product due to the volatility of acetic acid. Loss of acetic acid results in a pH shift when the product is reconstituted. The pH of solutions containing a phosphate buffer system have been shown to shift during cooling due to precipitation of sodium phosphate species. These pH shifts during freezing may cause damage to a protein. Since the specific buffer and the buffer capacity can contribute to injection pain, these effects should be evaluated in the selection of the buffer. Each species of the buffer system affects the tonicity of the final product; this influence must be considered during product development. For example, as the pH of a formulation containing monosodium phosphate is adjusted, the disodium salt is formed and contributes to product tonicity.

Antioxidants

Preformulation data will identify compounds sensitive to oxidation. Free radicals or molecular oxygen mediates oxidation, and several alternative stabilization approaches are available. In many cases, several approaches are utilized concurrently. One approach is lowering the product pH, which, according to the Nernst equation, increases the oxidation potential of the drug and thus increases stability. When oxygen contributes to degradation, it can be displaced during the filling operation by "bubbling" an inert gas such a nitrogen or argon gas through the solution prior to filling the vials. Additionally, the container headspace can be overlaid with the inert gas. An antioxidant may be useful if further protection is necessary. The specific antioxidant selected should have a lower oxidation potential than the drug. Several antioxidants and concentrations should be evaluated because, in many cases, a single agent is not sufficient. Sulfites are associated with allergic reactions in some patients. This reaction has a rapid onset and is not always confirmed by an oral challenge. Despite this reaction potential, sulfites may be used in a formulation if necessary to stabilize a life-saving product.

Examples of antioxidants include sodium bisulfite, ascorbic acid, glutathione, and propyl gallate. Sodium bisulfite tends to react irreversibly with the double bonds found in aldehydes and some ketones, and frequently results in a significant loss of biological activity. Epinephrine forms a bisulfite addition product, as do other sympathomimetic drugs having ortho- or para-hydroxybenzyl alcohol derivatives. The meta-hydroxy alcohol does not react with sodium bisulfite. Sulfites are converted to sulfates in the oxidation reaction, and if small amounts of barium are present, a precipitate will form.

Chelating Agents

Chelating agents are used to increase the solubility of a drug or to impart some product stability. Compounds such as ascorbic acid, citric acid, and ethylenediaminetetraacetic acid chelate metals, which would otherwise catalyze oxidation reactions, and provide measurable benefits for some products.

Surfactants

Surfactants are used to solubilize a drug and, for protein products, to minimize adsorption of the protein on surfaces. Most polysorbates are derived from animal sources, and their use in Europe is becoming problematic due to the increasing concerns with BSE. This concern is expanding to the rest of the world and will impact in the selection of excipients. Several suppliers are beginning to offer polysorbates from vegetable sources. Polysorbates can contain peroxides that may adversely affect product stability and, as for all excipients, specifications will need to be established.

Tonicity Agents

The active drug and each excipient contribute to the tonicity of the formulation. When the tonic contribution of these combined ingredients is not sufficient to provide an isotonic solution, then tonicity agents, such as dextrose, sodium chloride (NaCl), sodium sulfate, or mannitol can be added. Additional details are provided in the osmolality section below.

In summary, formulation activities focus on the selection of the solvent, the necessary excipients (buffers, antimicrobials, antioxidants, chelating agents, surfactants, and tonicity agents) with corresponding concentrations, the container/closure system, and on demonstrating adequate stability.

Focus on Osmolality, Cosolvents, Oils, and pH

The contribution of isotonicity in reducing injection pain is not always clear but, at a minimum, it may reduce tissue irritation. Injection pain may occur during and immediately following product administration but may be delayed or prolonged, with an increase in severity with subsequent injections. Pain can be difficult to assess because significant patient variation exists, and there are few preclinical methods for evaluation.

Literature describing pain associated with parenteral products has focused on three areas: osmolality, cosolvents, and pH. This is a pragmatic focus since osmolality and pH are easy to measure. Unfortunately, the adjustment of pH and osmolality may not be possible for some formulations due to physical or chemical stability of the product. In other products, the drug molecule may be inherently painful when injected. In both of these cases, formulations must be delivered at a low drug concentration or in complex formulations (such as emulsions or liposomes), in an attempt to "hide" the drug from pain receptors. Due to volume constraints, these are not always a viable alternative for IM or SC injections, leaving the formulator to design the best possible product and otherwise relying on the health professional to further minimize the injection pain at the time of administration. Since these formulations pose significant development issues, most formulators optimize the pH and isotonicity and provide information on appropriate dilution for administration.

Osmolality

The primary purpose for adjusting product osmolality is to minimize red blood cell lysis, tissue damage, and pain when the product is administered. An isotonic solution provides an electrolyte environment that allows human erythrocytes to maintain "tone." If cells are placed into a hypertonic solution, the cells may lose water and shrink (crenation). If placed in a hypotonic solution, the water moves into the cells, which can then swell to the point of breaking. Thus, the formulator's goal is to develop a product that, when administered, will be as close to isotonic as possible. In fact, the British Pharmacopoeia states that aqueous solutions for SC, intradermal, or IM injections should be made isotonic if possible. Unfortunately, there is no formulation solution for a product that is hypertonic. The necessity for administration in a diluted form or by slow infusion is appropriately noted in the product package insert.

Common agents used to adjust tonicity of a product include dextrose, NaCl, mannitol, and sodium sulfate. Care must be taken if sodium sulfate is selected for a product packaged in barium-containing glass, because even extremely small amounts of leached barium can lead to the precipitation of barium. Since all ingredients contribute to the tonicity of the product, it is necessary to measure or calculate the contribution of each and then, if necessary, adjust the product tonicity with additional agents.

Measuring Osmolality. Determination of osmolality is performed by measuring one of the four colligative properties, which depend only on the number of "particles" in the solution: (1) osmotic pressure elevation, (2) boiling point elevation, (3) freezing point depression, and (4) vapor pressure elevation. Of these methods, freezing point depression and vapor pressure elevation are most commonly utilized. These methods are relatively easy to perform and reasonably accurate. Commercial instruments are readily available.

Iso-osmolality, as determined by physical methods such as freezing point depression or vapor pressure reduction, is different from isotonicity determined by biological methods such as erythrocyte hemolysis. This difference is important since cells do not always behave as semipermeable membranes, and measuring biological compatibility by direct methods will identify problematic molecules that can cause lysis or tissue damage. Urea is the most frequently cited example of such a molecule; a 1.8 percent solution of urea has the same osmotic pressure as NaCl at 0.9 percent, but causes cell lysis. Other compounds that have specific cellular effects include glycerin, propylene glycol, and boric acid.

Although physical methods such as freezing point depression and vapor pressure are valuable tools in formulation development and quality control of the product, it is imperative to have direct methods to measure the effect of the product on red blood cells and tissue. Methods to evaluate cellular effects are given below, and methods to evaluate tissue effects are provided in other chapters of this book. The references provide additional information, and formulators are encouraged to include them in their library.

Determining Tonicity (Hemolysis). A common in vitro method to evaluate a product is by measuring erythocyte hemolysis. Typically the release of hemoglobin from the damaged cells is measured spectrophotometrically; however, a more sensitive method is to directly observe the changes in cell volume. An aqueous isotonic NaCl solution is used as the standard. Several protocols are available that describe incubating the product with erythrocytes suspended in defibrinated blood for a specified time, centrifuging to separate the erythrocytes and ghost cells, and then using a spectrophotometer to determine the absorbance of the supernatant versus a standard at 520 nm. Solution to blood ratios of 100:1 have been used. Concerns that this ratio is not realistic and can often give misleading results has lead investigators to use dilutions of 1:10—a complete reversal of proportions—with no hemolysis found.

Others have evaluated product effects by directly observing variations of red blood cell volume when suspended in solution. This method is more sensitive to small tonicity differences than the hemolysis method.

An alternative method to determine the compatibility of a product with blood is proposed by Ito et al. (1966). The coil planet centrifuge (CPC) method was originally developed to examine dynamic membrane properties of erythrocytes. The system comprises three instruments: the CPC itself, gradients for preparing the solution having an osmotic gradient in a coil, and a scanning spectrophotometer for recording a hemolytic pattern of the sample coil. The CPC is a specific centrifuge that rotates at 1,600 rpm around the main axis at a constant temperature of 37°C, while the coil holder fitted with coils rotates at 16 rpm. The design of this equipment ensures that the centrifugal force is constant irrespective of the distance from the main axis. It has been found that measuring the hemolysis of oil injections and those of high concentration or viscosity by this method is difficult, if not impossible.

The "osmogram" output shows red blood cell hemolysis as a function of the osmotic gradient. The hemolytic pattern of injections are divided into the following four patterns:

1. Hemolysis is remarkable, or erythrocyte is coagulated and does not move.

2.   Hemolysis takes place gradually and then continues or is shifted to the side of high osmotic pressure.

3.   No change is observed.

4.   Pattern is shifted to low osmotic pressure, indicating stabilization of the erythrocyte membrane.

This method may provide valuable information for the evaluation of parenteral products; however, the full potential of the method is unknown since there is little information available.

Calculating Tonicity. Several methods used to calculate tonicity are summarized below.

(1) The method of NaCl equivalents expresses tonicity in terms of the amount of drug equivalent to NaCl since, in most cases, when an aqueous solution is iso-osmotic with 0.9 percent NaCl, it will be isotonic with physiologic systems. The NaCl equivalent value, E, is defined as the weight of NaCl having the same osmotic effect as 1 g of the drug. A 1 percent NaCl solution has an equilibrium freezing temperature of -0.58°C and is given a NaCl E value of 1.00. The freezing temperature of serum is -0.52°C, equivalent to the freezing temperature of a 0.9 percent NaCl solution. Therefore, if a 1 percent solution of a specific compound has a freezing temperature of -0.058°C, then it has an E value of 0.1. Thus, 1.0 g of this compound will have the same tonic value as 0.1 g of NaCl; to prepare 100 mL of an isotonic solution containing 1 g of this substance, 0.8 g of NaCl must be added. *Remington's* (Gennaro 1995) has an extensive list of NaCl equivalents for specific excipients and drugs.

Different compounds can be used to adjust solution tonicity. For example, in the above calculation, 0.8 g of NaCl was needed to render the solution isotonic. If, however, dextrose is desired to adjust tonicity, then the amount of dextrose would be

$$(1 \text{ g dextrose}/0.16 \text{ g NaCl}) \times 0.8 \text{ g NaCl} = 5 \text{ g dextrose}$$

A comparison of measured osmolality to calculated values using the NaCl equivalent method shows agreement within 10 percent; for most systems this is sufficiently accurate.

(2) The freezing point depression method uses "D" values having units of °C per x percent of drug. The D values for some drug compounds can be obtained in the literature.

(3) The V value of a drug is the volume of water used to dissolve a specific weight of drug to prepare an isotonic solution. The purpose of this method is to prepare an isotonic solution of the drug and then to dilute this to the desired final concentration with a suitable isotonic vehicle. This method is most commonly used for ophthalmic preparations. Values for commonly used drugs are available in the literature.

(4) Other calculations such as the L_{iso} method can be used for estimations when values for a specific compound are not available. The mathematical relationship of L_{iso} to the NaCl equivalent, E, is:

$$E = 17 \, (L_{iso}/M)$$

where M is the molecular weight of the compound. Average L_{iso} values for different types of compounds are given in Table 17.4.

Cosolvents and Oils

Cosolvents are commonly used to enhance drug solubility and stability. Cosolvents may include ethanol, propylene glycol, polyethylene glycols, and glycerin. These components have intrinsic effects on biologic tissue and can alter the properties of other excipients, thus influencing the tissue damage or pain caused by the product. There is a dearth of literature on the pain caused by cosolvents, but there is also a growing body of knowledge on the tissue damage that they can cause. It is not certain that tissue damage is always directly correlated with injection pain, but minimization of both pain on injection and potential for tissue damage should be included in the product development plan.

In studies by Brazeau and Fung (1989a, b), moderate concentrations of organic cosolvents (20 to 40 percent v/v) show the following relative myotoxicity ranking: propylene glycol > ethanol > polyethylene glycol 400. These investigators also discovered that total myotoxicity equaled the sum of the individual myotoxicity of each component, with the exception of preparations containing polyethylene glycol 400, which apparently has a protective effect.

Table 17.4. Average L_{iso} Values for Different Types of Compounds

Compound Type	L_{iso}	Example
Nonelectrolyte	1.9	Sucrose
Weak electrolyte	2.0	Phenobarbital, boric acid
Di-divalent electrolyte	2.0	Zinc sulfate
Uni-univalent electrolyte	3.4	Sodium chloride
Uni-divalent electrolyte	4.3	Sodium sulfate, atropine sulfate
Di-univalent electrolyte	4.8	Calcium chloride
Uni-trivalent electrolyte	5.2	Sodium phosphate
Tri-univalent electrolyte	6.0	Aluminum chloride
Tetraborates	7.6	Sodium borate

Consideration must also be given to cosolvent effects on other product excipients. Since most buffers are conjugates of a weak acid or base, the polarity shift caused by cosolvents may shift the pK_a of the buffer species. It is best to evaluate biological compatibility using direct biological methods, because cosolvents may have both specific cellular effects and indirect excipient effects.

Another class of nonaqueous vehicles used in parenteral formulations are the fixed oils, including corn, cottonseed, olive, peanut, sesame, and soybean. Oils of vegetable origin are selected because they can be metabolized, are liquid at room temperature, and will not rapidly become rancid. To remain liquid at room temperature, a fixed oil must contain unsaturated fatty acids, which, when present in excessive amounts, can cause tissue irritation. The U.S. Pharmacopeia (USP) includes specifications for rancidity, solidification range of fatty acids, and free-fatty acids. The formulator may include antioxidants, such as tocopherol (a natural component of many fixed oils) to prevent the product from becoming rancid.

pH

A product buffer system is selected to help maintain an environment in which the drug is stable throughout the commercial shelf life of the product. These systems are composed of a weak acid or base and a corresponding salt. The ratio of these species determines the pH, and the concentration provides a buffer capacity to resist pH changes due to product degradation or container-closure interactions. A buffer system is most efficient at its pK_a, thus, buffers are generally chosen within one pH unit of the desired product pH.

The buffer concentrations typically chosen for a product range from 1 to 2 percent, although higher concentrations of up to 5 percent have been used with citrate buffers. The more a pH deviates from physiological conditions and the higher the buffer capacity, the more likely the product will contribute to tissue damage or injection pain. Table 17.3 provides a list of acceptable buffers with pK_a values and usual pH buffer ranges.

Buffer systems are in an equilibrium that is sensitive to temperature and the concentration of each species. Each species in this equilibrium may contribute differently to product osmolality. There may be an error in estimating the contribution to osmolality of each species at room temperature, since the most common method to measure osmolality is by freezing point depression. Cutie and Sciarrone (1969) demonstrated for boric acid, Sorensen, and Palitzsch buffers that if formulated to be isotonic as measured by freezing point depression, the solutions may be slightly hypertonic at 37°C. Sodium tetraborate has, in fact, been demonstrated to have a NaCl equivalent (E value) of 0.45 at 37°C but 0.35 at 0°C, a 23 percent change. For most formulations, this is not of physiological significance;

however, it should not be discounted for those formulations where close tolerance to isotonicity is necessary.

A vapor pressure osmometer provides an alternative to the freezing point method and may be particularly useful when the data for temperature and concentration effects on ionization constants are not available. A limitation of the vapor pressure method includes interference by volatile substances such as ethanol.

POST-FORMULATION PROCEDURES

Despite efforts to minimize or eliminate pain through formulation optimization, some products remain painful when injected. The literature is replete with suggestions on how to reduce pain during the administration of a product. Unfortunately, much of these data are incomplete or seemingly contradictory. Deficiencies in the research conducted on children's pain have been noted, and the point is frequently made that children are short-changed with respect to pain management. Post-formulation efforts to alleviate pain which are discussed in this chapter are included in the following categories: pH, additives or solvent adjustments; devices or physical manipulations, and psychological.

pH, Additives, and Solvents

Drugs stable only in acidic conditions are purposefully formulated to ensure an adequate commercial shelf life. Because these acidic products are associated with injection pain, sodium bicarbonate is extemporaneously added prior to administration to more closely match physiological pH (pH 7.3). This approach appears to successfully reduce the pain caused by local anesthetics; however, studies with other products have been equivocal. For anesthetics, this increased pH will alter the stability of the product and may result in the precipitation of the less soluble, nonionized species. The amount of sodium bicarbonate that can be safely added is variable given the range of anesthetic products (pH of 3.5 to 5.5), the concentration of sodium bicarbonate, and other variables.

The reduction in pain for anesthetic products does not appear to be entirely due to the increased pH of the solution. The indirect effect of increasing product pH is to shift the equilibrium of anesthetics to the uncharged species that may diffuse more rapidly and consequently inhibit pain perceptions. Individual drugs or drug species (charged or uncharged) may have different intrinsic pain induction potential, independent of pH. The study design and product ingredients must be considered when evaluating data, because some excipients such as benzyl alcohol have local anesthetic properties.

Another extemporaneous technique is to add lipids to the commercial formulation. This method shifts more of the drug from the aqueous phase and has been successful in reducing injection pain for methohexital and propofol. Such additions need to be supported by studies to verify product stability, similar pharmacokinetics, and efficacy.

Clinicians also minimize or eliminate injection pain by topical administration of local anesthetics, which decrease pain sensation, or nitroglycerin ointment, which dilates local blood vessels and promotes absorption of the irritating substance. Although of interest to the formulator, these topical approaches do not pose formulation issues.

Devices and Physical Manipulations

Parenteral administration techniques will affect the magnitude of the pain. These include the practical training received by healthcare professionals; proper selection of administration equipment; and manipulation of the injection rate, injection site, and temperature. The formulator should note how health professionals may use the product and consider the need for pertinent data during product development.

Parenteral administration techniques are part of a nurse's education. This practical training is aimed at increasing the comfort of the patient and efficiency of the nurse. The references given at the end of this chapter provide additional detail and information on less common parenteral routes of administration.

Subcutaneous Injection

Drugs recommended for SC injection include nonirritating aqueous solutions and suspensions contained in 0.5 to 2.0 mL (target 1 mL or less) of fluid. The needle sizes are 25 gauge 5/8 in. length for an average adult and 25 gauge 1/2 in. length for an infant, child, elderly, or thin patient. After cleaning the area with an alcohol sponge, allow the skin to dry before skin penetration to avoid the stinging sensation caused by the alcohol entering the subcutaneous tissue.

With the nondominant hand, grasp the skin around the injection site firmly to elevate the subcutaneous tissue, forming a 1 in. fat fold. This provides rigidity for needle entry. Tell the patient "you will feel a prick as the needle is inserted." Holding the syringe in the dominant hand with the needle bevel up, insert the needle quickly in one motion. Release the patient's skin to avoid injecting the drug into compressed tissue to minimize irritation of nerve fibers, confirm the needle is in the tissue, and inject slowly. After the injection, remove the needle quickly. Cover the skin and massage the site gently (unless contraindicated as with heparin or insulin) to help distribute the drug and reduce pain.

Intradermal Injection

Intradermal injections are typically used only for local effects or diagnostic purposes in volumes of 0.5 mL or less. Needles of 26 or 27 gauge and 1/2 to 5/8 in. in length are used. The injection is given at a 15° angle about 1/8 in. below the epidermis at sites 2 in. apart. Stop when the needle bevel tip is under the skin and inject slowly; some resistance should be felt. A wheal should form; if it does not, the injection is too deep. Withdraw the needle at the same angle as the entry. Do not massage the site, as this may cause irritation.

Intramuscular Injection

IM injections deliver medication into highly vascularized deep muscle tissue. Because there are few sensory nerves in these tissues, pain is minimized when injecting irritating drugs. The volume for IM injection can be up to 5 mL, although it is typically less than 3 mL. A 20 to 25 gauge needle of 1 to 3 in. in length is used. Once the appropriate injection site has been selected and properly prepared, gently tap it to stimulate nerve endings and minimize pain when the needle is inserted. The gluteal muscles should not be used for a child under the age of 3, nor for someone who has not been walking for the prior year. Never inject into sensitive muscles, especially those that twitch or tremble when you assess site landmarks. Injections in these trigger areas may cause sharp or referred pain, such as pain caused by nerve trauma.

Intravenous Bolus Injection

Bolus drug administration is used when immediate drug effects are necessary, when the drugs cannot be diluted (diazepam, digoxin, phenytoin), or for drugs that are too toxic or irritating for other routes of administration. A 20 gauge needle is typically used. Bolus injections are given through the largest vein suitable, since the larger the vein, the more dilute the drug becomes, thus minimizing vascular irritation. An in-depth discussion of specific routes of administration, techniques, equipment, and cautions is readily available in the literature referenced at the end of this chapter.

Devices

Devices offer significant opportunities to reduce the fear and increase the consistency of parenteral injections. Some of these devices are needle free, with the product propelled through the skin under pressure. Some studies have demonstrated reduced pain during administration. These devices may affect the quality of a shear-sensitive macromolecule or alter drug pharmacokinetics (PK) due to the pattern of drug deposition. For a given product, additional product or PK characterization may be necessary. These devices deliver subcutaneous injections; however, controversy remains on whether they can deliver an IM injection.

Other devices use "hidden" needles with guides that facilitate insertion of the needle and subsequent injection of the medication. These allow for reproducible injections. Their utility is dependent on the perception of the patient, the cost of the device, and the ease of use. These devices have been shown to be less painful and improve compliance for chronic administration of SC injections.

Temperature

Healthcare providers continually explore methods to increase the comfort of the patient by altering the temperature of the product or skin. Numbing the skin surface with ice or other means has successfully been used to reduce injection pain; in one case, injecting a cool solution before infusing the drug appeared to be successful in reducing pain. Changing the product temperature is more significant to the product formulator. Warming propofol to 37°C has been demonstrated to decrease the incidence of pain by 37 percent. Since both cooling and warming have been shown to reduce injection discomfort, it may be that some relief is provided by the quick, but transient temperature effects on the nociceptor receptors or pain mediators. The formulator should be aware that products might be either cooled or warmed by healthcare professionals and, therefore, consider the impact of temperature changes on the formulation during product development.

Psychological

The contribution of psychological factors to injection pain is substantial and has been considered in the design of the new devices mentioned previously. Psychology is used in the clinic to minimize injection pain, particularly in children. These are interesting and provided here for completeness.

The pain experience is influenced by age, physical, emotional, cultural, and, social factors as are the preferred control methods. A Gallup Poll stated that 58 percent of children rely on their own coping skills, such as thinking about something else to make shots bearable, and 47 percent said they specifically disliked needles. Perhaps we as healthcare providers can provide more assistance.

Several articles provide lists and examples of proactive psychological techniques shown to minimize injection pain, including distraction, honesty, and a demonstration of caring. Distraction asks the patient to focus on an image and and to use breathing techniques. The person giving the injection should be honest yet supportive while making general sympathetic statements that indicate the child can control pain. The child should be involved in discussions, and all actions should be described before or as they are being performed.

The psychology and perception of pain are important factors in pain management and both the healthcare provider and formulator can effectively utilize the techniques mentioned above in the development, support, and administration of therapeutic products.

REFERENCES

Brazeau, G., and H.-L. Fung. 1989a. An in-vitro model to evaluate muscle damage following intramuscular injections. *Pharm. Res.* 6:167–170.

Brazeau, G. A., and H.-L. Fung. 1989b. Use of an in-vitro model for the assessment of muscle damage from intramuscular injections: in-vitro/in-vivo correlation and predictability with mixed solvent systems. *Pharm. Res.* 6:766–771.

Brody, J. 1995. The pain-killing power of imagination. *Star Tribune (Minneapolis, Minn.),* 4 November, p. 10E.

Cleland, J. L., and R. Langer. 1994. *Formulation and delivery of proteins and peptides.* Washington, D.C. American Chemical Society, ACS symposium series 567.

Cutie, A. J., and B. J. Sciarrone. 1969. Re-evaluation of pH and tonicity of pharmaceutical buffers at 37 degrees. *J. Pharm. Sci.* 58:990–993.

Erramouspe, J. 1996. Buffering local anesthetic solutions with sodium bicarbonate: Literature review and commentary. *Hosp. Pharm.* 31:1275–1282.

Fletcher, G. C., J. A. Gillespie, and J. A. H. Davidson. 1996. The effect of temperature upon pain during injection of propofol. *Anaesthesia* 51:498–499.

Flynn, G. L. 1980. Buffers—pH control within pharmaceutical systems. *J. Parent. Drug Assoc.* 34:139.

Fowler-Kerry, S., and J. R. Lander. 1987. Management of injection pain children. *Pain* 30:169–175.

Gennaro, A. R. 1995. *Remington: The Science and Practice of Pharmacy.* Easton, Penn., USA: Mack Publishing Company.

Godschalk, M., D. Gheorghiu, P. G. Katz, and T. Mulligan. 1996. Alkalization does not alleviate penile pain induced by intracavernous injection of prostaglandin E1. *J. Urology* 156: 999–1000.

Hagan, C. 1996. No-pill pain relief: little tricks that can instantly sooth your child's hurt. *Good Housekeeping* 223:150–152.

Hammarlund, E. R., and G. L. V. Pevenage. 1966. Sodium chloride equivalents, cryoscopic properties, and hemolytic effects. *J. Pharm. Sci.* 55:1448–1451.

Husa, W. J., and O. A. Rossi. 1942. Isotonic solutions II: Permeability of red corpuscles to various cosolvents. *J. APhA. Sci. Ed* 31:270.

Ito, Y., M. A. Weinstein, I. Aoki, R. Harada, E. Kimura, and K. Nunogaki. 1966. Coil plant centrifuge. *Nature* 212:985–987.

Ito, Y., I. Aoki, E. Kimura, K. Nunogaki, and Y. Nunogaki. 1969. Micro liquid-liquid partition techniques with the coil plant centrifuge. *Anal. Chemist* 41:1579–1584.

Koenicke, A. W., M. F. Roizen, J. Rau, W. Kellermann, and J. Babl. 1996. Reducing pain during propofol injection: The role of the solvent. *Anesth. Analg.* 82:472–474.

Krzyzaniak, J. F., F. A. A. Nunez, D. M. Raymond, and S. H. Yalkowsky. 1997. Lysis of human red blood cells. 4. Comparison of in-vitro and in-vivo hemolysis data. *J. Pharm. Sci.* 86:1215–1217.

Lugo-Janer, G., M. Padial, and J. L. Sanchez. 1991. Less painful alternatives for local anesthesia. *J. Dermatol. Surg. Oncol.* 19:237–240.

Main, K. M., J. T. Jorgensen, N. T. Hertel, S. Jensen, and L. Jakobsen. 1995. Automatic needle insertion diminishes pain during growth hormone injection. *Acta. Paediatr.* 84:331–334.

Martin, A. N., J. Swarbrick, and A. Cammarata. 1969. *Physical pharmacy.* Philadelphia: Lea & Febiger.

Moriel, E. Z., and J. Rajfer. 1993. Sodium bicarbonate alleviates penile pain induced by intracavernous injections for erectile dysfunction. *J. Urology* 149:1299–1300.

Motola, S. 1992. *Pharmaceutical dosage forms: Parenteral medications,* vol. 1. New York: Marcel Dekker, Inc., pp. 59–113.

Piepmeier, E. H., and L. A. Gatlin. 1995. Ultrasonic vocalizations from rats following intramuscular administration of antimicrobials. *Proceedings of the AAPS Annual Meeting,* Miami Beach, Fla.

Queralt, C. B., V. Comet, J. M. Cruz, and C. Val-Carreres. 1995. Local anesthesia by jet-injection device in minor dermatologic surgery. *Dermatol. Surg.* 21:649–651.

Racz, I. 1989. *Drug Formulation.* New York: John Wiley and Sons.

Rubino, J. T. 1987. The effects of cosolvents on the action of pharmaceutical buffers. *J. Parent. Sci. Tech.* 41:45–49.

Rubino, J. T., and W. S. Berryhill. 1986. Effects of sovent polarity on the acid dissociation constants of benzoic acids. *J. Pharm. Sci.* 75:182–186.

Viele, C. 1994. Tips help to minimize injection-site pain from epoetin alfa therapy. *Oncology Nursing Forum* 21:781–782.

Wang, Y.-C. J., and R. R. Kowal. (1980) Review of excipients and pH's for parenteral products used in the United States. *J. Parent. Drug Assoc.* 14:452–462.

Wells, J. I. 1988. Pharmaceutical preformulation: The physiochemical properties of drug substances. In *Pharmaceutical technology.* Chichester, N.Y., USA: Halsted Press.

Westrin, P., C. Jonmarker, and O. Werner. 1992. Dissolving methohexital in a lipid emulsion reduces pain associated with intravenous injection. *Anesthesiology* 76:930–934.

Wiener, S. G. 1979. Injectable sodium chloride as a local anesthetic for skin surgery. *Cutis* 23:342–343.

Williams, J. M., and N. R. Howe. 1994. Benzyl alcohol attenuates the pain of lidocaine injections and prolongs anesthesia. *J. Dermatol. Surg. Oncol.* 20:730–733.

Index

T - #0315 - 101024 - C0 - 254/178/25 [27] - CB - 9781574910957 - Gloss Lamination